WOMEN AND CANCER

WOMEN AND CANCER

LAURIE ELIT
EDITOR

Nova Biomedical Books
New York

LIBRARY OF CONGRESS CATALOGING-IN-PUBLICATION DATA

Women and cancer / Laurie Elit (editor).
p. ; cm.
Includes bibliographical references and index.
ISBN-13: 978-1-60021-494-3
ISBN-10: 1-60021-494-0
1. Cancer in women. I. Elit, Laurie.
[DNLM: 1. Neoplasms. 2. Women's Health. QZ 200 W87151 2006]
RC281.W65W645 2006
616.99'40082--dc22

2006036345

Published by Nova Science Publishers, Inc. ✣ New York

CONTENTS

PREFACE

This new and timely book presents an in-depth overview of the medical, psychosocial and sexuality issues that confront women affected by cancer

Section 1, Chapter I - Lung cancer has reached nearly epidemic proportions in women; the incidence has quadrupled over the past 40 years. Multiple studies have been conducted to identify reasons for the dramatic increase in lung cancer over the past decades. Smoking behaviors, pathways of carcinogenesis and the impact of the hormonal milieu have all been examined as possible explanations. Although many studies have attempted to address these questions, they have been retrospective or case-control studies and results have been inconsistent. With the recognition that lung cancer may behave differently in men versus women, current studies are prospectively examining this question.

Section 2, Chapter I - This chapter reviews the surgical treatment options given various tissue diagnoses and the outcomes of each option in terms of local recurrence and survival.

Chapter II - This chapter reviews the treatment decision points concerning use of adjuvant hormones, chemotherapy or biologic agents. Anticipated outcome in terms of local recurrence, risk of contralateral breast cancer, disease free and overall survival and side effects are provided. Management options for women with metastatic disease and the goals of treatment are explored including bisphosphonates, chemotherapy, hormonal, and biologics such as Herceptin.

Chapter III - Radiation therapy is an important modality of treatment for breast cancers in the early as well as later stages of disease. Ongoing trials will help answer the questions of whether additional radiation to regional nodal areas is of benefit in node positive breast cancers as well as determine whether accelerated partial breast radiation is equivalent to whole breast radiation in early stage (node negative) disease. The use of new imaging and treatment modalities holds the promise of maintaining excellent control rates while further improving convenience and possibly further reducing morbidity.

Chapter IV - Breast reconstruction after breast cancer surgery is gaining popularity. The reported frequency has increased 3.5 fold to 35 percent from 8 to 10 percent a few years ago. This is anticipated to increase further with patient education and earlier detection.

Herein is provided a surgical algorithm for the approach to breast reconstruction that incorporates patient factors and surgical options. Patient factors include stage of disease, comorbidities and body habitus. Surgical options include consideration of timing of reconstruction, use of prosthesis versus autologous tissue and reconstruction of the nipple-areolar complex.

Finally a woman's perspective towards breast reconstruction is discussed.

Section 3, Chapter I - Colorectal cancer deaths are equally distributed among women and men. Prevention is possible using risk-stratified screening strategies and healthy lifestyle. Good outcomes are possible if the disease is discovered and treated at an early stage. Quality of life can be preserved but in rectal cancer patients, sexual function and changes in body image occur.

Section 4 - With recent advancements in the diagnosis and treatment of cancer there has been a focus to individualize treatment. This has been the result of growing knowledge of cancer genetics, improvement in imaging technology and increasing evidence about adjuvant treatments.

In this chapter the diagnosis and treatment of gynecologic cancers will be discussed. The chapter will be divided into sections by anatomic tumor site; ovary and fallopian tube, uterus, cervix and vagina, and vulva. Each section will be subdivided into two major headings: diagnosis and treatment. The subsection on diagnosis will cover familial cancer syndromes, screening, signs and symptoms of disease, imaging techniques specific to that cancer site, biopsies and genetic testing. The new developments in familial cancer syndromes, genetic testing, and imaging will be emphasized. Diagnosis will be followed by a discussion of treatment options, focusing on the treatment of the most common tumor types of that site. A short discussion on the treatment of the rare pathologies will also be made. Each treatment strategy will be discussed in the context of the use of surgery, radiotherapy, chemotherapy and novel biologic therapies for the disease. For each strategy the expectations of response as well as side effects will be covered. In summary, in this chapter we will highlight the recent advances in the diagnosis and treatment of gynecologic cancers orienting the contents to the scientific community who are involved in the education and treatment of these women.

Section 5, Chapter I - Objective: To provide an overview of the the major stressors related to having a cancer diagnosis and the emotional impact and quality of life issues associated with survivorship.

Results: The prevalence of distress following a cancer diagnosis and specific predictors of adjustment difficulties will be explored. In addition, a number of quality of life impacts and the specific impacts of cancer on body image , sexuality and identity are reviewed. The implications for assessment and treatment include psychosocial assessment, support resources and counseling approaches.

Conclusion: The diagnosis of cancer has psychosocial impacts on women and their families from the time of diagnosis, during treatment and recovery and through survivorship. Psychosocial screening, education and empirically-based treatment can address specific issues. Future work is needed to test innovative treatments.

Chapter II - When a woman learns she has cancer, she is confronted with the implications of the diagnosis, decisions about the treatment plan, and the often rigorous and physically demanding medical regimes. Following treatment, the identity of "cancer survivor" will be added to her life along with the 50% possibility of premature death. Cancer challenges a woman's roles in a patriarchal society, in which she is viewed as caretaker, nurturer and provider. Thus, a woman's ability to live well following a diagnosis of cancer is influenced not only by her understanding and beliefs about the disease, but by her self-perceptions about her multiple roles and how well a system of care meets her many needs. The ability of medical systems to provide equitable cancer care is challenged by the diversity and vulnerability of a woman's various identities and social situations. As a member of a cancer treatment team, social workers are trained from an ecosystemic perspective to assess the biopsychosocial needs of this vulnerable population. Personalised treatment plans are developed that consider a woman's identity and relational challenges in the face of cancer and lower both systemic and internal barriers to equitable care. Therefore, social workers provide a particular understanding of the unique and complex supportive care needs of their patients with the result of improved medical care and decreased costs to the medical system. The purpose of this chapter is to assess the identity challenges of women diagnosed with cancer and to address their supportive care needs. In order to accomplish this, we have three primary aims. First, we investigate how a cancer diagnosis can influence and infiltrate a woman's various identities and roles that have been constructed through the multiple relationships in her life. In this discussion we also consider the various supportive care needs that surface when a woman's self-perception and role responsibilities are confronted by cancer. Secondly, we propose how the perspective and practices of social work are uniquely qualified to address and provide for a woman's supportive care needs. Finally, we explore current gaps in oncological psychosocial interventions and suggest directions for future program development and research.

Chapter III - Objective: To review the importance of discussing sexuality with women at the time of treatment planning, and during the follow-up phase of managing gynecologic cancers.

Methods: Components of the sexual history, various barriers to discussing sexual function (ie., lack of knowledge) are reviewed using gynecologic cancers as an example. The interaction between quality of life and illness on sexual function is explored. Management strategies are discussed.

Conclusion: There may be sensitivities about broaching this topic for both the patient and the health care team. Usually the health care team can manage most of the issues; however, referral to sexual medicine may be required in complex situations.

Section 6, Chapter I - Objective: In an era where cancer is more and more often to be cured, strategies to preserve fertility in premenopausal women are becoming increasingly important.

Methods and Results: The impact of radiation and/or chemotherapy on ovarian function are reviewed. Both strategies are dependent on the age of the patient and dose of the agent. Strategies to preserve ovarian function such as GnRH agonists are discussed. Cryopreservations of embyos or ovarian tissue reimplantation are becoming options for those willing to pay. Fertility sparing surgical management such as radical trachelectomy for cervical cancer are becoming more widely available.

Conclusions: It is important to evaluate outcomes when challenging current cancer treatment strategies. It is important to ensure that fertility-sparing options are not just feasible but actually safe for the patient and her potential offspring.

Chapter II - Objectives: To address the many symptoms of menopause experienced by women as a result of treatment for their cancer.

Discussion: There is a relationship of premature ovarian failure with atherosclerosis and osteoporosis. Options for treating vasomotor symptoms may include environmental factors, physical activity, paced respiration, herbal and botanical, phytoestrogens, non-hormonal and hormonal therapy. Management of sleep disturbances will be reviewed. Risk factors for a depressed mood and management including conventional modalities and estrogen will be discussed. Vulvo-vaginal symptoms, joint pain and stiffness and sexuality concerns will be reviewed.

Conclusion: With increasing numbers of cancer patients living longer, quality of survivorship becomes an important issue. Menopausal symptoms are important for women and treatment options need to be made available.

Section 7, Chapter I - Objective: VTE is a common complication of patients with cancer.

Results: There are several techniques for diagnosing DVT: Doppler U/S is the preferred method due to low cost, high accuracy and high availability. There are several techniques for diagnosing PE: spiral CT scan is the preferred method. Treatment with LMWH or UFH in cancer is acceptable. Use of coumadin or long term LMWH is the subject of investigations.

Conclusion: VTE is a common complication in women with a diagnosis of cancer. Research continues into the optimal management strategy.

DEDICATION

Sometime the seeds of happiness are sewn in darkness.
Author unknown

This book is dedicated to those women who live with cancer. As health care staff, we have had the privilege to walk along side you in this journey of living with cancer. You have come to us looking for a cure. In some cases that has been realized. More often than naught, a cure was not possible, but we worked together to achieve relief from symptoms, for a time. We are in awe of your courage. We acknowledge the great lessons you have taught us on how to better care for those living with cancer.

FOREWARD

Laurie Elit *

Department of Obstetrics and Gynecology, McMaster University, Canada;
Juravinski Cancer Centre, Hamilton, Ontario, Canada.

In May 2004, I was asked to sit on the Women and Cancer Initiative at the Juravinski Cancer Centre in Hamilton. There are obvious differences between men and women when it comes to cancers related to gender specific organs. However, our group struggled to understand the differences between men and women in those cancers related to shared organs.

In 2005 the Ontario Women's Health Council in partnership with Cancer Care Ontario the Cancer Quality Council of Ontario funded through the Ministry of Health and Long-Term Care published a report titled "The Quality of Cancer Services for Women in Ontario 2005". Their key findings were that greater effort was needed in areas of prevention and screening (cervix, breast and colo-rectal) and there were few differences in cancer prevention and treatment by gender within the limitations of the data. More specifically in the area of primary prevention although the rates of smoking and obesity were lower in women than men, rates varied geographically and by age. In the area of treatment, there were no gender differences in terms of uptake of treatment guidelines, waiting times, and end of life care. Patient satisfaction with outpatient cancer care appeared to be lower in women. Recommendations were put forward on the need for population-based recruitment for screening, the importance of decreasing waiting times for everyone, the need to improve palliative care services, and hospital based understanding of the specific needs women with cancer face. Cancer Care Ontario was going to include gender in its performance measures and management activities into the future.

What is clear is that men and women have biological and physical differences related to the impact on health and illness. This can be clearly understood in gender specific organ

* Correspondence concerning this article should be addressed to Laurie Elit MD, Juravinski Cancer Centre 699 Concession Street, Hamilton, Ontario, Canada L8V 5C2. Phone: 905 389-5688; FAX: 575-6343; Email: laurie.elit@hrcc.on.ca.

issues. However, there can be different risk factors for the same disease, different symptoms for the same problem, different reactions to the same medication and different outcomes for the same condition. In addition to disease issues – men and women may interact differently to the health care system when offered the same treatments, use of services and satisfaction with care. There is emerging information that women and men differ in their psychological and social experience with cancer. How the woman's economic status, her caregiver role and age impact these experiences is an evolving area of research.

This book is an expansion of both disease specific issues as they pertain to women with cancer (ie. lung cancer) and modifiers (ie. effects of chemotherapy on fertility). The purpose of this book was to help health care professional better understand both the disease specific issues related to managing the leading causes of cancer in women; to understand those normal bodily functions that are influenced by cancer treatment; and to better appreciate those non-medical issues that may influence a woman's response to living with cancer.

Reference

Ontario Women's Health Council, Cancer Care Ontario, The Cancer Quality Council of Ontario. The Quality of Cancer Services for Women in Ontario 2005. 9/8/2005:1-103.

SECTION 1: WOMEN AND LUNG CANCER

In: Women and Cancer
Editor: Laurie Elit, pp. 3-20

ISBN: 978-1-60021-494-3

Chapter I

Women and Lung Cancer: A Neglected Epidemic

***C. Ho*[1], *P. N. Lara*[2,3], *D. R. Gandara*[2,3] *and A. M. Davies*[2,3,*]**

[1] British Columbia Cancer Agency, Vancouver, British Columbia, Canada
[2]UC Davis Cancer Center, Sacramento, California, USA;
[3]University of California, Davis School of Medicine, USA

Abstract

Lung cancer has reached nearly epidemic proportions in women; the incidence has quadrupled over the past 40 years. Multiple studies have been conducted to identify reasons for the dramatic increase in lung cancer over the past decades. Smoking behaviors, pathways of carcinogenesis and the impact of the hormonal milieu have all been examined as possible explanations. Although many studies have attempted to address these questions, they have been retrospective or case-control studies and results have been inconsistent. With the recognition that lung cancer may behave differently in men versus women, current studies are prospectively examining this question.

Introduction

Lung cancer is the leading cause of cancer-related death in both men and women. While lung cancer deaths in men have declined, they have risen for women [1]. Women will account for almost half (47%) of the projected new diagnoses of lung cancer (174,470) in the United States this year[1]. Mortality closely parallels incidence with an anticipated 162,460 deaths and an estimated 72,130 women's lives lost. In comparison, breast cancer accounts for

* Correspondence concerning this article should be addressed to Angela Davies, M.D. Assistant Professor of Medicine, UC Davis Cancer Center 4501 X Street, Suite 3016, Sacramento, California 95817. Phone: (916) 734-3771; Fax: (916) 734-7946; Email: Angela.davies@ucdmc.ucdavis.edu.

41,430 deaths per year, making lung cancer the leading cause of cancer death for women by a wide margin.

A significant increase in tobacco usage by women during and after World War II has been identified as the major contributor to this dramatic rise in incidence and mortality in lung cancer [2]. While changes in smoking behavior have been implicated, there has been much speculation about whether women have an increased susceptibility to develop lung cancer. Researchers have evaluated the role of sex, carcinogen metabolism, and the hormonal milieu as factors influencing lung cancer development and progression. This chapter will review the data currently available addressing these areas of interest in an effort to gain a better understanding of this disease in women.

SMOKING BEHAVIOR

Smoking and Lung Cancer

Although exposures to asbestos, arsenic, benzene, radon and radiation have been connected to lung cancer development, the agent with the most significant causal association is tobacco smoke. While only 20% of smokers develop this disease, the majority of lung cancer patients have a history of past or current tobacco use with a clear dose response curve for amount smoked and the development of lung cancer [3]. Although more difficult to quantify, secondhand or passive smoke exposure has also been linked to lung cancer. A meta-analysis of 37 published epidemiologic studies of lung cancer in non-smokers indicates that a woman who has never smoked has a 24% greater risk of developing lung cancer if she lives with a smoker [4]. Workplace smoke exposure is also associated with a 16-19% increase in risk to develop lung cancer [5]. With the delayed recognition of the perils of environmental smoke exposure, it is not surprising that non-smoking individuals represent approximately 15% of the lung cancer population [1].

Smoking and Lung Cancer Trends over Time

Smoking became a popular habit in the early 20th century due to mass production of cigarettes, increased marketing and subsequent social acceptability [2]. The epidemic began when smoking rates increased in men in higher socioeconomic groups in the 1940s-50s, with smoking in women lagging 10-20 years behind [6]. The impact of this negative behavior has manifested several years later due to a process of malignant transformation that occurs over decades. By 1987, lung cancer deaths began to exceed breast cancer mortality in women in the USA.

While overall rates have decreased, smoking is now paradoxically a habit of lower socioeconomic groups with less formal education [2]. The prevalence of smoking in 1965 in American women 18 years and older was 34% and over the years has declined; in 1970 the rate was 32%; 1980, 30%; 1990, 23% and in 2000, 22% [7]. Paralleling the prevalence of smoking, lung cancer incidence and mortality rates in women increased drastically in the 1970s through the mid-1990s and is only now finally beginning to stabilize [1].

Smoking and Youths

The National Survey on Drug Use and Health for 2004 [8] showed that while trends in smoking have declined overall, there was a significant and concerning rate of usage in younger populations. In youths aged 12 to 17, the rate of current smokers was 12.5% for females and 11.3% for males with young adults aged 18-25 having the highest rate of current tobacco use (44.6%). This trend of early smoking behavior was more prominently observed in young women. It was hypothesized that young women seek to emulate social images associated with glamour, independence and equality. A desire to bond with peers, improve self-image and maintain low body weight has also been suggested as factors.

Adolescents are clearly influenced by exposure through the media; a study noted that adolescents in the highest quartile of exposure to movie smoking were more likely to initiate smoking compared to those in the lowest quartile [9]. Recognizing the impact of media images, tobacco companies have spent over $200 million per year between 1995-2000 in marketing, with 50-60% of the funds directed towards youth-oriented magazines [10].

RISK OF LUNG CANCER

Smoke Exposure

The increase in the incidence of lung cancer observed in women has prompted epidemiological studies examining the relationship between sex, toxin exposure and disease development. While a number of large case-control and cohort studies have examined this relationship, it remains unclear whether women are more susceptible to the carcinogenic effects of cigarette smoke than men and even more difficult to determine susceptibility to second hand smoke exposure.

Harris et al, used the American Health Foundation data to perform a case-control study of over 8,000 patients examining race and sex differences in lung cancer risk for smokers (Table 1) [11]. Women were at increased risk (RR 1.7) compared to men for a given level of smoke exposure. Zang et al updated this in 1996, adding more than 600 cases, equivalent controls and with more precise information regarding histological classification, smoking exposure and body size [12]. Similar to the initial study, women had a 1.5 fold higher relative risk of developing lung cancer compared to men given the same level of cigarette smoke exposure. Case control analysis of data collected by the Cancer Surveillance Program in Orange County California found an age and ethnicity adjusted odds ratio for ever smokers compared to never smokers of 19.7 for women and 15 for men [13]. Risch et al performed a case control study in Canada; the risk of lung cancer for both sexes was associated with cigarette consumption and increased with the number of pack years [14]. The odds ratio for 40 pack year smokers compared to lifelong non-smokers was 27.9 for women and 9.6 for men, indicating a substantially higher risk for women than men. A CT lung cancer screening study also found an increased risk of lung cancer for women; after controlling for age and smoking history, the odds ratio was 2.7 for females compared to males [15]. All of these studies, the majority of which are case-control in design, suggest that women are more susceptible than men to the negative effects of cigarette smoking, resulting in higher lung cancer rates.

In contrast, in the Cancer Prevention Study II (CPS II) the relative risk of a smoker developing lung cancer compared to a never smoker was 22.3 for men and 11.9 for women [16]. Kreuzer et al, using pooled data from 6 European case-control studies from 1988-94, found that the risk of lung cancer in ever smokers compared to never smokers was higher in men than women [17]. However, when controlled for duration of smoking, average daily consumption and time since quitting, the risk was the same for both genders. Two other large cohort studies have demonstrated similar results; the Carotene and Retinol Efficacy trial (n=18,172) had a hazard ratio of 0.9 (female compared to male smokers) when adjusted for age, asbestos exposure, smoking duration, dose and time since quitting [18]. In the data extracted from the Nurse Health Study of women and the Health Professionals Follow-up study of men (total n=85,693), the hazard ratio in women ever-smokers compared to men was 1.08, adjusted for pack years and time since quitting [19]. These latter studies have demonstrated no increased risk of lung cancer in women compared to men when variables like dose and duration are taken into account.

Table 1. Summary of studies evaluating the risk of lung cancer in women versus men

Year	Author	Source Data	Study design	n	Women increased risk
1973-1993	Harris	American Health Foundation	Case-control		Yes
1981-1985	Risch	Canada	Case-control	1617	Yes
1981-1994	Zang	American Health Foundation	Case-control	3959	Yes
1982-1988	Halpern	American Cancer Society's Cancer Prevention Study II	Cohort	1.2 million	No
1984-1986	Osann	Cancer Surveillance Program Orange County	Case-control	5493	Yes
1985-1994	Bach	Carotene and Retinol Efficacy Trial	Cohort	18,172	No
1986-2000	Bain	Nurses Health Study and Health Professionals Follow up study	Cohort	85,693	No
1988-1994	Kreuzer	European	Case-control	9792	No
1993-2001	Henschke	CT screening study	Screening	2490	Yes

Sex difference in susceptibility to lung cancer with smoke exposure continues to be a topic of controversy. These differences were initially observed in case-control studies but are not supported by subsequent cohort observations. All of these studies are confounded by the retrospective nature of reporting smoking history. In addition, they were unable to account for environmental smoke exposure. While this debate will likely never be settled, it has prompted investigations into biological variations in lung cancer between sexes.

CARCINOGEN METABOLISM

A model of carcinogenesis proposes that activation of pro-carcinogens in smoke leads to the formation of DNA adducts which, if unrepaired, leads to critical mutations resulting in cancer. Sex differences in carcinogen metabolism have been proposed at multiple levels in this model including pro-carcinogen activation, carcinogen neutralization, DNA repair and mutagenesis of key cell signaling proteins (Figure 1).

Cytochrome P450

The first step of the carcinogenesis process involves the metabolism of polycyclic aromatic hydrocarbons (PAH) in cigarette smoke by the cytochrome P450 pathway. The CYP1A1 isoform activates aryl hydrocarbon hydroxylase, an enzyme that metabolizes PAH into highly reactive diol-epoxides. Cigarette smoking induces gene expression of CYP1A1 leading to pro-carcinogen activation [20,21]. Mollerup et al observed that female smokers had a higher expression of CYP1A1 and aromatic DNA adducts than their male counterparts in their non-tumor lung tissue [22]. Consistent with this observation, women had higher levels of DNA adducts per pack years as compared to men indicating a higher degree of DNA damage for the amount of exposure.

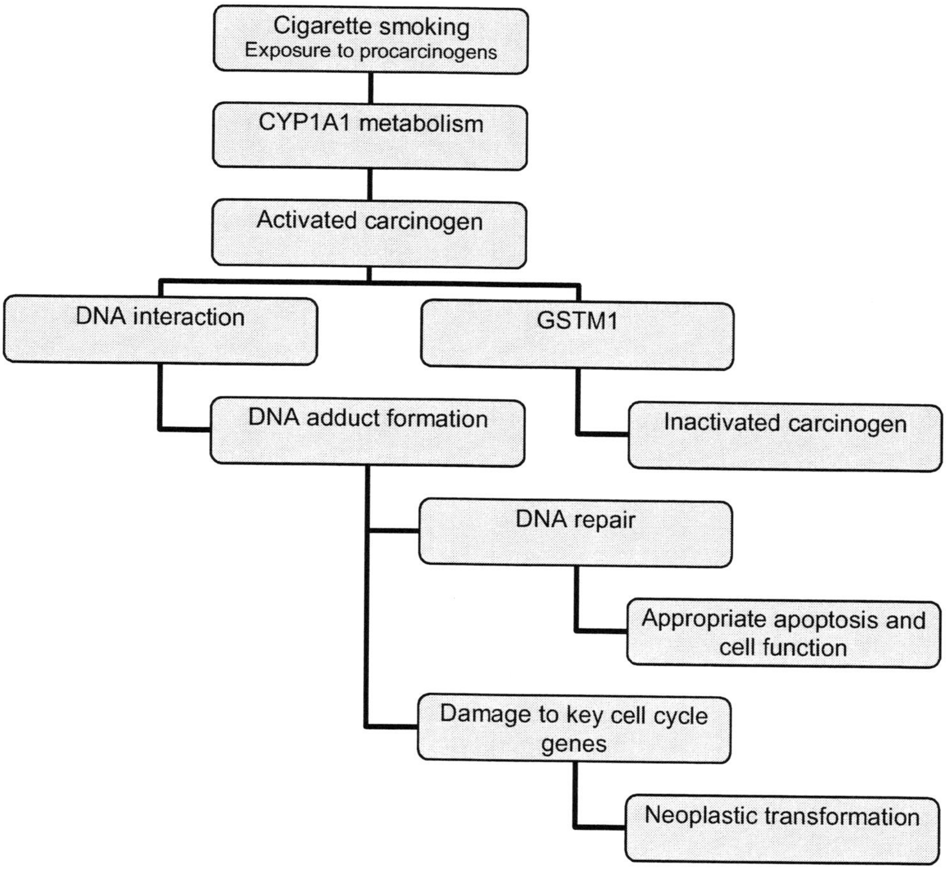

Figure 1. Mechanism of cigarette smoke carcinogenesis.

Glutathione-- Transferase M1 (GSTM1)

Reactive PAH species generated by cytochrome P450 enzymes can be neutralized by Phase II detoxification enzymes that include glutathione-S-transferase. These enzymes catalyze the conversion of the electrophilic metabolites to inactive conjugates, preventing adduct formation with DNA. In 40-50% of the general population, the GSTM1 gene is absent [23]. Molecular epidemiologic case-control studies have noted that the GSTM1 null genotype is significantly associated with lung cancer for women but not men [24]. In a study evaluating DNA extracted from peripheral mononuclear cells, the combined genotype of CYP1A1 exon 7 mutation and null GSTM1 in women has an odds ratio of 6.54 for the development of lung cancer as compared to 2.36 in men [25]. Polymorphisms in cytochrome P450 and GSTM1 may be a contributing factor to the increased risk of lung cancer in women.

DNA Repair Capacity

Observational studies have consistently shown higher levels of DNA adducts in women than men [22.26.27]. The impact of these adducts and their association with the development of malignancy is dependent on the ability of the cells to repair DNA damage. DNA repair capacity (DRC) has been evaluated in a case-control study of patients with lung cancer. The DRC of patients' cultured lymphocytes was determined by measuring the activity of a reporter gene exposed to a reactive intermediate of PAH metabolism, B(a)P diol epoxide [28]. In this study, women had a lower DNA repair capacity than men. A statistically significant trend of increased lung cancer risk with lower levels of DRC was observed, suggesting that women are at higher risk of disease development.

p53

The impact of DNA adduct formation depends on the location of damage and the disruption of key cell cycle genes. Specifically, p53 and K-ras have been examined as a target of PAH cigarette damage. Cigarette smoke and PAH exposure associated p53 mutations are typically G:C to T:A transversions and have been linked to several hotspots in the p53 gene [29]. An analysis of the 2002 International Agency for Research on Cancer mutational database demonstrated that 36% of smoking women had a G to T transversion mutation as compared to 13% of non-smoking women with lung cancer indicating the mutational impact of smoking [30]. In contrast, 31% of smoking and 27% of non-smoking men with lung cancer were observed to have this type of mutation. This suggests that susceptibility to DNA damage is increased in women exposed to tobacco smoke.

K-Ras

Activation of K-ras causes downstream signaling via the MAP kinase cascade, amongst others, resulting in cell proliferation and tumor growth. Codon 12 of K-ras is frequently mutated in lung adenocarcinomas and is associated with cigarette smoke exposure and poor outcomes. A prospective study evaluating K-ras mutational status in 200 lung cancer patients found that mutations were only present in current or former smokers. In addition, a higher proportion of women (26.2%) had the mutation as compared to men (17.4%) [31]. Even after controlling for pack years of smoking, there was a statistically significant association between K-ras mutation and female sex. In contrast, a retrospective analysis of K-ras mutational status in patients treated on the TRIBUTE trial (carboplatin and paclitaxel with or without erlotinib, n=264) demonstrated that the mutation rate was the same in men and women (approximately 20%). However, similar to the previous study, K-ras mutations were only observed in smokers.

Overall, environmental exposure to cigarette smoke and its toxins appears to have a greater impact at the biological level in women than in men. This appears to be due to differences at multiple steps along the carcinogen pathway. Women have increased metabolism of PAH resulting in increased DNA adducts and have a lower capacity for DNA repair. In addition, essential proteins for regulated cell growth are targeted and altered by the PAH adducts resulting in an even higher propensity for cancer development. Dose for dose, these studies suggest the carcinogenic effects of cigarettes are greater for women.

HORMONE RECEPTORS IN LUNG CANCER

While the importance of hormones and their receptors have long been recognized in breast and prostate cancer, the potential role of a hormonal influence on lung cancer has not been as well studied. Estrogen receptors (ER α and ER β) regulate transcription processes by binding at the estrogen response element (ERE) and the AP1 response element (Figure 2). Interaction of estrogen-bound ER α and β with the ERE results in increased transcription of key proteins; in contrast, anti-estrogens causes transcription downregulation [32]. Responses differ at the AP1 site with ER α binding of estrogen and anti-estrogens increasing transcription and ER β binding of estrogens causing transcription inhibition, while anti-estrogen binding results in transcription activation. This suggests that ER α and β have different roles in transcription modification.

It has been hypothesized that the presence of ER β, the most common ER detected in lung tissue, is a negative prognostic indicator in women with lung cancer because of endogenous estrogen binding resulting in transcription activation. Retrospective studies examining pathological specimens, found that 45-67% of lung tumors were ER β positive [33,34,35]. In a retrospective, population-based, case-control study (n=278), for women with ER β positive tumors, there was a non-significant trend towards increased mortality compared to ER β negative tumors [35]. Approximately 40% of the women had used HRT; however, the analysis did not look at outcomes in this subset of women or specifically define HRT use. In contrast, men with ER β positive tumors had a reduction in mortality compared to their negative counterparts. Overall, women had better survival rates than men, regardless of ER β status. Expression of ER β may be related to histology, with one report indicating higher levels of ER β expression in adenocarcinoma (85%) compared to squamous cell carcinoma (30%) [33]. Wu et al did not find a correlation between histology and ER β status but noted increased ER β expression in females, non-smokers, smaller tumors ($\leq$ 3 cm), well-differentiated tumors and absence of lymph node metastasis [34]. The prognostic implications of ER β status are unclear, possibly due to the dual mechanism of transcription modification through the ERE and AP1 pathways.

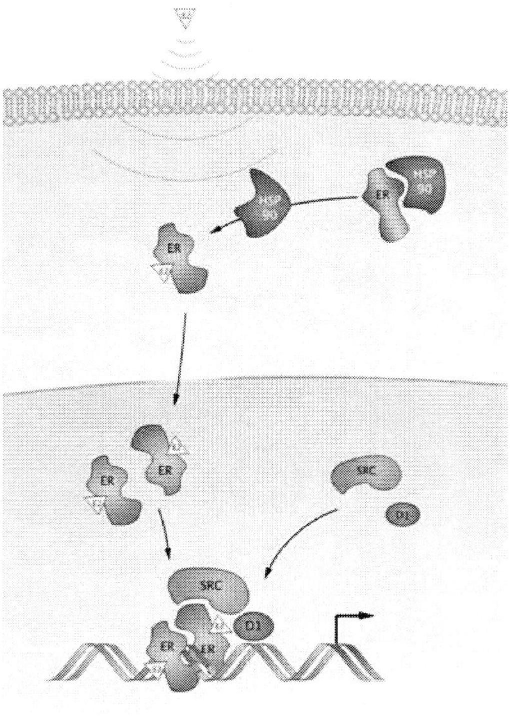

Figure 2. Estrogen receptor signaling and transcription activation (ER - estrogen receptor, E2 - estrogen, HSP 90 - heat shock protein 90, D1 – cyclin D1).
From: http://mekentosj.com/science/er/overview.html

Progesterone receptors (PR) have been detected in NSCLC and have been identified as a positive prognostic indicator in both sexes. In a study by Ishibashi et al, 46% of tumors were PR positive, and PR were more commonly observed in females and adenocarcinoma histology [36]. Their pre-clinical models demonstrated that progesterone inhibited cell proliferation *in vitro* and in tumor xenografts. Tumor xenografts growth inhibition by progesterone was associated with increase p21 and p27 levels with decreased cyclin A, cyclin D1, cyclin E and Ki-67. Endogenous progesterone may have a role in suppressing progression of PR positive NSCLC tumors. The positive prognostic role of PR and the impact of progesterone needs validation in future studies as it may provide therapeutic options for patients with PR positive tumors.

In addition to the presence of ER and PR, immunohistochemistry of archival NSCLC tissue has demonstrated expression of aromatase, the enzyme that converts androgens (testosterone) into estrogens, in 86% of samples [37]. Higher levels of aromatase activity were found in tumor cells compared to adjacent normal lung tissue. Evidence to support a potential therapeutic intervention includes the *in vitro* application of an aromatase inhibitor, anastrazole, which reduces enzyme activity, cell growth and causes tumor growth inhibition in A549 tumor xenografts in ovariectomized nude mice [37].

The hormone mediated proliferation pathway may overlap with the epidermal growth factor receptor (EGFR) cascade, a well recognized pathway, important in the growth of lung cancer. In studies of lung tumor cell caveolae, ER and EGFR have been localized in close proximity [38] and *in vitro*, estrogen and epidermal growth factor are known to stimulate cell proliferation. Thus, both ER and EGFR pathways have been targeted together in lung cancer cell models. NIH N23 lung adenocarcinoma cells were treated with fulvestrant, an ER antagonist and gefitinib, an EGFR tyrosine kinase inhibitor *in vitro* [38,39]. Marked inhibition of cell growth was noted with this combination compared to the hormonal agent alone. Similarly, Stabile et al found that in A549 (bronchioloalveolar), 201T (adenocarcinoma) and 273T (squamous) cell lines and mouse 201T xenografts, there was improved anti-tumor effect with the combination therapy [39]. This correlated with evidence of increased apoptosis, decreased phospho-MAPK, a downstream proliferation-signaling molecule, and decreased Ki-67, a proliferation index, compared to single agent therapy. This pre-clinical work has been translated to the clinic, where a small trial (n=22) was conducted in post-menopausal women combining gefitinib and fulvestrant [40]. Thus far there is no apparent correlation between ER α, ER β, EGFR expression and response to treatment. The treatment was well tolerated with 6 patients experiencing stable disease and an additional 2 with confirmed partial responses.

The presence of hormone receptors and aromatase activity in lung cancer tissue raise interesting questions regarding the role of endogenous and exogenous estrogens in NSCLC growth and development. There are clearly complex interactions between hormones and hormone receptors that warrant further investigation to increase our understanding for potential therapeutic interventions in lung cancer.

Table 2. Summary of studies evaluating the association between hormone replacement therapy and lung cancer risk in women

Year published	Author	Source	Study design	n	Hormonal therapy and lung cancer risk
1988	Wu	Southern California database	Case-control	336	Same
1994	Taioli	American Health Foundation	Case-control	483	Increased
1996	Persson	Sweden	Cohort	22,597	Same
2002		Women's Health Initiative	Cohort	16,608	Same
2002	Blackman	Four centres United States	Case-control	662 cases	Same
2003	Kreuzer	Germany	Case-control	1,723	Decreased
2003	Olsson	Sweden	Cohort	29,508	Decreased
2004	Schabath	MD Anderson	Case-control	1018	Decreased
2005	Ganti	US community based teaching hospital	Case-control	498	Detrimental effect on overall survival

Hormone Replacement Therapy

The impact of hormone replacement therapy (HRT) on lung cancer risk has been examined in multiple studies. Data has been collected from case-control and cohort studies without reaching a consensus on risk (Table 2). Three studies have demonstrated a decreased risk of lung cancer with HRT, including a case-control study by Kreuzer et al performed in Germany [41]. After adjusting for the age, region, pack years, time since smoking cessation and education level, the odd ratio (OR) for lung cancer associated with the use of exogenous hormones was 0.69 for oral contraceptives and 0.83 for HRT. However, the study lacked information regarding the composition and dose of the hormone therapy. A second study, a population-based cohort study involving over 29,000 women, noted a protective benefit from HRT [42]. Long-term HRT users had a decreased incidence of all smoking related malignancies including lung cancer. This advantage was observed in progestin and non-progestin users, regardless of smoking dose. Similarly, in a study conducted at MD Anderson, HRT, estrogen alone and estrogen with progesterone, was associated with a reduction in the risk of lung cancer with an odds ratio of 0.66 [43]. Their model incorporated age, ethnicity, smoking status, education, body mass index and menopausal status.

Several studies have shown no change in lung cancer risk with the use of HRT. A population-based case-control series in the United States found, after accounting for other risk factors including HRT, that only personal smoking, personal and family history of lung disease were associated with increased risk [44]. A large cohort study in Sweden found no adverse or protective effects against lung cancer with the use of HRT after 13 years of follow-up [45]. In 662 female lung cancer patients in four American centers, comparing use $<$ 3 months of HRT to $\geq$ 3 months, the odds ratio was 1.0 [46]. The Women's Health Initiative, designed primarily to assess the impact of HRT on cardiovascular and breast cancer outcomes, found no HRT influence on the incidence of lung cancer (hazard ratio 1.04) [47]. According to these analyses, HRT is not associated with increased or decreased incidence of lung cancer.

One study suggests that the incidence of lung cancer is increased in women taking HRT. Taioli et al, in a case-control study, observed that the use of HRT was significantly associated with the incidence of adenocarcinoma (OR 1.7) [48]. The risk of adenocarcinoma was significant higher in women who smoked and used HRT compared to those who only smoked. Like other studies, there are limitations to this study with the absence of information regarding dose and composition of HRT.

Multiple studies have conflicting results regarding the use of HRT and risk of lung cancer; perhaps the more important question is not about the impact of HRT in incidence but rather outcomes of women on HRT with lung cancer. Ganti et al performed a hypothesis-generating retrospective chart review of almost 500 women with lung cancer [49]. The use of HRT was defined as 6 continuous weeks of estrogen and progestin or estrogen alone prior to the diagnosis of lung cancer, excluding oral contraceptive use. In comparing non-hormone and hormone user, the only statistically significant difference was the median age at diagnosis, with the non-hormone users being slightly older (68 versus 63 years); histologic and stage distribution was similar in both groups. The overall survival was significantly reduced in patients treated with HRT compared to those that were not (39 versus 79 months,

HR 1.97, 95% CI, 1.14-3.39). This raises the possibility of estrogen promoting tumor growth or contributing to more aggressive tumor behavior. Further evaluation of the potential detrimental effect of HRT on survival outcomes in women with lung cancer is required.

While multiple studies have attempted to evaluate biological differences between men and women in the development and progression of lung cancer it is difficult to draw solid conclusions based on the data to date. Recognizing the importance of this issue, the Southwest Oncology Group (SWOG) is conducting a molecular epidemiology case series study in smoking and non-smoking women and men diagnosed with lung cancer (S0424). This study will assess DNA adducts, alterations in specific genes, proteins and receptors (eg. ER, HER2, p53, k-ras), in tumor tissue and peripheral blood. Over 700 patients will be enrolled with the hope of gaining greater knowledge regarding the relationship between sex, smoking status and lung cancer.

Clinical Observations in Lung Cancer

Stage at Diagnosis

SEER data indicate that women and men have the same stage distribution at diagnosis [50]. From 1995-2001, 16% of individuals presented with localized lung cancer, 37% regional, 39% distant and 8% were unstaged. However, when diagnosed women are more likely to be younger, non-smokers, have better pulmonary function and less cardiovascular disease than men [51-55]. In keeping with this observation, women, stage for stage, appear to do better than men. The 5 year survival rates for men with localized, regional and distant disease are 44.8%, 14.2% and 1.7% compared to women, 53.5%, 17.1% and 2.2% respectively (Table 3).

Histology

Retrospective reviews of lung cancer patients have identified consistent trends in histological diagnoses [51-56]. The rates of squamous cell carcinoma are proportionally higher in men. In contrast, women proportionally had higher rates of adenocarcinoma and bronchioloalveolar carcinoma. Rates of small cell lung cancer, most closely associated with smoking, was also higher in women, approximately 25% compared to men, 20% [54]. The reason for these differences is unknown, although it has been hypothesized that smoking behaviors and hormone receptors may play a role. This variation in histological distribution however, may contribute to the differences observed in survival between sexes.

Table 3. 5 year overall survival rates by stage and gender, SEER data

Stage	Male 5 year OS	Female 5 year OS
Localized	44.8%	53.5%
Regional	14.2%	17.1%
Distant	1.7%	2.2%

Treatment

Surgery

The primary modality of treatment for early stage NSCLC is surgery. Several retrospective studies have examined prognostic factors in resected NSCLC and female sex consistently bodes for better survival [51,53-55]. Reviews that controlled for other factors including age, smoking status, pulmonary function, stage, histology and type of surgery continue to demonstrate a better outcome in women with surgically resected NSCLC.

Systemic Therapy

In advanced stage NSCLC, similar to early stage disease, female sex is a positive prognostic factor [56-59]. This may reflect a different underlying biology of advanced disease in women and may be related to likelihood of response to treatment. Studies utilizing chemotherapy and newer molecularly targeted therapies have examined the impact of sex on outcomes.

Chemotherapy(further subheading of systemic therapy)

Eastern Cooperative Oncology Group study, E1594, was a large Phase III trial comparing four platinum-based chemotherapy regimens in advanced NSCLC [60]. All treatment groups had similar outcomes with response rates of 17-22% and median survivals of 8 months. A retrospective analysis, including 437 women and 726 men, evaluated outcomes according to sex [61]. There was no statistically significant difference in performance status, weight loss > 10%, stage or incidence of brain metastasis. While response rates were similar (19%) median survival, accounting for known prognostic indicators, was prolonged in women compared to men (9.2 versus 7.3 months respectively, p=0.004). In addition, women had greater rates of toxicity with respect to nausea, vomiting, alopecia, neurosensory and neuropsychiatric symptoms.

Targeted Therapy(further subheading of systemic therapy)

The EGFR pathway plays a pivotal role in the development and progression of NSCLC and has become a key target in the treatment of advanced NSCLC. The epidermal growth factor receptor tyrosine kinase inhibitors (EGFR TKIs) block the signaling cascade initiated by activation of the EGFR, inhibiting cell proliferation, angiogenesis and metastasis. This pathway may be particularly important in the growth of NSCLC in women, and thus women may be more likely to benefit from EGFR-targeted therapies. Sensitivity to EGFR TKIs has been associated with activating EGFR mutations [64,65] and initially it was thought that these mutations were more common in women. However, larger series have demonstrated a similar incidence of these mutations in men and women [63,65,66]. Thus, presence of EGFR mutations does not explain the apparent increased benefit women obtain from treatment with these agents compared to men.

A recent phase II trial (Southwest Oncology Group study, S0126) evaluated gefitinib, an EGFR TKI, in advanced bronchioloalveolar carcinoma (a histological subtype of NSCLC) [62]. An unplanned subgroup analysis demonstrated that women (n=70) had a significantly longer median survival compared to men (n=67) (19 months versus 8 months, respectively, p=0.007). This benefit in survival was maintained in a multivariate model that incorporated rash (a common side effect of this class of drugs), smoking history and performance status. In a phase III National Cancer Institute of Canada (NCIC) led trial (BR 21) patients with advanced NSCLC that had progressed after front line therapy were randomized to erlotinib, another EGFR-TKI, or placebo. While women had higher response rates compared to men (14% vs 6%, p=0.007) [63], there was no difference in survival.

In contrast, a recent trial incorporating the novel antibody directed against vascular endothelial growth factor (VEGF), bevacizumab, did not show a survival benefit for women in an unplanned subgroup analysis. The ECOG 4599 trial compared carboplatin/paclitaxel -/+ bevacizumab (PC vs PCB) in 855 chemo-naïve advanced stage NSCLC patients [67]. The bevacizumab containing arm demonstrated an improved response rate (10% versus 27.2%, p<0.0001) and median survival (10.2 versus 12.5 months, p=0.007). In an unplanned subgroup analysis, the survival benefit with the addition of bevacizumab was only seen for men; hazard ratio for death PC vs PCB in men 0.69 (p=0.003) and women 0.96 (p=0.80). The reason for this lack of benefit in women is unclear; it may reflect differences in second and third line treatment, imbalances in unmeasured baseline prognostic factors or may in fact represent a true difference.

Outcomes

Despite the body of evidence that, at a biologic level, women may be more susceptible to the negative effects of cigarette smoke and estrogens may contribute to increase tumor proliferation, studies indicate that overall, women have a better prognosis once diagnosed with lung cancer than men. Women diagnosed with lung cancer are more likely to be younger, non-smokers, with better pulmonary function and less cardiovascular disease than their male counterparts [51-55]. When analyses have controlled for these potential confounding prognostic indicators, women still have a better survival. The 5 year survival rate from data compiled by the NIH from 1995-2001 was 13.6% for women compared to 5% for men, for all stages combined [68]. This observation may be the result of both different underlying disease biology and increase likelihood of response to current therapies.

Conclusion

Lung cancer in women is a significant health issue, responsible for more cancer related mortality than breast and colorectal cancer combined. There appear to be biological differences in lung cancer related to sex. Women seem to be more susceptible to the negative effects of smoke exposure possibly due to differences in carcinogen metabolism. The presence of hormone receptors may also impact the natural history of disease, playing a role in tumor proliferation and growth. Yet, despite this, once diagnosed with lung cancer women have a better overall prognosis than men. Clearly there are complex mechanisms involved and a better understanding of sex-related biology will enable us to more effectively direct research and apply treatments for both women and men.

References

[1] Society AC: *Cancer Facts and Figures* 2006, 2006.

[2] Giovino, GA. Epidemiology of tobacco use in the United States. *Oncogene*, 2002 21, 7326-40.

[3] Khuder, SA. Effect of cigarette smoking on major histological types of lung cancer: a meta-analysis. *Lung Cancer*, 2001 31, 139-48.

[4] Hackshaw, AK; Law, MR; Wald, NJ. The accumulated evidence on lung cancer and environmental tobacco smoke. *Bmj,* 1997 315, 980-8.

[5] Sasco, AJ; Secretan, MB; Straif, K. Tobacco smoking and cancer: a brief review of recent epidemiological evidence. *Lung Cancer 45 Suppl 2*, 2004, S3-9.

[6] Bolego, C; Poli, A; Paoletti, R. Smoking and gender. *Cardiovasc Res*, 2002 53, 568-76.

[7] WHO, 2006.

[8] Services USDoHaH: *National Survey on Drug Use and Health* 2004, 2006.

[9] Dalton, MA; Sargent, JD; Beach, ML; et al. Effect of viewing smoking in movies on adolescent smoking initiation: a cohort study. *Lance*t, 2003 362, 281-5.

[10] King, C, 3rd; Siegel, M. The Master Settlement Agreement with the tobacco industry and cigarette advertising in magazines. *N Engl J Med*, 2001 345, 504-11.

[11] Harris, RE; Zang, EA; Anderson, JI; et al. Race and sex differences in lung cancer risk associated with cigarette smoking. *Int J Epidemiol*, 1993 22, 592-9.

[12] Zang, EA; Wynder, EL. Differences in lung cancer risk between men and women: examination of the evidence. *J Natl Cancer Inst*, 1996 88, 183-92.

[13] Osann, KE; Anton-Culver, H; Kurosaki, T; et al. Sex differences in lung-cancer risk associated with cigarette smoking. *Int J Cancer*, 1993 54, 44-8.

[14] Risch, HA; Howe, GR; Jain, M; et al. Are female smokers at higher risk for lung cancer than male smokers? A case-control analysis by histologic type. *Am J Epidemiol*, 1993 138, 281-93.

[15] Henschke, CI; Miettinen, OS. Women's susceptibility to tobacco carcinogens. *Lung Cancer*, 2004 43, 1-5.

[16] Halpern, MT; Gillespie, BW; Warner, KE. Patterns of absolute risk of lung cancer mortality in former smokers. *J Natl Cancer Inst*, 1983 85, 457-64.

[17] Kreuzer, M; Boffetta, P; Whitley, E; et al. Gender differences in lung cancer risk by smoking: a multicentre case-control study in Germany and Italy. *Br J Cancer*, 2000 82, 227-33.

[18] Bach, PB; Kattan, MW; Thornquist, MD; et al. Variations in lung cancer risk among smokers. *J Natl Cancer Inst*, 2003 95, 470-8.

[19] Bain, C; Feskanich, D; Speizer, FE; et al. Lung cancer rates in men and women with comparable histories of smoking. *J Natl Cancer Inst*, 2004 96, 826-34.

[20] Kouri, RE; Rude, TH; Curren, RD; et al. Biological activity of tobacco smoke and tobacco smoke-related chemicals. *Environ Health Perspect*, 1979 29, 63-69.

[21] McLemore, TL; Adelberg, S; Liu, MC; et al. Expression of CYP1A1 gene in patients with lung cancer: evidence for cigarette smoke-induced gene expression in normal lung tissue and for altered gene regulation in primary pulmonary carcinomas. *J Natl Cancer Inst*, 1990 82, 1333-9.

[22] Mollerup, S; Ryberg, D; Hewer, A; et al. Sex differences in lung CYP1A1 expression and DNA adduct levels among lung cancer patients. *Cancer Res*, 1999 59, 3317-20.

[23] Bell, DA; Taylor, JA; Paulson, DF; et al. Genetic risk and carcinogen exposure: a common inherited defect of the carcinogen-metabolism gene glutathione S-transferase M1 (GSTM1) that increases susceptibility to bladder cancer. *J Natl Cancer Inst*, 1993 85, 1159-64.

[24] Tang, DL; Rundle, A; Warburton, D; et al. Associations between both genetic and environmental biomarkers and lung cancer: evidence of a greater risk of lung cancer in women smokers. *Carcinogenesis*, 1998 19, 1949-53.

[25] Dresler, CM; Fratelli, C; Babb, J; et al. Gender differences in genetic susceptibility for lung cancer. *Lung Cancer*, 2000 30, 153-60.

[26] Ryberg, D; Hewer, A; Phillips, DH et al. Different susceptibility to smoking-induced DNA damage among male and female lung cancer patients. *Cancer Res*, 1994 54, 5801-3.

[27] Haugen, A. Women who smoke: are women more susceptible to tobacco-induced lung cancer? *Carcinogenesis*, 2002 23, 227-9.

[28] Wei, Q; Cheng, L; Amos, CI; et al. Repair of tobacco carcinogen-induced DNA adducts and lung cancer risk: a molecular epidemiologic study. *J Natl Cancer Inst*, 2000 92, 1764-72.

[29] Kure, EH; Ryberg, D; Hewer, A; et al. p53 mutations in lung tumours: relationship to gender and lung DNA adduct levels. *Carcinogenesis*, 1996 17, 2201-5.

[30] Toyooka, S; Tsuda, T; Gazdar, AF. The TP53 gene, tobacco exposure, and lung cancer. *Hum Mutat*, 2003 21, 229-39.

[31] Nelson, HH; Christiani, DC; Mark, EJ; et al. Implications and prognostic value of K-ras mutation for early-stage lung cancer in women. *J Natl Cancer Inst*, 1999 91, 2032-8.

[32] Paech, K; Webb, P; Kuiper, GG; et al. Differential ligand activation of estrogen receptors ERalpha and ERbeta at AP1 sites. *Science*, 1997 277, 1508-10.

[33] Omoto, Y; Kobayashi, Y; Nishida, K; et al. Expression, function, and clinical implications of the estrogen receptor beta in human lung cancers. *Biochem Biophys Res Commun*, 2001 285, 340-7.

[34] Wu, CT; Chang, YL; Shih, JY; et al. The significance of estrogen receptor beta in 301 surgically treated non-small cell lung cancers. *J Thorac Cardiovasc Surg*, 2005 130, 979-86.

[35] Schwartz, AG; Prysak, GM; Murphy, V; et al. Nuclear estrogen receptor beta in lung cancer: expression and survival differences by sex. *Clin Cancer Res*, 2005 11, 7280-7.

[36] Ishibashi, H; Suzuki, T; Suzuki, S; et al. Progesterone receptor in non-small cell lung cancer--a potent prognostic factor and possible target for endocrine therapy. *Cancer Res*, 2005 65, 6450-8.

[37] Weinberg, OK; Marquez-Garban, DC; Fishbein, MC; et al. Aromatase inhibitors in human lung cancer therapy. *Cancer Res*, 2005 65, 11287-91.

[38] Pietras, RJ; Marquez, DC; Chen, HW; et al. Estrogen and growth factor receptor interactions in human breast and non-small cell lung cancer cells. *Steroids*, 2005 70, 372-81.

[39] Stabile, LP; Lyker, JS; Gubish, CT; et al. Combined targeting of the estrogen receptor and the epidermal growth factor receptor in non-small cell lung cancer shows enhanced antiproliferative effects. *Cancer Res*, 2005 65, 1459-70.

[40] Traynor, AM; Schiller, JH; Stabile, LP; et al. Combination therapy with gefitinib and fulvestrant (G/F) for women with non-small cell lung cancer (NSCLC*). J Clin Oncol (Meeting Abstracts)*, 2005 23, 7224-.

[41] Kreuzer, M; Gerken, M; Heinrich, J; et al. Hormonal factors and risk of lung cancer among women? *Int J Epidemiol*, 2003 32, 263-71.

[42] Olsson, H; Bladstrom, A; Ingvar, C. Are smoking-associated cancers prevented or postponed in women using hormone replacement therapy? *Obstet Gynecol*, 2003 102, 565-70.

[43] Schabath, MB; Wu, X; Vassilopoulou-Sellin, R; et al. Hormone replacement therapy and lung cancer risk: a case-control analysis. *Clin Cancer Res*, 2004 10, 113-23.

[44] Wu, AH; Yu, MC; Thomas, DC; et al. Personal and family history of lung disease as risk factors for adenocarcinoma of the lung. *Cancer Res*, 1988 48, 7279-84.

[45] Persson, I; Yuen, J; Bergkvist, L; et al. Cancer incidence and mortality in women receiving estrogen and estrogen-progestin replacement therapy--long-term follow-up of a Swedish cohort. *Int J Cancer*, 1996 67, 327-32.

[46] Blackman, JA; Coogan, PF; Rosenberg, L; et al. Estrogen replacement therapy and risk of lung cancer. *Pharmacoepidemiol Drug Saf*, 2002 11, 561-7.

[47] Rossouw, JE; Anderson, GL; Prentice, RL; et al. Risks and benefits of estrogen plus progestin in healthy postmenopausal women: principal results from the Women's Health Initiative randomized controlled trial. *Jama*, 2002 288, 321-33.

[48] Taioli, E; Wynder, EL. Re: Endocrine factors and adenocarcinoma of the lung in women. *J Natl Cancer Inst*, 1994 86, 869-70.

[49] Ganti, AK; Sahmoun, AE; Panwalkar, AW; et al. Hormone replacement therapy is associated with decreased survival in women with lung cancer. *J Clin Oncol*, 2006 24, 59-63.

[50] SEER: *SEER data for lung and bronchus cancer*, 2006.

[51] Ferguson, MK; Wang, J; Hoffman, PC; et al. Sex-associated differences in survival of patients undergoing resection for lung cancer. *Ann Thorac Surg*, 2000 69, 245-9, discussion 249-50.

[52] Radzikowska, E; Langfort, R; Giedronowicz, D; Estrogen and progesterone receptors in non small cell lung cancer patients. *Ann Thorac Cardiovasc Surg*, 2002 8, 69-73.

[53] Alexiou, C; Onyeaka, CV; Beggs, D; et al. Do women live longer following lung resection for carcinoma? *Eur J Cardiothorac Surg*, 2002 21, 319-25.

[54] Chatkin, JM; Abreu, CM; Fritscher, CC; et al. Is there a gender difference in non-small cell lung cancer survival? *Gend Med*, 2004 1, 41-7.

[55] Batevik, R; Grong, K; Segadal, L; et al. The female gender has a positive effect on survival independent of background life expectancy following surgical resection of primary non-small cell lung cancer: a study of absolute and relative survival over 15 years. *Lung Cancer*, 2005 47, 173-81.

[56] Radzikowska, E; Glaz, P; Roszkowski, K. Lung cancer in women: age, smoking, histology, performance status, stage, initial treatment and survival. Population-based study of 20 561 cases. *Ann Oncol*, 2002 13, 1087-93.

[57] Albain, KS; Crowley, JJ; LeBlanc, M; et al. Survival determinants in extensive-stage non-small-cell lung cancer: the Southwest Oncology Group experience. *Journal of Clinical Oncology*, 1991 9, 1618-26.

[58] Paesmans, M; Sculier, JP; Libert, P; et al. Prognostic factors for survival in advanced non-small-cell lung cancer: univariate and multivariate analyses including recursive partitioning and amalgamation algorithms in 1,052 patients. The European Lung Cancer Working Party. *Journal of Clinical Oncology*, 1995 13, 1221-30.

[59] Visbal, AL; Williams, BA; Nichols, FC, 3rd; et al. Gender differences in non-small-cell lung cancer survival: an analysis of 4,618 patients diagnosed between 1997 and 2002. *Ann Thorac Surg*, 2004 78, 209-15, discussion 215.

[60] Schiller, JH; Harrington, D; Belani, CP; et al. Comparison of four chemotherapy regimens for advanced non-small-cell lung cancer. *New England Journal of Medicine*, 2002 346, 92-8.

[61] Wakelee, H WW; Schiller, J; Langer, C; Sandler, A; Belani, C; Johnson, D. Survival differences by gender for patients with advanced non-small cell lung cancer in Eastern Cooperative Group trial 1594. *J Thoracic Oncology In press*, 2006.

[62] West, H; Franklin, WA; Gumerlock, P; et al. *Gefitinib (ZD1839) therapy for advanced bronchioloalveolar lung cancer: Southwest Oncology Group Study S0126.*, ASCO. New Orleans, 2004.

[63] Tsao, MS; Sakurada, A; Cutz, JC; et al. Erlotinib in lung cancer - molecular and clinical predictors of outcome. *N Engl J Med*, 2005 353, 133-44.

[64] Pao, W; Miller, V; Zakowski, M; et al. EGF receptor gene mutations are common in lung cancers from "never smokers" and are associated with sensitivity of tumors to gefitinib and erlotinib. *PNAS* 101:13306-13311, 2004.

[65] Paez, JG; Janne, PA; Lee, JC; et al. EGFR Mutations in Lung Cancer: Correlation with Clinical Response to Gefitinib Therapy. *Science*, 2004 304, 1497-1500.

[66] Eberhard, DA; Johnson, BE; Amler, LC; et al. Mutations in the Epidermal Growth Factor Receptor and in KRAS Are Predictive and Prognostic Indicators in Patients

With Non-Small-Cell Lung Cancer Treated With Chemotherapy Alone and in Combination With Erlotinib. *J Clin Oncol*, 2005 23, 5900-5909.

[67] Sandler, AB; Gray, R; Brahmer, J; et al. Randomized phase II/III trial of paclitaxel (P) plus carboplatin (C) with or without bevacizumab (NSC #704865) in patients with advanced non-squamous non-small cell lung cancer (NSCLC): An Eastern Cooperative Oncology Group (ECOG) Trial - E4599. *J Clin Oncol (Meeting Abstracts)*, 2005 23, LBA4-.

[68] Health USNIo: *Surveillance Epidemiology and End Results (SEER)*, 2005.

In: Women and Cancer
Editor: Laurie Elit, pp. 21-48
ISBN: 978-1-60021-494-3

Chapter II

WOMEN AND LUNG CANCER: A SECOND OPINION

***Jyoti D. Patel*[1,*] *and Joan H. Schiller*[2]**
[1]Division of Hematology/Oncology, Feinberg School of Medicine, Northwestern University, Robert H. Lurie Comprehensive Cancer Center, Chicago, USA;
[2]Division of Hematology and Oncology, Deputy Director of Simmons Comprehensive Cancer Center, Andreas L. Simmons Distinguished Chair in Cancer Research, University of Texas Southwestern Medical School, Dallas, USA.

LUNG CANCER IN WOMEN

Lung cancer is the leading cause of cancer death in the United States and throughout the world. It is estimated that 84,470 new lung cancers will be diagnosed in United States women in 2006 [1] resulting in 73,230 deaths of from progressive disease. Lung cancer accounts for 26% of all cancer deaths in United States women, far surpassing deaths caused by breast and gynecologic cancers. In 1987, lung cancer surpassed breast cancer to become the leading cause of cancer death among women (Figure 1). There has been a fourfold increase in lung cancer in women over the past 30 years, and it is estimated that this rise will not plateau until after 2010. Birth cohorts of women characterized by the highest smoking prevalence have yet to reach the age of highest lung cancer risk. It is projected that mortality from lung cancer in women will continue to increase as the at-risk population increases [2].

* Correspondence concerning this article should be addressed to:
Jyoti D. Patel, M.D. Division of Hematology/Oncology, Feinberg School of Medicine, Northwestern University Robert H. Lurie Comprehensive Cancer Center, 676 N. St. Clair Street, Suite 850, Chicago, IL 60611; Tel: 312-695-4549; Fax: 312-695-4530; Email: jd-patel@northwestern.edu.
Joan H. Schiller, MD. Chief, Division of Hematology and Oncology, Deputy Director of Simmons Comprehensive Cancer Center, Andreas L. Simmons Distinguished Chair in Cancer Research, University of Texas Southwestern Medical School 214-648-4180. FAX: 214-648-1955; Email: joan.schiller@utsouthwestern.edu. University of Texas Southwestern, Division of Hematology/Oncology 5323 Harry Hines Blvd, Dallas, Texas 75390-8852.

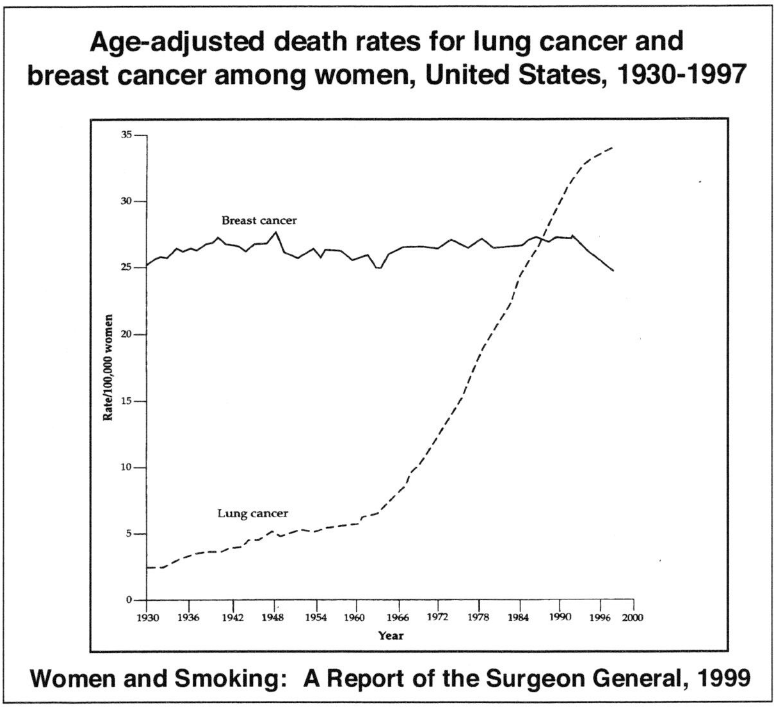

Figure 1.

EPIDEMIOLOGY AND ETIOLOGY

Changes in smoking habits in the United States, and in particular in women, have directly resulted in the death rates from lung cancer in women increasing more rapidly that any other cancer death rate. Cigarette smoking is known to be the major cause of lung cancer in both men and women, with 85% to 90% of all lung cancer patients having smoked cigarettes at some time in their lives. Despite significant declines in smoking prevalance, almost one quarter of US women continue to smoke. Approximately 22 million US women smoke and at least 500,000 teenage girls use tobacco products [3].

Smoking

Lung cancer incidence and mortality patterns follow, after a latency interval of 20 or more years, the temporal patterns of cigarette smoking. The risk of dying from lung cancer from lung cancer is associated with age of initiation and duration of cigarette smoking, and the number of cigarettes smoked each day or as a regular pattern. The cumulative probability of lung cancer in the general population for individuals up to 74 years of age is 10% to 15% in those who smoke one or more packs of cigarettes per day [4].

The complexity of tobacco smoke, with over 3,000 different chemicals, has made it difficult to identify the contribution of the more than 40 putative carcinogens. The carcinogens in tobacco smoke include the polynuclear aromatic hydrocarbons, N-nitrosamines, aromatic amines, other organic (benzene, acrylonitrile) and inorganic (aresenic, acetaldehyde) compunds and polonium 210. Side stream smoke emitted from a smoldering cigarette between puffs contains virtually all the carcinogenic compounds that have been identified in the mainstream smoke inhaled by smokers.

Unfortunately, young women and girls continue to smoke and are specifically targeted in tobacco advertising, which is dominated by themes of social desirability and independence. The belief that smoking will help control weight motivates many young women to smoke [5]. Up to 30% of high school girls report having smoked cigarettes in the past 30 days [6]. In addition, despite the clear health consequences to the fetus of smoking during pregnancy, estimates of women smoking during pregnancy range from 13% to as high as 22% [7]. Although smoking rates in US women have stabilized in the past decade, just less than one quarter of all women are active smokers (Figure 2).

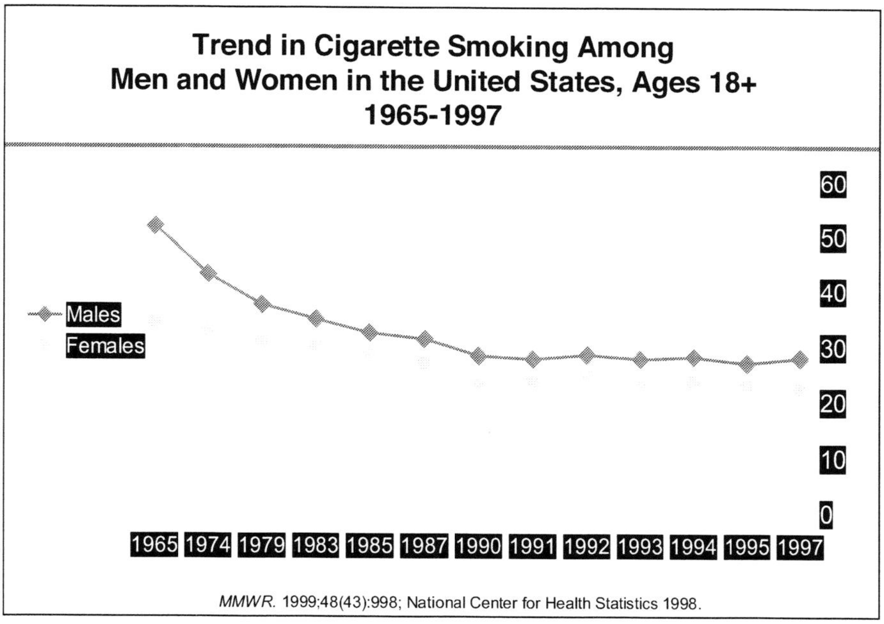

Figure 2.

Finally, once women begin to smoke, several reports indicate that they are less successful than men in their attempts to stop smoking [8-10]. Population studies indicate that more men than women report ever smoking however, the quit ratio (former smokers to current smokers) is consistently lower for women than for men. Moreover, although men and women are equally likely to attempt to self quit, women have more difficulty maintaining abstinence after a smoking quit attempt [11,12]. Bohadana et al found cessation rates among male smokers to be 16% higher than among female smokers (62% vs. 46%) [13]. In this study, behavioral factors, rather than nicotine dependence alone, correlated with cessation rates of female smokers. Several factors may contribute to the gender disparity in smoking cessation outcomes. Research suggests that women are more likely to than men to smoke to manage negative affect [14]. Moreover negative affect, weight gain issues, and depression are more common precipitants to relapse for women than men [15-17]. Bupriopion is an antidepressant that has shown to be effective as a treatment for smoking cessation by attenuating post quit negative affect and reducing postcessation appetite and weight gain [18]. Bupropion may attenuate the gender disparity seen in smoking cessation rates [19]. These findings suggest that smoking cessation programs that emphasize behavioral counseling alone may not adequately address the needs of women who wish to stop smoking, and that they also may benefit pharmacological intervention.

Smoking rates in Europe and in Asian are generally not as high as those in North American women. In Europe, smoking rate among women over 15 years vary widely, with the highest rates in found Serbia and Montenegro (42%) to just 1% of women smoking in Armenia and 2% in the Republic of Moldova. Regardless, lung cancer accounts for 10% of all cancer deaths in European women [20]. Trends of cigarette use in developing countries have been less well documented. An estimated 20 million women have started smoking in China since the 1990s [21], and after aggressive promotional campaigns targeting women and girls, smoking among women in Japan doubled from 9% to 18% in just five years from 1986 to 1991 [22]. Available evidence suggests that increasing rates of cigarette smoking in developing countries will in time be reflected in lung cancer mortality.

Controversy exists as to whether women are more or less susceptible to the carcinogenic effects of cigarette smoke than men. Several case control studies from the 1990's have argued that women are more susceptible to the carcinogens in cigarette smoke than men. A 1993 study of 800 Canadians found that compared with nonsmokers, the odds ratio of developing lung cancer for those with a 40-pack year history was 27.9 in women and 9.6 in men [23]. This study was followed by a 1996 American Health Foundation study of almost 4000 patients and control subjects that found that female smokers had a 1.5-fold higher estimated relative risk of developing lung cancer than did male smokers [24]. More recently, Henschke and Miettinene evaluated the absolute risk for lung cancer in men and women smokers undergoing baseline computed tomography (CT) screening for lung cancer [25]. 1200 women and 1200 men who were over 40 years old and had at least a 10 pack year tobacco history were included. The diagnostic protocol for positive CT scans (1-6 noncalcified nodules) included biopsy and diagnosis by pathologists with expertise in thoracic malignancies. With use of logistic regression analysis, and controlling for age and smoking history, the risk for lung cancer in women versus men was 2.7. They concluded that for a given level of smoking, more women than men developed lung cancer.

On the other had, multiple carefully conducted cohort studies have reported that women are not more susceptible to the harmful effects of tobacco smoke than are men. The American Cancer Society follow up prevention study, which enrolled 1.2 million men and women in 1982 and followed them until 1988, demonstrated that although the overall risk of lung cancer in women smokers was 11.9, male smokers had an even greater relative risk (22.3) of developing lung cancer. In the Carotene and Retinol Efficacy Trial (CARET), a randomized study with over 18,000 participants, Bach et al found no association between sex and lung cancer risk [26]. Most recently, an analysis of the of the Nurses' Health Study of over 60,000 women and the Health Professionals Follow-up Study of over 25,000 men showed no convincing evidence of increased lung cancer risk in women [27].

Although the differences in sex risk have been widely touted, the methods in studies by Risch [23] and Zang [28] have been challenged [29]. Various biases, such as the underreporting of smoking habits and the confounding effects of passive smoking, can affect comparisons of sex differences in risk, and it is likely that this debate will continue.

Other Risks

The risk of dying from lung cancer in 30% higher for a nonsmoker living with a smoker compared with a nonsmoker living with a nonsmoker. Increases in lung cancer risk exposure accompany exposure to carcinogens such as asbestos, radon, chromium, chloromethylethers, nickels, mustard gas and radiation (including radon). Exposure to other environmental and occupational respiratory carcinogens may be interactive with cigarette smoking, and may influence trends of lung cancer incidence and mortality.

Although tobacco smoke and environmental exposures account for the vast majority of lung cancer, only 10-15% of all smokers develop lung cancer and 10-15% of all lung cancers occur among nonsmokers. It is probable that there are individual differences in susceptibility, some of which have a genetic component. Variations in the metabolism of carcinogens have been implicated by many, and it appears that there are sex based variations in risk.

Sex Based Differences in Lung Cancer Biology

Genetic Differences

Genetic variation between men and women is present in some genes that encode carcinogen metabolizing enzymes. The *CYP1A1* gene codes for an enzyme that is central to the metabolism of carcinogenic polycyclic aromatic hydrocarbons [30]. Activation of polycyclic aromatic hydrocarbons by the *CYP1A1* gene product leads to highly reactive substances that bind to DNA, forming adducts [31]. Increased expression of the *CYP1A1* gene in the lung has been demonstrated in female smokers compared with male smokers [32]. Increased CYP1A1 enzymes expression may be the result of induction by hormones, notable estrogen. Previous work in the breast cancer cell line MDA-MB-2131 has suggested that cross-talk between the estrogen receptor and the aryl hydrocarbon receptor may exist. This could in turn modulate the expression of polycyclic aromatic hydrocarbon metabolizing enzymes, specifically the CYP1A1 enzyme [33].

Although the *CYP1A1* gene codes for phase 1 enzymes that metabolically activate carcinogens, phase 2 enzymes compete with phase 1 carcinogen-activating enzymes to inhibit the formation of free radicals and also catalyze the conversion of reactive intermediates to inactive conjugates that are more water soluble and more readily excreted [34]. The most common polymorphism in the phase 2 detoxification enzymes is the glutathione S-transferase M1 (*GSTM1*) null genotype, which is present in 40% to 60% of the general population due to a gene deletion [35]. Expression of the null phenotype may be a marker of susceptibility, and the effects of *GSTM1* gene deletion may be heightened among female smokers [36]. The effect of polymorphisms in both *CYP1A1* and *GSTM1* gene could contribute to differences in the etiology of lung cancer in women.

Other lines of evidence for sex-related differences in lung cancer come from studies on the gastrin-releasing peptide receptor (GRPR). A number of studies have shown that gastrin-releasing peptide (GRP), a bombesin-like peptide, plays a role in neoplasia by stimulating cell proliferation [37,38]. In normal tissues, this peptide stimulates the growth of bronchial epithelial cells and has been implicated as regulator of human lung development. The effect of these peptides is mediated mainly through and interaction with the gastrin releasing peptide receptor (GRPR). The gene for GRP's receptor (GRPR) is X-linked, located on chromosome Xp22, near a cluster of genes that escape X-inactivation. Women, therefore, can have two actively transcribed alleles of the GRPR gene, compared with only one in men. It has been reported that GRPR mRNA expression was noted in 55% of female "nonsmokers" but only 0% of male "nonsmokers" and that 75% of women who were short-term smokers (1-25 pack years) had GRPR mRNA expression compared with 20% of male short-term smokers [37]. Subsequently it was demonstrated that expression of GRPR mRNA in lung fibroblasts was elevated following exposure to nicotine, and hypothesized that women may be increased risk to the carcinogenic effects of nicotine through the induction of GRPR expression [39]. There is increased expression of the GRPR gene when human airway cells were exposed to estrogen, suggesting that GRPR could also be regulated by the hormone [37].

Molecular Differences

Carcinogens, such as polycyclic aromatic hydrocarbons (PAH) and nitrosamines, are present in tobacco smoke and exert their biologic effects after transformation through the formation of DNA adducts in target tissues and mutations in transforming genes [40]. The extent of DNA adduct formation depends on the balance between rates of oxidation or the compounds and the rates of detoxification of the reactive products by way of conjugation and DNA repair capacity. Although there is considerable variation between tobacco exposure and adduct level [41], high levels of stable adducts in lung tissue are believed to play a role in the initiation of carcinogenesis [42]. Higher smoking-related DNA adduct levels in female patients with lung cancer, when adjusted for smoking dose, have been reported in tumors and adjacent lung tissue [31,41]. DNA adduct levels in a series of non-smoking Taiwanese women were also significantly higher than those in non-smoking men and may reflect the burden of environmental carcinogen exposure in Asian women [43]. Reduced DNA repair capacity is associated with an increased risk of lung cancer, and women are reported to have lower DNA repair capacity than men [44].

Multiple studies suggest that women may be more predisposed than men to molecular aberrations that result from the carcinogenic effects of tobacco smoke. p53 is a tumor suppressor gene that is often mutated in lung cancer (ranging from 70% in small cell lung cancer to 33% in lung adenocarcinoma) [45]. The dominant mutation in the p53 gene is a G:C→T:A transversion [46]. A higher frequency this mutation in the p53 gene and a higher average DNA adduct level in the lung tumors of women and men has been found, even though the level of exposure to carcinogens from cigarette smoking was lower among women (mean, 23-pack years) than among men (mean, 39 pack years) [47]. Similarly, the International Agency for Research on Cancer database has been studied for the mutation G:C→T:A in the p53 gene. In the 705 cases for which smoke exposure data were available, they found that although subtle differences in the p53 gene mutational spectrum existed between men and women smokers, there was a significantly higher frequency of the transversion in women smokers compared to women who had never smoked. The authors concluded that lung cancers in women smokers demonstrate significantly more tobacco-related mutations than women who had never smoked and than male smokers.

The K-ras oncogene encodes a protein that is oncogenic when mutated or overexpressed in lung tumors. One study attempted to define the patient characteristics that are associated with K-ras gene mutation and to determine whether mutation of the gene correlated with patient prognosis [48]. Mutations in codon 12 of the K-ras oncogene occurred predominantly in adenocarcinomas were found only in patients who had a history of smoking, and were more common in women than men (26% and 17%, respectively). The investigators concluded that cigarette smoking induces K-ras mutations and the resultant clones could be further expanded by a second event that may be specific for adenocarcinoma histology. Given the sex difference in the mutation patterns, this event could involve the growth-promoting effects of hormones such as estrogen.

Hormonal Differences

There are significant sex differences in lung cancer at the genetic and biochemical levels. It is therefore reasonable to postulate that these effects are mediated in some way by circulating estrogen. Classical estrogen receptor (ERαβ) is a ligand-activated transcription factor that is associated with the development of estrogen-dependent cancers such as breast and endometrial carcinoma. A second estrogen receptor, estrogen receptor β(ERβ), was identified in 1996 and localized to chromosome 14 [49]. Both receptors possess several distinct functional domains, including a central DNA binding domain that is highly conserved between ERα and ERβ [50]. The C-terminus encodes the ligand-dependent tanscription activation function (AF-2) of the protein. Located at the N-terminus is a second transcription activation function (AF-1), which is ligand independent and is activated by growth factor-mediated phosphorylation. ERβ has biologic roles that are distinct from those of ERα. Whereas ERα is required for ovulation, ERβ is required for the differentiation of estrogen sensitive tissues. The tissue distribution of these two receptors also varies. Relative quantities of estrogen receptor β mRNA are highest in human granulosa cells, endothelial cells, the ovary, and the lung [49]. In tissues that express both ERα and ERβ, there is potentially very complex gene regulation via formation of ERα and ERβ heterodimers. Alternatively spliced variants of both ERα and ERβ have been identified in lung tissue [51]. Finally, estrogen can bind to either estrogen responsive elements (ERE) or AP-1 enhancer elements in the promoter of a variety of target genes and activate transcription be recruiting coactivator proteins. ERα and ERβ have been shown to signal in opposite ways when complexed with estradiol from an AP1 site. With ERα, estradiol activates transcription, whereas with ERβ, estradiol inhibits transcription [52].

Although several investigators have reported presence of estrogen receptor α in human lung cancer, the results are inconsistent, of uncertain clinical significance, and expression by immunohistochemistry ranges from 7-97% [53-56]. More recently, investigators have shown that ERα mRNA and protein are expressed at extremely low levels in the lung and that splice variants with questionable functionality represent the majority of the ERα transcripts in the lung [57]. It has been shown, however, that lung tumors from women are more likely to express ERα than those from men [58] and could thus contribute to differences in disease development and progression in men and women.

ERβ is expressed in both normal lungs as well as in lung tumors and appears to have biological function [59]. Omoto et al have reported higher ER□ expression in lung adenocarcinomas than squamous cell carcinomas [59]. Stabile and colleagues have shown that β-estradiol causes proliferation in non-small cell lung cancer cells and that antiestrogens can block this effect [60]. More recently, Patrone et al demonstrated the ERβ regulates lung development, in particular alveolar formation and surfactant homeostasis, in mouse models [61]. ERβ expression in the lung has also been shown to correlate with the expression of certain phase I and II carcinogen metabolizing enzymes, such as CYP1B1 and GSTT1, implicating sex-related differences in lung cancer susceptibility [62].

In addition to the classic estrogenic effects in the nucleus, it is increasingly clear that estrogen signaling effects may take place via estrogen receptors in the plasma membrane, causing interactions between ERs and growth factors [63]. Growth factors such as epidermal growth factor (EGF) and insulin-like growth factor (IGF-1), stimulate the transcriptional activity of ERs in an estrogen-independent manner. Recent studies suggest the existence of a nonnuclear ER that can activate PI3 kinase and the EGF family of receptors [63]. In cells that express EGFR and ER, estrogen may stimulate cellular proliferation and survival through these alternate pathways.

Taioli and Wynder presented evidence that exogenous and endogenous estrogens may play a role in the development of lung adenocarcinoma in women [64]. Using case control data, they showed the following: 1) early age at menopause (40 years or younger) is associated with a reduced risk of adenocarcinoma of the lung (OR = 0.3); 2) the use of estrogen replacement therapy is associated with a higher risk of adenocarcinoma of the lung (OR = 1.7); and 3) there is a positive interaction between estrogen replacement, smoking, and the development of adenocarcinoma of the lung (OR = 32.4). Blackman et al investigated the use of estrogen replacement therapy and lung cancer in another case control trial [65]. The OR for lung cancer among women who used estrogen replacement therapy for > 3 months was 1.0, independently of duration or type of estrogen. In this study, estrogen use alone appeared not to be an independent risk factor for lung cancer. In another study, Schabath and colleagues, again using a case-control design, evaluated the association between hormone replacement therapy and lung cancer risk in 499 women with lung cancer and 519 age-matched control subjects [66]. In this study, hormone replacement therapy was associated with a 34% overall reduction in lung cancer risk after controlling for age, ethnicity, tobacco exposure, body mass index, and menopausal status. However, because the hypothesis of the study was to identify molecular markers for lung cancer, the authors urged caution in interpretation as the dose and duration of hormone use was not rigorously obtained.

More recently, endocrine effects in lung cancer outcome were suggested by a retrospective study of the impact of postmenopausal hormone therapy on the natural history of lung cancer in 498 women [67]. Multivariable analysis showed that overall survival was significantly longer in women who had not been postmenopausal hormone therapy compared to those who had received such treatment (79 versus 39 months; hazard ratio 1.97, 95% CI 1.14-3.39). In addition, patients who had not received postmenopausal hormone therapy were significantly older at the time of diagnosis (68 versus 63 years of age). The older age of onset and longer survival in those not receiving postmenopausal hormone therapy are consistent with the hypothesis that endocrine factors either accelerate the transition of preneoplastic lesions to overt malignancy or promote tumor growth once a malignancy is evident. Although these data require confirmation, consideration should be given to discontinuing postmenopausal hormone therapy in women diagnosed with lung cancer. Additional prospective studies are needed to gain better understanding of the relationship among cigarette smoke, estrogen use, and lung cancer.

Estrogens may be involved in lung tumorigenesis at many different levels. They may act as ER ligands, activating cellular proliferation pathways. Alternatively, they may undergo metabolic activation to reactive intermediates than can produce DNA adducts or cause oxidative damage. This potential role of estrogens in lung cancer is understudied and only more research can yield new insights into the mechanisms underlying its effects.

The epidermal growth factor receptor (EGFR) is a transmembrane glycoprotein that is expressed in the majority of non-small cell lung cancers. Binding of ligands to the extracellular domain results in tyrosine kinase activation with downstream effects including cell proliferation, differentiation, migration, motility, resistance to apoptosis, enhanced survival and gene transcription [68]. Inhibition of the tyrosine with small molecule drugs such as erlotinib and gefitinib has caused tumor regressions in select patients with non-small cell lung cancer. In the monotherapy trials of gefitinib, radiographic response correlated with female sex as well as adenocarcinoma histological type [69,70]. This differential effect was confirmed in the pivotal erlotinib monotherapy trial as well [71]. It has been learned that mutations in the tyrosine kinase domain of *EGFR* are associated with sensitivity of non-small cell lung cancer to gefitinib and erltonib [72,73]. In total, deletions or amino acid substitutions in exons 18, 19, and 21 of *EGFR* were found in 13 of 14 tumors sensitive to the drug, but in none of 11 tumors with no response. Lynch and colleagues found mutations in another 2 of 25 primary NSCLCs, and Paez et al found *EGFR* mutations in 16 of 119 unselected tumors, with a striking predominance of mutations found in 15 of 58 (28%) specimens from Japan as compared to 1 of 61 from the US(2%). Strikingly, the mutation was much more common in women (9/45 or 20%) than in men (7/74 or 9%). The highest fraction of *EGFR* mutations was observed in Japanese women with adenocarcinoma (8/14 or 57%).

In another recent study, Huang et al performed mutational analysis of the *EGFR* coding sequence on 101 fresh frozen lung tumor tissues [74]. Among the 101 patients, 39% carried *EGFR* mutations within the tumor. Of the 69 patients with adenocarcinoma, 56% had at least 1 mutation in exons 18 to 21 of the EGFR gene. In this study, there was no significant difference in the *EGFR* mutation rate between male (18 of 33, 54.5%) and female (20 of 36, 55.5%) patients with adenocarcinoma, and the mutation patterns were also similar between the two groups. It remains to be determined whether sex might play a role in gefinitib or erlotinib response in patients with *EGFR* mutations or whether the effect is more related to never smoking status as often these clinical characteristics overlap.

Pathology

The World Health Organization (WHO) classification of lung cancer is accepted worldwide (Figure 3). Small cell lung cancer constitutes approximately 15% to 20% of all lung cancers, whereas non-small cell lung cancer is much more common and includes carcinoma, adenocarcinoma, and large cell (undifferentiated) carcinoma. Small cell lung cancer and adenocarcinoma are more common in women than in men (27% vs 20%, $p<0.001$ and 22% vs 10% $p<0.001$) [75]. Furthermore, it appears that squamous cell carcinoma and small cell carcinoma have a distinct dose-response relation, with increasing tobacco exposure producing increasing numbers of these histologic types. Worldwide, however, adenocarcinoma appears to be increasing, especially in women, despite the fact that it does not have this significant dose-response relation with smoking. This increasing incidence of adenocarcinoma is seen especially in the United States.

World Health Organization Histologic Classification of Epithelial Tumors of the Lung

I. Squamous cell Carcinoma
   - I. Epidermoid
   - II. Spindle cell variant

II. Small Cell Carcinoma
   - I. Combined small cell carcinoma

III. Adenocarcinoma
   - I. Acinar
   - II. Papillary
   - III. Bronchioloalveolar carcinoma (BAC)
   - IV. Solid carcinoma with mucin

IV. Large Cell Carcinoma
   - I. Giant cell
   - II. Clear Cell

Figure 3.

Small Cell Lung Cancer

The origin of SCLC is undefined but is believed to be the peptide hormone-secreting basal neuroendocrine or Kulchitsky's cell. SCLC is composed of neoplastic cells that are arranged in clusters or sheets. They tend to have scant cytoplasm, have high mitotic rates and areas of necrosis. There can be variants with interspersed large cells or adenosquamous cells. It is unclear whether survival in patients with mixed morphology is better or worse than those with typical SCLC.

The tumor typically arises in the central airways and initially infiltrates the submucosa, gradually obstructing the lumen by extrinsic or endobronchial spread. SCLC is distinguished from all other cancers by its high incidence of tumor suppressor gene inactivation. More than

90% of SCLCs inactivate p53 function, which is an important sensor of DNA damage and regulates progression through cell-cycle checkpoints. More than 90% inactivate Rb function, a major determinant of the G1/S cell-cycle checkpoint. More that 90% show deletions of the short arm of chromosome 3, suggesting the presence of additional important candidate tumor-suppressor genes for SCLC. SCLC also shows overexpression of many dominant oncogenes including the following: Myc, kit, kit ligand, and telomerase.

Non-Small Cell Lung Cancer

Non-small cell lung cancer (NSCLC) accounts for 85% of all lung cancers.

Squamous Cell Carcinoma

Although at one time the most frequent of lung cancers in the North America, squamous cell carcinoma now accounts for 29% of newly diagnosed lung cancer. Squamous cell lung cancer arises most frequently in proximal segmental bronchi and is associated with squamous metaplasia. In its earliest form, carcinoma *in situ*, stratified squamous epithelium is replaced by malignant squamous cells without invasion through the basement membrane. This tumor can be detected at a very early stage through sputum cytology. With continued growth, the tumor invades the basement membranes and extends into the endobronchial lumen, producing obstruction with resultant atelecatasis or pneumonia. Histologically, the squamous cell tumor is composed of sheets of epithelial cells. Well-differentiated tumors can contain keratin pearls. Even poorly differentiated cells should have keratin staining. These tumors tend to be slow growing, and it is estimated that up to 3 or 4 years are required from the development of *in situ* carcinoma to a clinically apparent tumor.

Adenocarcinoma

Adenocarcinoma is the most frequent lung tumor, accounting for 40% of cases. Most of these tumors are peripheral in origin, arising from alveolar surface epithelium or bronchial mucosal glands. Histologically, they can be divided by the WHO classification. However, the only division with clinical relevance is that of bronchioloalveolar carcinoma. Bronchioloalveolar carcinoma appears to be a distinct clinicopathological entity that appears to arise from type II pneumocytes, grows along alveolar septa by lepidic growth, and shows little, if any, desmoplastic or gladular change. These tumors are interesting in that they present in three different forms: a solitary peripheral nodule, multifocal disease, or a rapidly progressive pneumonic form. Furthermore, they appear to be less frequently associated with smoking, occur more often in women, have a propensity for intrapulmonary metastases, and tend to have a more indolent course than other non-small cell lung cancer [76].

Large Cell Carcinoma

Large cell carcinoma is the least common of all NSCLC tumors, accounting for approximately 15% of all lung cancers. Large cell lung cancer represents an extremely poorly differentiated NSCLC without features that permit assignment to one of the more usual and better-differentiated forms of lung carcinoma. These tumors often have some neuroendocrine features, and may have slightly worse prognosis that other NSCLC.

CLINICAL FEATURES

The signs and symptoms manifested by patients suffering from lung cancer depend upon the location of the tumor, its locoregional spread, the effects of metastatic spread, or those related to paraneoplastic syndromes. A minority of patients have an asymptomatic lesion that is discovered incidentally on a chest radiograph (Figure 4). Locoregional manifestations include cough, hemoptysis, and dyspnea (Figure 5).

Clinical Presentation

Less than 10% of patients are asymptomatic

Symptoms at Diagnosis of NSCLC	
Cough	45-75%
Dyspnea	40-60%
Weight loss	20-70%
Chest pain	30-45%
Hemoptysis	25-35%

Chute, Cancer 1985: 56:2107
Beckles, Chest 2003;123(1 Suppl): 97S-104S
Ferguson Hematol Oncol Clin N Am 1990:4:1053-68

Figure 4.

Metastatic Disease

Patients with metastatic disease tend to have more than one symptom at the time of diagnosis. In fact, fatigue and decreased activity were reported by 80%, and most patients also experienced cough, dyspnea, decreased appetite, and weight loss [77]. Although lung cancer can metastasize to any organ, the most common clinically apparent sites of spread are the pleura, lung, bone, brain, pericardium, and liver [78]. Adrenal metastases are common, and have been reported in up to 40% of autopsy series [79]. Adrenal and intra-abdominal lymph node metastases are usually detected on CT scans performed to evaluate lung cancer. In most cases, these lesions are asymptomatic. Large adrenal masses may cause pain. Adrenal insufficiency is usually not observed but should be considered in patients with bilateral adrenal metastases who present with appropriate clinical symptoms and laboratory abnormalities.

Symptoms and Signs of Lung Cancer

- Primary disease
  - Central or endobronchial tumor growth
    - Cough
    - Sputum production
    - Hemoptysis
    - Dyspnea
    - Wheeze (classically unilateral)
    - Stridor
  - Peripheral
    - Pain, from pleural or chest wall involvement
    - Cough
    - Dyspnea
- Regional involvement (either direct or metastatic)
  - Hoarseness (recurrent laryngeal nerve paralysis)
  - Tracheal obstruction
  - Dysphagia
  - Dyspnea (pleural effusion, tracheal/bronchial obstruction, pericardial effusion, phrenic nerve palsy, lymphatic infiltration, superior vena cava obstruction
  - Horner's syndrome
- Metastatic (common sites)
  - Bone involvement—Pain, often worse at night
  - Liver involvement—RUQ pain, icteris, altered mentation
  - Brain metastases—altered mental status, seizures, motor and sensory deficits

Figure 5.

Paraneoplastic Syndromes

Carcinomas of the lung most often present with symptoms related to locoregional spread or to the manifestation of extrathoracic spread. However, patients can also present with paraneoplastic syndromes, which are remote effects of the primary tumor that can result in organ dysfunction. Several different paraneoplastic syndromes are clinically apparent in 10%-20% of patients with bronchogenic carcinoma. These syndromes occur with greater frequency in SCLC (Figure 6). The anorexia-cachexia syndrome and generalized weakness and fatigue are the most common and least understood non-metastatic complications of lung cancer. Hypertrophic osteoarthopathy occurs frequently in patients with NSCLC. Symptoms of bone and joint pain herald the onset of the condition and can be the presenting signs of the lung cancer. Clubbing of the digits is observed, and the alkaline phosphatase is generally elevated. Plain films demonstrate periosteal inflammation and elevation, and radionuclide bone scans reveal symmetric and intense uptake of the radio label, especially in the long bones. Symptoms usually respond dramatically to aspirin and other nonsteriodal antiinflammatory agents and often disappear after treatment of the primary lesion. Approximately 10% of patients with SCLC can develop the syndrome of inappropriate antidiuretic hormone, and symptoms are present in about 5%. Patients can also develop Cushing's syndrome from increased levels of adrenocorticotropic hormone. Other neurologic paraneoplastic syndromes that are observed in SCLC include cerebellar ataxia, subacute sensory neuropathy, and Eaton-Lambert myasthenic like syndrome which is characterized by proximal muscle weakness that improves with continued use. The cause is related to autoantibody impairment of acetylcholine release form the cholinergic nerve terminals.

Paraneoplastic Syndromes in Lung Cancer

- Clubbing
- Hypertrophic pulmonary osteoarthropathy
- Hypercalcemia
- Dermatomyositis
- Eaton-Lambert syndrome
- Hypercoagulable state
- Gynecomastia

Figure 6.

Diagnosis and Staging

The worldwide tumor, node, metastasis (TNM) staging system is a standardized system that is useful in estimating prognosis, selecting treatment and in reporting data. The primary tumor is subdivided in four categories (T1-4), depending upon size, site, and local involvement. Lymph node spread has been subdivided into bronchopulmonary (N1), ipsilateral mediastinal (N2), and contralateral or supraclavicular disease (N3), and metastatic spread is absent (M0) or present (M1) (Figure 7). Four stages of lung cancer have been identified with significant differences found in 5 –year survival, depending upon the stage at diagnosis (Figure 8).

Staging

T1	**≤ 3cm**
T2	**> 3cm, involves mainstem bronchus, invades visceral pleura**
T3	**CW, diaphragm, parietal/mediastinal pleura, pericardium, < 2cm from carina, lung collapse**
T4	**Mediastinum, carina, vertebral body, satellite nodules in same lobe, pleural/pericardial effusion**
N1	**Lobar, segmental, subsegmental**
N2	**Ipsilateral mediastinal, subcarinal**
N3	**Contralateral mediastinal, ipsilateral supraclavicular**
M1	**Metastatic**

Figure 7.

Staging, cont'd

		5 YEAR SURVIVAL	
		CLINICAL	PATHOLOGIC
IA	T1N0	67%	61%
IB	T2N0	57%	38%
IIA	T1N1	55%	34%
IIB	T2N1, T3N0	39%	29%
IIIA	T3N1, T1-2N2	25%	13%
IIIB	T4, T1-3N3	5%	5%
IV	M1	<1%	<1%

Figure 8.

NSCLC Staging
Current Treatment and Survival Rates[1]

Stage	Treatment	5-Year Survival, %*
I	Surgery/Chemotherapy?	60-70
II	Surgery/Chemotherapy	30-50
IIIA	Surgery/Chemotherapy/ Radiation?	10-30
IIIB	Chemotherapy/ Radiation	5
IV	Chemotherapy	<1

*Overall 5-year survival is 14%.[2]
1. Mountain CF. *Semin Surg Oncol.* 2000;18:106-115.
2. National Cancer Institute: SEER Cancer Statistics Review;1973-1998.

Figure 9.

History and Physical Examination

A detailed history and accurate physical examination are the most important steps in assessing a patient with lung cancer. Smoking history, past exposure to environmental carcinogens, and family history may suggest a higher probability of lung cancer. New cough, recurrent respiratory infections and symptoms of local or metastatic disease should be of concern.

Pathologic Diagnosis

If disease is suspected, a noninvasive method of confirming the diagnosis is sputum cytology. However, the yield of sputum cytology depends upon many factors including the ability of the patient to produce sufficient sputum, the size of the tumor, and the location of the tumor. Up to 80% of central tumors can be diagnosed from sputum cytology, whereas less than 20% of peripheral tumors less than 3 cm will yield positive cytology.

Other invasive techniques for establishing pathologic diagnosis include bronchoscopy (with brushings, washings), transthoracic biopsy, CT-guided transthoracic biopsy, thoracentesis for pleural effusions, and mediastinoscopy with mediastinal node biopsy.

In some cases, such as a patient with an asymptomatic, solitary pulmonary nodule, tissue diagnosis may be made at the time of definitive surgical resection.

Radiologic Studies

Computed Tomography

The majority of lung cancers are visible on plain films, but detection of mediastinal lymph node metastases and invasion of the chest wall or mediastinum are suboptimal. A chest CT should be obtained in all patients with lung cancer. The CT scan should survey an area from above the apices to the lungs to below the adrenal glands, with inclusion of the contiguous chest wall. CT scanning facilitates staging by allowing precise measurements of tumor diameter and demonstrating pleural effusion and atelectasis. CT scanning, however, has limitations in evaluation of the mediastinum. One meta-analysis of 42 studies examining the accuracy of CT in detecting malignantly infiltrated mediastinal lymph nodes reported a sensitivity and specificity of 79 and 78 percent, respectively [80]. Although CT scanning is useful for directing biopsy of suspicious lymph nodes, it is not definitive.

Brain Imaging

Lung not infrequently metastasizes to the brain. In a meta-analysis of 16 published trials, head CT discovered unexpected metastases in only 26 of 785 patients (3%) [81]. Brain MRI provides higher resolution of intracranial structures and is probably more sensitive that CT for the early detection of metastases [82]. Currently, most recommend that a head CT or brain MRI is performed in asymptomatic patients with stage III NSCLC who are being considered for aggressive local therapy [83]. PET is not useful in detecting brain metastasis because of the high rate of glucose metabolism in normal brain tissues [84].

PET

Positron emission tomography (PET) with 18-fluor-2-deoxyglucose (FDG) is a noninvasive method to assess for mediastinal or distant metastases by detecting areas of high FDG uptake (ie, increased metabolic activity). When added to CT, the information gained from PET can alter patient management, most often by detecting unsuspected sites of distant metastases, and altering the treatment intent from curative to palliative.

The role of PET scanning in noninvasive staging of the mediastinum is controversial. In several studies using surgery as the gold standard of comparison, the accuracy of PET alone is consistently superior to that of CT, particularly with regard to the negative predictive value, which ranges from 87 to 100%. The positive predictive value is somewhat lower, 75 to 80 percent in many studies. In one prospective trial involving 102 patients with NSCLC, the sensitivity, specificity, negative predictive value, positive predictive value rates for detecting mediastinal metastases with PET alone were 91, 86, 95, and 74 percent while the corresponding values for CT alone were 75, 66, 85, and 50 percent, respectively [85].

A positive PET scan of the mediastinal nodes is considered sufficiently nonspecific by most clinicians that sampling of the mediastinal lymph nodes to confirm malignant involvement is generally still recommended [83,84].

Pretreatment Prognostic Factors

After establishing the diagnosis and clinical stage of NSCLC, it is desirable to determine the likely course and survival outcome. This is important for both the patient and the treating physician, because this estimate is essential to guide the choice of therapy. Stage is the most important determinant of prognosis. Multiple groups have assessed host factors to assess prognosis. Good performance status (overall well being) appears to be the most important clinical determinant of improved survival. Other factors including presence of bone metastases and weight loss are also important (Table 7).

Interestingly, female sex is correlated with improved survival regardless of histological type or stage of disease [75,86-91].

Pathologic features including histologic type and molecular and genetic markers have also been studied, but have not been reliably associated with prognosis. No single molecular marker or molecular profile has emerged that consistently identifies patients who would be predicted to have a worse prognosis, or derive greater (or lesser) benefit from adjuvant therapies, although early data from gene expression profiling holds promise.

Management: Treatment Modalities According to Stage of Disease

Early Stage NSCLC

Patients who are medically fit and can undergo resection with clinical stage IA/B or IIA/B are usually treated with surgery, since this is the treatment that has produced the vast majority of long-term survivors.

These patients are best served by referral to a thoracic surgeon with a special interest in lung cancer surgery. Despite complete surgical excision, patients with stage IB, II, or IIIA NSCLC are at substantial risk for recurrence and death. As many as 50 percent of patients with stage IB, 70 percent of stage II, and a greater percentage of those with stage IIIA NSCLC recur and die of their disease despite potentially curative surgery. Patients with stage I disease more frequently have distant recurrence as whereas those with stage II disease have increased proportion of local recurrence.

In recent years the idea of chemotherapy after surgery, or adjuvant therapy, has evolved rapidly. The results of several large randomized trials using modern platinum-based regimens suggest that adjuvant chemotherapy can significantly improve survival in these populations.

Until the publication of the International Adjuvant Lung Cancer Trial (IALT) in early 2004 [92], virtually all authorities had concluded that there was insufficient evidence to recommend adjuvant chemotherapy in any subgroup of patients with respected NSCLC. In dramatic contrast, the results of the IALT and Canadian JBR 10 trials [93], as well as preliminary reports of the Cancer and Leukemia Group B (CALGB) trial 9633 [94], and the ANITA trial [95] have led to a remarkable reversal in practice trends, with most authorities now recommending that adjuvant chemotherapy be considered in all patients with completely resected NSCLC, except those with IA disease. These three recent randomized studies in more homogeneous patient populations, utilizing contemporary platinum-based doublet regimens, suggest that the magnitude of benefit may significant (8 to 12 percent).

Because prognosis is relatively favorable, and in view of the absence of any data-suggesting efficacy, most experts explicitly recommend against adjuvant therapy for stage IA NSCLC, except in the context of a well-designed randomized controlled trial targeting this subgroup.

Stage III NSCLC

The optimal treatment of stage III NSCLC is uncertain and many aspects are controversial; while there are many potential treatment options, none yields a high probability of cure. Due to the clinical heterogeneity that is inherent in stage III disease, no single approach can be recommended for all patients.

Initial nonoperative treatment is generally recommended for patients with mediastinal nodal involvement that is documented prior to resection (Table 9). Approaches have included preoperative induction therapy (ie, chemotherapy, radiation therapy [RT], chemoradiotherapy) or definitive chemoradiation without surgery.

Surgical resection after chemotherapy is favored in patients with minimal N2 disease. This approach requires an experienced and skilled thoracic surgeon. Chemotherapy prior to surgery, "neoadjuvant" therapy has the theoretic advantage of diminishing nodal involvement, thus making surgical intervention less difficult, more likely to have an impact on survival, and more likely to provide immediate systemic therapy in patients at high risk for distal relapse. However, it should be noted that local therapy is delayed by this approach, and that a potentially resectable tumor may become unresectable. Furthermore, the continued presence of N2 nodal disease after surgery is associated with poorer outcome. Patients with T4 lesions, bulky multilevel N2 or N3 involvement are not eligible for curative surgical resection. The most appropriate scheduling of chemotherapy and radiation therapy as well as the most appropriate chemotherapy agents to use with radiation remain under active investigation.

Advanced NSCLC (Stage IIIB with Malignant Pleural Effusions, and Stage IV)

The survival of patients with advanced NSCLC remains poor. Fully ambulatory patients have increased survival and palliation of symptoms with platinum containing chemotherapy. A clear advantage for the use of chemotherapy has been demonstrated in patients with metastatic disease who have good performance status. The median survival of patients with "best supportive care" alone is approximately 4 months, and the 1 –year survival rate is 10%. Newer chemotherapy regimens (carboplatin plus paclitaxel, cisplatin plus gemcitabine, cisplatin plus vinorelbine) have resulted in median survivals of 9 to 10 months and 1-year survivals of 30% to 40% in large multicenter randomized trials [83,96-99]. Furthermore, it has been shown that it is cost-effective to treat patients with chemotherapy because of the reduced need for hospitalization, radiation therapy, and other interventions [100].

Several cytotoxic drugs have single agent activity in NSCLC. The most active are the platinum salts (cisplatin and carboplatin), etoposide, ifosfamide, irinotecan, vinorelbine, taxanes, gemcitabine, and pemetrexed. In general, combination therapy is preferred as first-line treatment for younger patients with advanced NSCLC and a good performance status. The main utility of single agent therapy is in elderly patients, those with a poor performance status, or for second line salvage treatment after failure of initial combination therapy. Multiple combination regimens are reasonable for fit patients, although no single regimen has emerged as the best choice for the treatment of advanced NSCLC.

Novel Agents in NSCLC

The desire to provide less toxic therapeutic alternatives for patients with advanced NSCLC has led to the exploration of novel targeted therapies. Because targeted therapies seek to differentiate between malignant and nonmalignant cells, they lack many of the side effects associated with systemic chemotherapy. Furthermore, they presumably do not share the same pathways of drug resistance, and many have synergistic or additive effects when added to conventional chemotherapeutic agents.

Abnormalities in several cell-signaling pathways have been identified in NSCLC, and increasingly, these are being exploited for therapeutic purposes. One of the most promising approaches focuses upon pathways involving receptor tyrosine kinases. Tumor growth and progression depends largely upon the activity of cell surface membrane receptors that control the intracellular signal transduction pathways regulating proliferation, apoptosis, angiogenesis, adhesion and motility. One such family of receptors are the receptor tyrosine kinases, which include the epidermal growth factor receptor (EGFR, also called HER-1 or erbB-1). EGFR exists as a monomer on the cell surface, and it must dimerize to activate the TK. While receptor tyrosine kinase activity is tightly controlled in normal cells, the genes encoding these receptors have escaped from their usual intracellular control through amplification, overexpression or mutation.

This pathway has become an important focus for the development of new drugs in NSCLC. One such drug that specifically targets the EGFR TK domain is erlotinib. The clinical efficacy and safety profile were established in a phase III study in patients previously treated with one or two chemotherapy regimens. In this study, 731 patients were randomized to receive treatment with erlotinib or placebo. Increased response rate (9% versus <1%), increased overall survival (6.7 months versus 4.7 months) and greater reductions in the cancer related symptoms of dyspnea, pain, and cough were all noted on the erlotinib arm.

Both clinical and molecular parameters have been analyzed to predict which patients benefit from treatment with EGFR tyrosine kinase inhibitors. Observations from multiple studies have suggested that patients with adenocarcinoma (and particularly bronchoalveolar carcinoma), women, nonsmokers and Asians were more likely to benefit from treatment. However, even for the poor prognosis subsets (ie men, non-adenocarcinoma histology, non-Asian ethnicity, and current or former smokers) there was a reduction in the hazard ratio for death among patients treated with erlotinib.

From the phase III trial comparing erlotinib to placebo, tissue was available from 325 of 731 patients [101]. Samples were analyzed for overexpression of the EGFR protein, gene amplification, and the presence of mutations in the tyrosine kinase domain of the receptor; the results were correlated with objective response and overall survival. On multivariate analysis, the molecular markers were not independent predictors of improved responsiveness to erlotinib. The predictors of increased survival were the clinical parameters noted above (Asian ethnicity, women, never having smoked, and adenocarcinoma). It is clear that women are more likely than men to have response to erlotinib, but the basis of this is not completely understood.

Vascular endothelial growth factor (VEGF) is an endothelial-specific mitogen, and a potent angiogenic factor that is expressed on a wide array of tumors. In NSCLC, as in other tumors, high levels of VEGF are associated with poor prognosis, suggesting that interference with this pathway might be useful therapeutically. One approach to inhibiting the VEGF pathway is with bevacizumab, a recombinant humanized monoclonal antibody which binds to VEGF. A randomized phase II study suggested that this approach merited further investigation, but also suggested that those patients with squamous cell histology were at increased risk of severe, fatal hemoptysis [102]. A phase trial in 878 previously untreated patients with advanced, non-squamous NSCLC comparing bevacizumab plus paclitaxel and carboplatin to the same chemotherapy alone was conducted. Patients had to have good performance status; those with a history of brain metastases or hemoptysis were excluded. Patients receiving chemotherapy plus bevacizumab had a significantly increased objective response rate (27 versus 10 percent), overall survival (12.5 versus 10.2 months), and one-year and two-year survival rates (58 versus 44 and 22 versus 17) [103]. Interestingly, in subgroup analysis, men derived greater benefit from the addition of bevacizumab than did women. It is unclear at this juncture whether this represents a true difference or rather is statistical chance or the effect of second line therapy with erlotinib.

Treatment of Small Cell Lung Cancer

Small cell lung cancer represents 15-20% of lung cancer. It is distinguished from non-small cell lung cancer (NSCLC) by its rapid doubling time, high growth fraction, and the early development of metastases. Although considered highly responsive to chemotherapy and radiotherapy, SCLC commonly relapses within months despite treatment.

Limited Stage Small Cell Lung Cancer

Combined therapy with chest irradiation and chemotherapy are generally recommended to well patients with limited stage disease. Combination therapy is often associated with considerable toxicity.

Although several single agents show activity against SCLC, significantly superior response rates and survival with multiagent therapy have made combination therapy the standard approach in initial treatment. Optimal regimens yield 80% to 90% response rates, 50% to 60% complete response rates, and 2-year survival rates of 15% to 40%. Although several regimens have been used successfully, the most commonly used regimen currently is etopside and cisplatin because of its overall favorable toxicity profile.

Thoracic radiation provides a marginal survival advantage and reduced local recurrence rates when added to chemotherapy in limited-stage disease. Most regimens incorporating radiation therapy use a total dose of 45 to 50 Gy. The optimal timing of radiotherapy is unclear, but concurrent is favored over sequential regimens.

Extensive Stage Disease

Combination therapy without thoracic irradiation is the cornerstone of therapy. Combination chemotherapies identical to those used in limited stage disease are used with overall response rates of 60% to 80%, complete response rates of 15% to 20%, and median survival of 7 to 11 months. Two-year survival is uncommon with currently available therapies.

CONCLUSION

Lung cancer is now the leading cancer killer of women, having surpassed breast cancer in 1987. Almost twice as many women in the United States are expected to die from lung cancer compared to breast cancer this year (73,020 versus 40,400). There is accumulating evidence suggesting that the development of lung cancer is different in women compared with men. Women smokers are more likely than men to develop adenocarcinoma of the lung. Women who have never smoked are more likely to develop lung cancer than men who have never smoked. These differences are due to hormonal, genetic and metabolic differences between the sexes.

A more thorough understanding of the heterogeneity of lung cancer may lead to innovations in treatment and prevention strategies. It seems likely that estrogens are involved in lung carcinogenesis; either by acting as ER ligands and activating cellular proliferation pathways or by metabolic activation to reactive intermediates that can produce DNA adducts and cause oxidative damage. These estrogenic pathways may act disproportionately in women and could be responsible for sex differences in lung carcinogenesis.

Smoking remains the primary cause of lung cancer, and nearly 14 million U.S. women in their reproductive years still smoke [7]. Although lung cancer death rates have plateaued in recent years, the number of women who will die from lung cancer remains alarmingly high. It is incumbent upon us to have a better understating of the genetic, metabolic and hormonal factors that affect the way women react to carcinogens and lung cancer. This information could affect the way patients who smoke are screened and evaluated and the way smoking cessation and lung cancer prevention programs are directed. Finally, future lung cancer research must include a proportion of women that reflects the true incidence of lung cancer in women.

REFERENCES

[1] Jemal, A; Siegel, R; Ward, E; et al. Cancer statistics, 2006. *CA Cancer J Clin*, 2006 56(2), 106-30.

[2] Jemal, A; Tiwari, R; Murray, T; et al. Cancer Statistics, 2004. *CA*, 2004 54, 8-29.

[3] Control CfD. Cigarette smoking among adults. *Morb Mortal Wkly Rep*, 2004 53(20), 427-31.

[4] Ezzati, M; Lopez, AD. Measuring the accumulated hazards of smoking: global and regional estimates for 2000. *Tob Control*, 2003 12(1), 79-85.

[5] French, SA; Perry, CL; Leon, GR; Fulkerson, JA. Weight concerns, dieting behavior, and smoking initiation among adolescents: a prospective study. *Am J Public Health*, 1994 84(11), 1818-20.

[6] Johnston, L; Bachman, J. PM OM. *Monitoring the Future: Questionnaire Responses From the Nation's High School Seniors 1997*. Ann Arbor: Institute for Social Research, University of Michigan, 2001.

[7] General US. *Women and Smoking: A Report of the Surgeon General*. Washington, DD: US Dept of Health and Human Services, Public Health Service, Office of the Surgeon General, 2001.

[8] Brauch, H; Johnson, B; Hovis. J; et al. Molecular analysis of the short arm of chromosome 3 in small-cell and non-small cell carcinoma of the lung. *N Engl J Med*, 1987 317(18), 1109-13.

[9] Westmaas, J; Wild, T; Ferrence, R. Effects of gender in social control of smoking cessation. *Health Psychol*, 2002 21, 368-76.

[10] Husten, C; Shelton, D; Chrismon, J. Cigarette smoking and smoking cessation among older adults: United States, 1965-1994. *Tob Control*, 1997 6, 175-80.

[11] Osler, M; Prescott, E; Godtfredsen, N; Hein, HO; Schnohr, P. Gender and determinants of smoking cessation: a longitudinal study. *Prev Med*, 1999 29(1), 57-62.

[12] Royce, JM; Corbett, K; Sorensen, G; Ockene, J. Gender, social pressure, and smoking cessations: the Community Intervention Trial for Smoking Cessation (COMMIT) at baseline. *Soc Sci Med*, 1997 44(3), 359-70.

[13] Bohadana, A; Nilsson, F; Rasmussen, T. Gender differences in quit rates following smoking cessation with combination nicotine therapy: influence of baseline smoking behavior. *Nicotine Tob Res*, 2003 5, 111-16.

[14] Livson, N; Leino, EV. Cigarette smoking motives: factorial structure and gender differences in a longitudinal study. *Int J Addict*, 1988 23(6), 535-44.

[15] Jarry, JL; Coambs, RB; Polivy, J;, Herman, CP. Weight gain after smoking cessation in women: the impact of dieting status. *Int J Eat Disord*, 1998 24(1), 53-64.

[16] Perkins, KA; Marcus, MD; Levine, MD; et al. Cognitive-behavioral therapy to reduce weight concerns improves smoking cessation outcome in weight-concerned women. *J Consult Clin Psychol*, 2001 69(4), 604-13.

[17] Niaura, R; Abrams, DB. Stopping smoking: a hazard for people with a history of major depression? *Lancet*, 2001 357(9272), 1900-1.

[18] Lerman, C; Shields, PG; Wileyto, EP; et al. Pharmacogenetic investigation of smoking cessation treatment. *Pharmacogenetics*, 2002 12(8), 627-34.

[19] Collins, BN; Wileyto, EP; Patterson, F; et al. Gender differences in smoking cessation in a placebo-controlled trial of bupropion with behavioral counseling. *Nicotine Tob Res*, 2004 6(1), 27-37.

[20] Boyle, P; Ferlay, J. Cancer incidence and mortality in Europe, 2004. *Ann Oncol*, 2005 16(3), 481-8.

[21] Tomlinson, R. Smoking death toll shifts to Third World. *BMJ*, 1997 315(7108), 565.

[22] Chaloupka, FJ; Laixuthai, A. Cigarette smoking in Pacific Rim countries: The impact of U.S. trade policy: National Bureau for Economic Research, Inc.

[23] Risch, HA; Howe, GR; Jain, M; Burch, JD; Holowaty, EJ; Miller, AB. Are female smokers at higher risk for lung cancer than male smokers? A case-control analysis by histologic type. *Am J Epidemiol*, 1993 138(5), 281-93.

[24] Zang, E; Wynder, E. Differences in lung cancer risk betweem men and women: examination of the evidence. *J Natl Cancer Inst*, 1996 88(3-4), 183-92.

[25] Henschke, CI; Miettinen, O. Women's susceptibility to tobacco carcinogens. *Lung Cancer*, 2004 43(1), 1-5.

[26] Bach, PB; Kattan, MW; Thornquist, MD; et al. Variations in lung cancer risk among smokers. *J Natl Cancer Inst*, 2003 95(6), 470-8.

[27] Bain c, D F; Speizer, FE;, et al. Lung cancer rates in men and women with comparable histories of smoking. *J Natl Cancer Inst*, 2004 96(11), 826-34.

[28] Zang, EA; Wynder, EL. Differences in lung cancer risk between men and women: examination of the evidence. *J Natl Cancer Inst*, 1996 88(3-4), 183-92.

[29] Perneger TV. Sex, smoking, and cancer: a reappraisal. *J Natl Cancer Inst*, 2001 93(21), 1600-2.

[30] McLemore, TL; Adelber, S; Liu, MC; et al. Expression of CYP1A1 gene in patients with lung cancer: Evidence for cigarrette smoke-induced gene expression in normal lung tissue and for altered gene regulation in primary pulmonary carcinomas. *J Natl Cancer Inst*, 1990 82(16),1333-9.

[31] Guengerich FP. Characterization of human cytochrome P450 enzymes. *The FASEB Journal*, 1992 6, 745-8.
[32] Mollerup, S; Ryberg, D; Hewer, A; Phillips, DH; Haugen, A. Sex differences in lung CYP1A1 expression and DNA adduct levels among lung cancer patients. *Cancer Res*, 1999 59(14), 3317-20.
[33] Thomsen, JS; Wang, X; Hines, RN; Safe, S. Restoration of aryl hydrocarbon (Ah) responsiveness in MDA-MB-231 human breast cancer cells by transient expression of the estrogen receptor. *Carcinogenesis*, 1994 15(5), 933-7.
[34] Daniel, V. Glutathione S-transferases: gene structure and regulation of expression. *Crit Rev Biochem Mol Biolo*, 1993 28(3), 173-207.
[35] Bell, D; Taylor, J; Paulson, D; Robertson, C; Mohler, J; Lucier, G. Genetic risk and carcinogen exposure: A common inherited defect of the carcinogen-metabolism gene glutathione S-transferase M1 (GSTM1) that increases susceptibility to bladder cancer. *J Natl Cancer Inst*, 1993 85, 1159-64.
[36] Tang, DL; Rundle, A; Warburton, D; et al. Associations between both genetic and environmental biomarkers and lung cancer: evidence of a greater risk of lung cancer in women smokers. *Carcinogenesis*, 1998 19(11), 1949-53.
[37] Shriver, SP; Bourdeau, HA; Gubish, CT; et al. Sex-specific expression of gastrin-releasing peptide receptor: relationship to smoking history and risk of lung cancer. *J Natl Cancer Inst*, 2000 92(1), 24-33.
[38] Balsara, BR; Sonoda, G; du Manoir, S; Siegfried, JM; Gabrielson, E; Testa JR. Comparative genomic hybridization analysis detects frequent, often high-level, overrepresentation of DNA sequences at 3q, 5p, 7p, and 8q in human non-small cell lung carcinomas. *Cancer Res*, 1997 57(11), 2116-20.
[39] Siegfried, JM; DeMichele, MA; Hunt, JD; Davis, AG; Vohra, KP; Pilewski, JM. Expression of mRNA for gastrin-releasing peptide receptor by human bronchial epithelial cells. Association with prolonged tobacco exposure and responsiveness to bombesin-like peptides. *Am J Respir Crit Care Med*, 1997 156(2 Pt 1), 358-66.
[40] Rom, W; Hay, J; Lee, T. Molecular and genetic aspects of lung cancer. *Am J Resp Crit Care Med*, 2000 161, 1355-67.
[41] Ryberg, D; Hewer, A; Phillips, DH; Haugen, A. Different susceptibility to smoking-induced DNA damage among male and female lung cancer patients. *Cancer Res*, 1994 54(22), 5801-3.
[42] Swenberg, J; Richardson, F; Boucheron, J. Dyroff M. Relationships between DNA adduct formation and carcinogenesis. *Environ Health Perspect*, 1985 62, 177-83.
[43] Cheng, YW; Hsieh, LL; Lin, PP; et al. Gender difference in DNA adduct levels among nonsmoking lung cancer patients. *Environ Mol Mutagen*, 2001 37(4), 304-10.
[44] Wei, Q; Cheng, L; Amos, CI; et al. Repair of tobacco carcinogen-induced DNA adducts and lung cancer risk: a molecular epidemiologic study. *J Natl Cancer Inst*, 2000 92(21), 1764-72.
[45] Greenblatt, M; Bennett, W; Hollstein, M; Harris, C. Mutations in the p53 tumor suppressor gene: clues to cancer etiology and molecular pathogenesis. *Cancer Res*, 1994 54(18), 4855-78.

[46] Denissenko, M; Chen, J; Tang, M; Pfeifer, GP. Cytosine methylation determines hot spots of DNA damage in the human p53 gene. *Proc Natl Acad Sci*, 1997 94(8), 3893-8.
[47] Toyooka, S; Shimizu, N; Gazdar, A. The TP53 gene, tobacco exposure, and lung cancer. *Hum Mutat*, 2003 21(March (3)), 229-39.
[48] Nelson, HH; Christiani, DC; Mark, EJ; Wiencke, JK; Wain, JC; Kelsey KT. Implications and prognostic value of K-ras mutation for early-stage lung cancer in women. *J Natl Cancer Inst*, 1999 91(23), 2032-8.
[49] Enmark, E; Pelto-Huikko, M; Grandien, K; et al. Human estrogen receptor beta-gene structure, chromosomal localization, and expression pattern. *J Clin Endocrinol Metab*, 1997 82(12), 4258-65.
[50] Pettersson, K; Gustafsson, J. Role of estrogen receptor beta in estrogen action. *Annu Rev Physiol*, 2001 63, 165-92.
[51] Fasco, M; Hurteau, G; Spivack, S. Gender-dependent expression of alpha and beta estrogen receptors in human nontumor and tumor lung tissue. *Mol Cell Endocrinol*, 2002 188(1-2), 125-40.
[52] Paech, K; Webb, P; Kuiper, GG; et al. Differential ligand activation of estrogen receptors ERalpha and ERbeta at AP1 sites. *Science*, 1997 277(5331), 1508-10.
[53] Canver, CC; Memoli, VA; Vanderveer, PL; Dingivan, CA; Mentzer, RM, Jr. Sex hormone receptors in non-small-cell lung cancer in human beings. *J Thorac Cardiovasc Surg*, 1994 108(1), 153-7.
[54] Cagle, PT; Mody, DR; Schwartz, MR. Estrogen and progesterone receptors in bronchogenic carcinoma. *Cancer Res*, 1990 50(20), 6632-5.
[55] Ollayos, CW; Riordan, GP; Rushin, JM. Estrogen receptor detection in paraffin sections of adenocarcinoma of the colon, pancreas, and lung. *Arch Pathol Lab Med*, 1994 118(6), 630-2.
[56] Beattie, CW; Hansen, NW; Thomas PA. Steroid receptors in human lung cancer. *Cancer Res*, 1985 45(9), 4206-14.
[57] Matsuda, S; Kadowaki, Y; Ichino, M; Akiyama, T; Toyoshima, K; Yamamoto, T. 17 beta-estradiol mimics ligand activity of the c-erbB2 protooncogene product. *Proceedings of the National Academy of Science*, 1993 90(20), 10803-7.
[58] Kaiser, U; Hofmann, J; Schilli, M; et al. Steroid-hormone receptors in cell lines and tumor biopsies of human lung cancer. *Int J Cancer*, 1996 67(3), 357-64.
[59] Omoto, Y; Kobayashi, Y; Nishida, K; et al. Expression, function, and clinical implications of the estrogen receptor beta in human lung cancers. *Biochem Biophys Res Commun*, 2001 285(2), 340-7.
[60] Stabile, LP; Davis, AL; Gubish, CT; et al. Human non-small cell lung tumors and cells derived from normal lung express both estrogen receptor alpha and beta and show biological responses to estrogen. *Cancer Res*, 2002 62(7), 2141-50.
[61] Patrone, C; Caseel, T; Pettersson, K; et al. Regulation of postnatal lung development and homeostasis by estrogen receptor beta. *Mol Cell Biol*, 2003 23(23), 8542-52.
[62] Spivack, S; Hurteau, G; Fasco, M; Kamisky, L. Phase I and II carcinogen metabolism gene expression in human lung tissue and tumors. *Clin Cancer Res*, 2003 9, 6002-11.
[63] Levin, E. Bidirectional signaling between the estrogen receptor and the epidermal growth factor receptor. *Mol Endocrinol*, 2003 17(3), 309-17.

[64] Taioli, E; Wynder, EL. Re: Endocrine factors and adenocarcinoma of the lung in women. *J Natl Cancer Inst*, 1994 86(11), 869-70.

[65] Blackman, J; Coogan, P; Rosenberg, L; Strom, B; Zauber, A; Palmer, J. Estrogen replacement therapy and risk of lung cancer. Pharmacoepidemiol Drug Saf, 2002 11(7), 561-7.

[66] Schabath, M; Wu, X; Vassilopoulou-Sellin, R; Vaporiciyan, A, MR. Hormone replacement therapy and lung cancer risk: A case-control analysis. *Clin Cancer Res*, 2004 10, 113-23.

[67] Ganti, AK; Sahmoun, AE; Panwalkar, AW; Tendulkar, KK; Potti, A. Hormone replacement therapy is associated with decreased survival in women with lung cancer. *J Clin Oncol*, 2006 24(1), 59-63.

[68] Olayioye, M; Neve, R; Lane, H; Hynes, N. The erbB signaling network: receptor heterodimerization in development and cancer. *EMBO J*, 2000 19, 3159-67.

[69] Kris, M; Natale, R; Herbst, R; et al. Efficacy of gefitinib, an inhibitor of the epidermal growth facotr receptor tyrosine kinase, in symptomatic patients with non-small cell lung cancer. *JAMA*, 2003 290(16), 2149-58.

[70] Fukuoka, M; Yano, S; Giaccone, G; et al. Multi-institutional randomized phase II trial of gefitinib for previously treated patients with advanced non-small cell lung cancer. *J Clin Oncol*, 2003 21(12), 2237-46.

[71] Shepherd, FA; Pereira, J; Ciuleanu, T; Tan, E. A randomized placebo-controlled trial of erlotinib in patients with advanced non-small cell lung cancer (NSCLC) following failure of 1st line or 2nd line chemotherapy. A National Cancer Institute of Canada Clinical Trials Group (NCIC CTG) trial. In: *Proc Amer Soc Clin Onco*; 2004. New Orleans: 2004; 14S.

[72] Lynch, T; Bell, D; Sordella, R; et al. Activating mutations in the epidermal growth factor receptor underlying responsiveness of non-small cell lung cancer to gefitinib. *N Engl J Med*, 2004 350(21), 2129-39.

[73] Paez, J; Janne, P; Lee, J; et al. EGFR mutations in lung cancer: correlation with clinical response to gefitinib therapy. *Science*, 2004 304, 1497-500.

[74] Huang, S; Liu, H; Ling-Hui, L; et al. High frequency of epidermal growth factor receptor mutations with complex patterns in non-small cell lung cancers related to gefitinib responsiveness in Taiwan. *Clin Cancer Res*, 2004 10, 8195-203.

[75] Radzikowska, E; Glaz, P; Roszkowski, K. Lung cancer in women: age, smoking, histology, performance status, stage, initial treatment and survival. Population based study of 20561 cases. *Ann Oncol*, 2002 13(7), 1087-93.

[76] Breathnach, O; Ishibe, N; Williams, J; Linnoila, R; Caporaso, N; Johnson, B. Clinical features of patients with stage IIIB and IV bronchioloalveolar carcinoma of the lung. *Cancer*, 1999 86(7), 1165-73.

[77] Kris, MG; Gralla, RJ; Potanovich, LM; Marks, LD; Heelan, RT. Assessment of pretreatment symptoms and improvement after EDAM+mitomycin+vinblastine in patients with inoperable non-small cell lung cancer. *Proc Am Soc Clin Oncol*, 1990 9, 229 (Abstract).

[78] Chute, CG; Greenberg, ER; Baron, J; Korson, R; Baker, J; Yates, J. Presenting conditions of 1539 population-based lung cancer patients by cell type and stage in New Hampshire and Vermont. *Cancer*, 1985 56(8), 2107-11.

[79] Matthews, MJ. Problems in morphology and behavior of bronchopulmonary malignant disease. In: Israel, L; Chahinian, AP; eds. *Lung Cancer: Natural History, Prognosis, and Therapy*. New York: Academic Press; 1976; 23-62.

[80] Dales, RE; Stark, RM; Raman, S. Computed tomography to stage lung cancer. Approaching a controversy using meta-analysis. *Am Rev Respir Dis*, 1990 141(5 Pt 1), 1096-101.

[81] Hillers, TK; Sauve, MD; Guyatt, GH; Analysis of published studies on the detection of extrathoracic metastases in patients presumed to have operable non-small cell lung cancer. *Thorax*, 1994 49(1), 14-9.

[82] Yokoi, K; Kamiya, N; Matsuguma, H et al. Detection of brain metastasis in potentially operable non-small cell lung cancer: a comparison of CT and MRI. *Chest*, 1999 115(3), 714-9.

[83] Pfister, DG; Johnson, DH; Azzoli, CG; et al. American Society of Clinical Oncology treatment of unresectable non-small-cell lung cancer guideline: update 2003. *J Clin Oncol*, 2004 22(2), 330-53.

[84] Spiro, SG; Porter, JC. Lung cancer--where are we today? Current advances in staging and nonsurgical treatment. *Am J Respir Crit Care Med*, 2002 166(9), 1166-96.

[85] Pieterman, RM; van Putten, JW; Meuzelaar, JJ; et al. Preoperative staging of non-small-cell lung cancer with positron-emission tomography [comment]. *N Engl J Med*, 2000 343(4), 254-61.

[86] Alexiou, C; Onyeaka, CV; Beggs, D; et al. Do women live longer following lung resection for carcinoma? *Eur J Cardiothorac Surg*, 2002 21(2), 319-25.

[87] Ferguson, MK; Wang, J; Hoffman, PC; et al. Sex-associated differences in survival of patients undergoing resection for lung cancer. *Ann Thorac Surg*, 2000 69(1), 245-9, discussion 9-50.

[88] de Perrot, M; Licker, M; Bouchardy, C; Usel, M; Robert, J; Spiliopoulos, A. Sex differences in presentation, management, and prognosis of patients with non-small cell lung carcinoma. *J Thorac Cardiovasc Surg*, 2000 119(1), 21-6.

[89] O'Connell, J; Kris, MG; Gralla, RJ; et al. Frequency and prognostic importance of pretreatment clinical characteristics in patients with advanced non-small cell lung cancer treated with combination chemotherapy. *J Clin Oncol*, 1986 4, 1604-14.

[90] Albain, KS; Crowley, JJ; LeBlanc, M; Livingston, RB. Survival determinants in extensive-stage non-small-cell lung cancer: The Southwest Oncology Group experience. *J Clin Oncol*, 1991 9, 1618-26.

[91] Johnson, BE; Steinberg, SM; Phelps, R; Edison, M; Veach, SR; Ihde DC. Women small cell lung cancer patients live longer than men. *Am J Med*, 1988 85, 194-6.

[92] Arriagada, R; Bergman, B; Dunant, A; Le Chevalier, T; Pignon, JP; Vansteenkiste, J. Cisplatin-based adjuvant chemotherapy in patients with completely resected non-small-cell lung cancer. *N Engl J Med*, 2004 350(4), 351-60.

[93] Winton, T; Livingston, R; Johnson, D; et al. Vinorelbine plus cisplatin vs. observation in resected non-small-cell lung cancer. *N Engl J Med*, 2005 352(25), 2589-97.

[94] Strauss, GM; Herndon, JE; Maddaus, MA. Randomized clinical trial of adjuvant chemotherapy with paclitaxel and carboplatin following resection in stage IB non-small cell lung cancer (NSCLC): Report of Cancer and Leukemia Group B (CALGB) Protocol 9633. In: *Am Soc Clin Oncol*; 2004, 2004. p. pp621a.

[95] Douillard, J-Y; Rosell, R; Delena, M. ANITA: Phase III adjuvant vinorelbine and cisplatin versus observation in completely resected (stage I-III) non-small cell lung cancer patients: final results after 70-month median follow-up. *J Clin Oncol*, 2005 23(Suppl 16S), 624s.

[96] Schiller, J; Harrington, D; Belani, C; et al. Comparison of four chemotherapy regimens for advanced non-small-cell lung cancer. *New Engl J Med*, 2002 346(2), 92-8.

[97] Sandler, A; Nemunaitis, J; Dehnam, C; et al. Phase III study of cisplatin (C) with or without gemcitabine (G) in patients with advanced nonsmall cell lung cancer (NSCLC). *Proc Am Soc Clin Oncol*, 1998 17, 454a.

[98] Chemotherapy in non-small cell lung cancer: a meta-analysis using updated data on individual patients from 52 randomised clinical trials. *BMJ*, 1995 311(7 October), 899-909.

[99] Shanafelt, TD; Loprinzi, C; Marks, R; Novotny, P; Sloan, J. Are chemotherapy response rates related to treatment-induced survival prolongations in patients with advanced cancer? *J Clin Oncol*, 2004 22(10), 1966-74.

[100] Evans, WK; Will, BP; Berthelot, JM; Wolfson, MC. Estimating the cost of lung cancer diagnosis and treatment in Canada: the POHEM model. *Can J Oncol*, 1995 5(4), 408-19.

[101] Tsao, MS; Sakurada, A; Cutz, JC; et al. Erlotinib in lung cancer - molecular and clinical predictors of outcome. *N Engl J Med*, 2005 353(2), 133-44.

[102] Johnson, D; Fehrenbacher, L; Novotny, P. Randomized phase II trial comparing bevacizumab plus carboplatin and paclitaxel with carboplatin and paclitaxel alone in previously untreated locally advanced or metastatic non-small-cell lung cancer. *J Clin Oncol*, 2004 22(11), 2184-91.

[103] Sandler, A; Gray, R; Brahmer, J. Randomized phase II/III trial of paclitaxel plus carboplatin with or without bevacizumab in patients with advanced non-squamous non-small cell lung cancer: An Eastern Cooperative Oncology Group Trial-E4599. In: *Proc Amer Soc Clin Onco*; 2005. Orlando, FL; 2005; p. LBA4.

SECTION 2: WOMEN AND BREAST CANCER

In: Women and Cancer
Editor: Laurie Elit, pp. 51-57

ISBN: 978-1-60021-494-3

Chapter I

SURGICAL MANAGEMENT OF BREAST CANCER

*Nicole C. Hodgson**
Assistant Professor, Department of Surgery, McMaster University, Juravinski Cancer Centre, Hamilton, Ontario, Canada.

ABSTRACT

This chapter reviews the surgical treatment options given various tissue diagnoses and the outcomes of each option in terms of local recurrence and survival.

INTRODUCTION

Breast cancer is a common malignancy in women with a 1 in 9 lifetime risk for women and the risk increases with age. Breast cancer incidence has risen since the early 1980's and this increase has been attributed to increased mammographic screening. There has been some plateauing of the incidence since the 1990's with the exception of the 55-74 age group. There is also regional variation across Canada and the US [1]. The mortality rates have fallen. The early detection of breast cancer by mammographyin women over the age of 50 has been shown by many studies to reduce mortality approximately 30%. [2] There is considerable evidence that the etiology of breast cancer is related largely to reproductive hormones, although most reported associations are relatively weak and not always consistent. Risk factors include early age at menarche, late menopause and nulliparity and reduced risk for women with early removal of ovaries or onset of menopause and higher numbers of pregnancies.

* Correspondence concerning this article should be addressed to Nicole Hodgson MD, Division of Surgical Oncology, Juravinski Cancer Centre, 699 Concession Street Hamilton, Ontario Canada. L8V 5C2 Phone 905 387-9495; Email: Nicole.hodgson@hrcc.on.ca.

Breast cancer surgery has evolved dramatically, from radical mastectomies to less extensive procedures. Breast conserving surgery (BCS) and mastectomy, have equivalent therapeutic benefits that have been confirmed by randomized clinical trials, the largest the, National Surgical Adjuvant Breast and Bowel Project (NSABP) B-06 protocol. Local recurrence rates after lumpectomy and radiation are in the range 5-10% over 10 years for early breast cancer [3]. The NSABP trial has recently been updated with a 25 year follow-up [3]. The 1991 National Cancer Institute (NCI) position statement clearly denotes BCS as an oncologically safe treatment and also as the preferred surgical option for women diagnosed with breast cancer [4]. However, despite this there is still considerable surgical practice variation with BCS underutilized in the United States and some areas of Canada [5]. This variation may be secondary to numerous factors including patient age, socioeconomic status, surgeon bias, geographic distance from radiation facilities, and treatment at teaching/cancer centres. Enabling patients to make a treatment choice on type of surgery was evaluated in a study using a decision aid outlining the details of mastectomy versus radiation [6]. Patients who used the decision board were more likely to choose BCT (94% vs 76%) treatment. Such instruments may be considered by surgeons when communicating the different surgical options to women with breast cancer.

Preoperative Assessment

A preoperative core biopsy to confirm tissue diagnosis is important to determine surgical therapy. Core biopsies are more accurate than fine needle aspirates, and also have the advantage of providing tissue for determining if the lesion is invasive or in situ. Most breast cancers are of ductal origin and noninvasive ductal carcinoma in situ (DCIS) lesions are diagnosed more frequently due to increased surveillance. DCIS, given its noninvasive nature does not require lymph node surgery, whereas invasive cancers require axillary lymph node sampling. Extensive preoperative staging is not recommended as less than 2% of operable breast cancer harbour metastatic disease at diagnosis.

Patients with dense fibroglandular tissue may present with mammographically occult lesions. The false negative rates of mammography range from 5-15%. Breast magnetic resonance imaging (MRI) is a new diagnostic tool used as an adjunct in further delineating occult lesions as well as lobular histologic types (Figure 1 and 2). MRI has the advantage of visualizing the breast in three dimensions and using nonionizing radiation. MRI has superior sensitivity than mammography for invasive cancers but its detection for DCIS is limited, as microcalcifications are not reliably identified [7]. Breast MRI may also have utility in optimizing surgical planning for patients with multifocal disease, positive margins after lumpectomy, or treatment response to neoadjuvant chemotherapy. Communication between radiologist and surgeon for appropriate surgical planning is paramount.

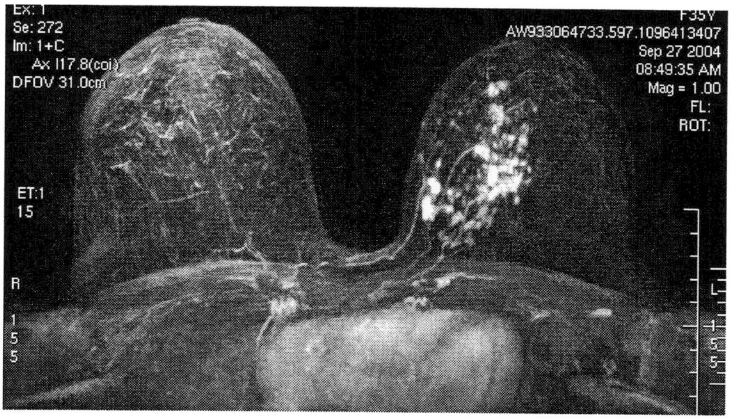

Figure 1. Breast MRI

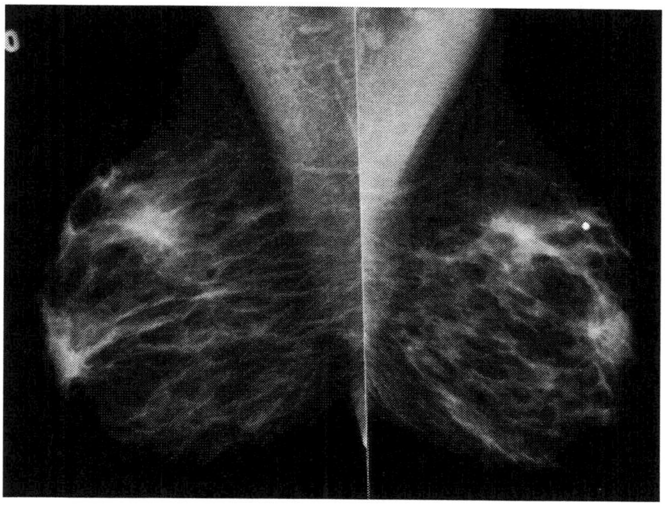

Figure 2. Mammogram In same patient as Figure 1

Breast Conserving Surgery and Mastectomy

With smaller breast cancers and in situ cancers being diagnosed due to mammographic screening. Radiographic wire localizations are used with increasing frequency to help the surgeon localize the area. Although this technique is used worldwide, it is not without some technical problems such as wire dislodgement or difficulty locating the lesion if the wire entry or incision is distant from the lesion. Extensive tunneling during lumpectomy is discouraged as it may compromise margin status. Radical incisions for lumpectomy are no longer considered appropriate. With smaller tumor volumes being resected, and little or no skin being removed, transverse incisions or cicrumareaolar incisions leave the best cosmetic outcome. Newer oncoplastic techniques such as triangle incisions, relocation of the nipple areolar complex and inframmary incisions are also performed.

Clear lumpectomy margins are important for optimal local control and decreased local recurrence. Definitions of clear margins vary from center to center. The NSABP criteria states no tumor at the inked margin, other definitions include tumor at least 1 mm from the inked margin, or >2 mm from the margin. The surgeon must label the lumpectomy specimen orientation (i.e. superior, lateral and deep), using sutures or ink, in order for accurate pathologic examination. Many series report increased risk of local recurrence for positive margins, 2, to 3 fold increased rates [8-10]. Margin status and tumor recurrence may be linked to tumor histology, presence of extensive intraductal component, patient age and the addition of systemic therapy. Location of the margin may also be important, as posterior or deep margins close to the chest wall and anterior margins where little or no breast tissue remains may not represent an increased risk of residual tumor burden.

Indications for mastectomy include multicentric tumors, tumor volume greater than breast volume, locally advanced and inflammatory cancers post neoadjuvant chemotherapy, history of previous radiation, recurrent cancer and patient preference.

Surgical Management of the Axilla

Axillary lymph node dissection, removal of the underarm lymph nodes, for accurate staging and excellent local control has been the standard of care for many years. Axillary lymph node surgery involves removing level I and II lymph nodes. This surgery is not without morbidity, which includes: postoperative pain, numbness under the arm, parasthesias, shoulder immobility and a risk of lymphedema. Lymphedema is a sequela of axillary node dissection and occurs in about 15-20% of patients (Figure 3)[11]. It is often exacerbated by infection or radiation.

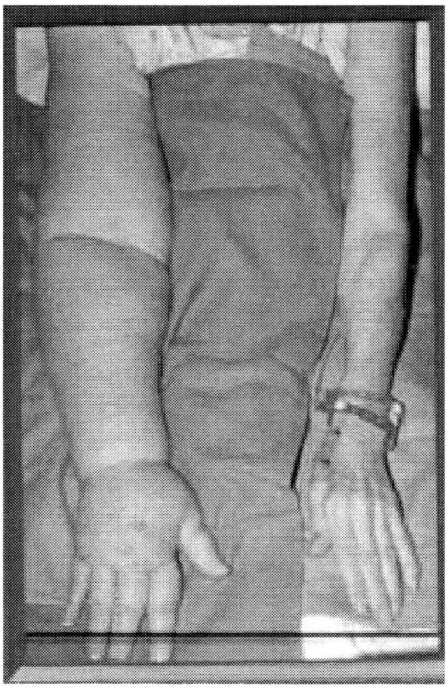

Figure 3. Lymphedema in a woman's right hand after axillary node dissection

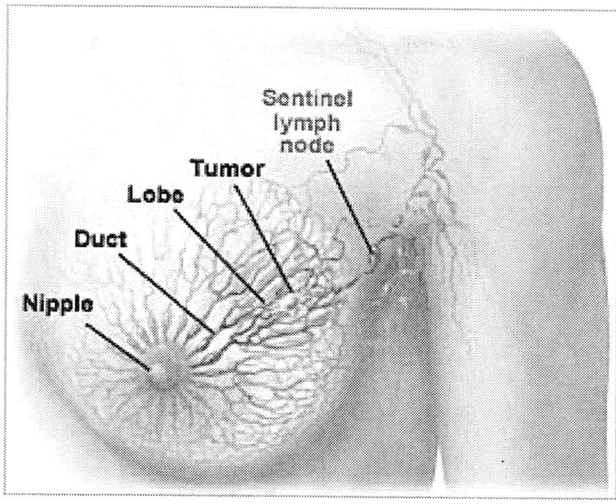

Figure 4. Concept behind the sentinel node

The sentinel lymph node (SLN) concept states that the sentinel node is the first node in the regional basin to receive lymphatic drainage from a primary breast cancer and therefore the most likely to contain metastatic tumor cells (Figure 4). If the SLN is negative then the remainder of the lymph nodes are negative versus if the SLN is positive for tumor then other nodes may be involved (Figure 5). The technique for identification of the correct sentinel lymph node requires an experienced team comprising of surgeon, nuclear medicine physician and pathologist. A radiocolloid injection and intraoperative blue dye injection is performed and an intraoperative gamma probe is used to localize and remove the sentinel node [12]. The radioactivity is minimal and a low 1% allergic reaction risk due to the blue dye. The SLN identification rate using the double dye technique is 98% and in experienced hands the false negative rate is less than 5% [13]. Studies have shown that learning curves are necessary in order to achieve a low false negative rate [14]. The technique allows for smaller incisions, no postoperative drain, and less pain and parasthesias. Longterm results are not yet available and randomized trials, the NSABP-32 [15]and ACOSOG trials will address overall mortality and disease free survival. Secondary outcomes include lymphedema rates and other potential side effects. Information from these three trials will offer: (1) survival data on sentinel node negative patients who undergo no further axillary therapy; (2) prognostic information on the importance of immunohistochemistry (IHC) positive sentinel lymph nodes and ICC positive bone marrow, which will lead to further studies on selective distribution of adjuvant chemo-hormonal therapy; and (3) survival data on sentinel node-positive patients who undergo no further axillary therapy. The ALMANAC randomized multicenter trial of SLN biopsy has reported lymphedema rates of 5-7%, this study's specific objective was to assess shoulder and arm morbidity [16].

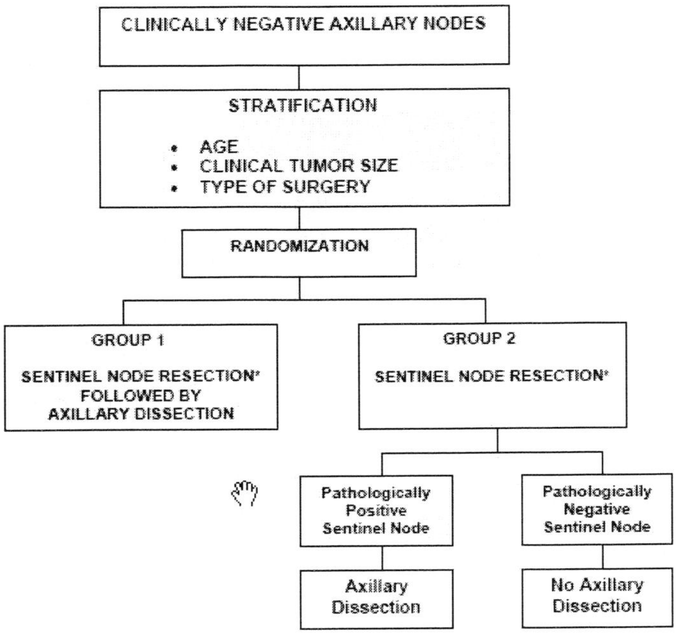

Figure 5. Algorithm for Sentinel Node dissection

More detailed pathologic examination of the sentinel node with the addition of immunohistochemistry has led to upstaging of cases and an increased incidence of micrometastases. Current guidelines are to proceed with completion axillary dissection if the sentinel node is found to be positive, as residual disease may be seen in 10-40% of cases [17]. Isolated tumor cells on immunohistochemistry are of unknown significance and further surgery and or adjuvant chemotherapy is not recommended in this scenario. The continued participation of surgeons in clinical trials contributes to the advancement of evidence-based therapeutic strategies for patients diagnosed with breast cancer.

For DCIS, lymph node sampling is not usually indicated as the lymphatic metastatic potential of DCIS low if not negligible. However, if there is suspicion for microinvasion in high grade DCIS, palpable DCIS, extensive DCIS measuring greater than 3-4 cm on mammography, or patients electing to have mastectomy which may preclude further lymphatic mapping, SLN biopsy can be considered[17]. Further evaluation of SLN utility in DCIS requires study in clinical trials.

Surgery in BRCA1/2 Mutation Carriers

Hereditary breast cancer represents approximately 5-10% of all breast cancers. The BRCA1 and BRCA2, (BReast CAncer) genes were identified in 1994 and 1995. Carriers of either gene have an 80% lifetime risk of developing breast cancer and a 40-60% risk of developing ovarian cancer [18]. Prevention choices for women diagnosed with either gene is surveillance, prophylactic surgery or chemoprevention.

Prophylactic mastectomy, usually a total or simple mastectomy, (no axillary dissection versus a subcutaneous mastectomy are described. Subcutaenous mastectomy differs from a total mastectomy in that the nipple arealar complex is not removed; therefore breast tissue is remaining and may portend a higher risk for development of breast cancer. It is important to note that mastectomy does not reliably remove all breast tissue as microscopic cells may remain beneath the skin flaps or in the axillary tissue. In 1991, Toth and Lappert [19] introduced the concept of skin sparing mastectomy (SSM), these patients had limited resection of skin with only the nipple areola resected and the biopsy site. The skin sparing mastectomy has been used primarily for patients with Stage 0, 1 and early Stage II disease when eligible for immediate reconstruction. Indications for prophylactic mastectomy include: carrier of BRCA1 or BRCA2 gene, a personal history of breast cancer, a family member with premenopausal breast cancer, family member with bilateral breast cancer, lobular or ductal carcinoma in situ, atypical hyperplasia. Prophylactic surgery may also be considered in women with a family history, multiple breast biopsies, difficult to monitor mammograms (obscured by fibrosis) or an extreme fear of cancer.

A retrospective cohort study at the Mayo clinic followed women who underwent bilateral prophylactic mastectomies and found a 90% risk reduction in development of cancer as well as a reduction in mortality 20]. Options of primary or secondary prevention and breast reconstructive options are important discussion points for surgeons and their patients. Genetic counseling and accurate risk assessment is vital for women at hereditary risk of breast cancer. These women face difficult decisions, advantages and disadvantages of surveillance, preventative surgery or chemoprevention need to be extensively reviewed.

Breast cancer statistics continue to show increasing incidence and decreasing mortality, this will ultimately result in more survivorship. Breast cancer surgery and treatment has profound impact on women's body image, sexuality, emotional and social well-being. Surgeons are often the first physician encounter for women diagnosed with breast cancer and their role in enabling patient decisions and care paths as well as enrollment in clinical trials is instrumental.

References

[1] Chen VW, Wu XC and Andrews PA, eds. Cancer Incidence in North America, 1996-2000. Volume One: Incidence. Sacramento, CA: North American Association of Central Cancer Registries, April 2003.

[2] Feuer E, Wun L-M. How much of the recent rise in breast cancer incidence can be explained by in crease in mammography utilization? Am J Epidemiol. 1992,136:1423-36.

[3] Ischer Twenty-year follow-up of a randomized trial comparing total mastectomy, lumpectomy, and lumpectomy plus irradiation for the treatment of invasive breast cancer. *N Engl J Med*, 2002 Oct 17 347(16), 1233-41.

[4] NIH consensus conference. Treatment of early-stage breast cancer. *JAMA* 265:391-395, 1991.

[5] Tarbox, BB et al. Are modified radical mastectomies done for T1 breast cancers because of surgeons advice or patient's choice? *AM J Surg*, 1992 164, 417.

[6] Whelan et al. Effect of a decision aid on knowledge and treatment decision making for breast cancer surgery: a randomized trial. *JAMA*, 2004 Jul 28 292(4), 435-41.

[7] Esserman, L. et al. Utility of magnetic resonance imaging in the management of breast cancer. Evidence for improved preoperative staging. *J Clin Oncol*, 1999 17, 110-119.

[8] Park CC et al. Outcome at 8 years after breast conserving therapy surgery and radiation therapy for invasive therapy: influence of margin status and systemic therapy on local recurrence. *J. Clin Oncol*, 2000 18, 1669.

[9] Scnitt, SJ. et al. The relationship between microscopic margins of resection and the risk of local recurrence in patients with breast cancer treated with breast conserving surgery and radiation therapy. *Cancer*, 1994 74, 1746.

[10] Pittinger, TP et al: Importance of margin status in outcome of breast conserving surgery for carcinoma. *Surgery*, 1994 116, 605.

[11] Ganz, PA. The quality of life after breast cancer-solving the problem of lymphedema. *N Engl J Med*, 1999 340, 383-385.

[12] Schwarz, GF et al. *For the Consensus Conference Committee: proceedings of the consensus conference on the role of sentinel lymph node biopsy in carcinoma of the breast.* April 19-22, 2001, Philadelphia, Pennsylvania

[13] Giuliano, AE et al. Lymphatic mapping and sentinel lymphadenectomy for breast cancer. *Ann Surg*, 1994 220, 391.

[14] Krag et al. The sentinel node in breast cancer: a multicenter validation study. *N Engl J Med*, 1998 339, 941.

[15] Harlow SP Prerandomization surgical training for the NSABP B-32 trial, A randomized phase III clinical trial to compare sentinel node resection to conventional axillary dissection in clinical node-negative breast cancer. Ann Surg 2005 24(1) 48-54.

[16] Mansel Re, Randomized multicenter trial of sentinel node biopsy versus standard axillary treatment in operable breast cancer: the ALMANAC trial. J Natl Cancer inSt. 2006: 98(9) 599-609.

[17] Lyman, GH et al. American Society of Clinical Onncology guideline recommendation for sentinel lymph node biopsy in early stage breast cancer. J Clin Oncol 2005:23(30):7703-20.

[18] Antoniou, A. Average risks of breast cancer and ovarian cancer associated with BRCA1 and BRCA2 mutations detected in case series unselected for family history: A combined analysis of 22 studies. *AM J of Hum Genetics*, 2003 72, 1117-1130.

[19] Toth BA, Lappert P. Modified skin incisions for mastectomy: the need for plastic surgical input in preoperative planning. Plast reconstr Surg 1991: 87(6) 1048-57.

[20] Meijers-Heijboer, H; van Geel, B; van Putten, WL; et al. Breast cancer after prophylactic bilateral mastectomy in women with BRCA1 and BRCA2 mutation. *N Engl J Med*, 2001 345, 159-164.

[21] Hartmann, LC et al. Efficacy of bilateral prophylactic mastectomy in women with a family history of breast cancer. *N Engl J Med*, 1999 340, 77-84.

In: Women and Cancer
Editor: Laurie Elit, pp. 59-74
ISBN: 978-1-60021-494-3

Chapter II

MEDICAL MANAGEMENT OF BREAST CANCER

Sukhbinder Dhesy-Thind*
Department of Medicine, McMaster University, Juravinski Cancer Centre, Hamilton, Ontario, Canada.

ABSTRACT

This chapter reviews the treatment decision points concerning use of adjuvant hormones, chemotherapy or biologic agents. Anticipated outcome in terms of local recurrence, risk of contralateral breast cancer, disease free and overall survival and side effects are provided. Management options for women with metastatic disease and the goals of treatment are explored including bisphosphonates, chemotherapy, hormonal, and biologics such as Herceptin.

INTRODUCTION

The mortality rate from breast cancer is decreasing in many countries, likely due to increased awareness, organized screening programs leading to earlier detection and the increasing use of effective adjuvant therapies [1-3]. The medical management of invasive breast cancer includes a number of hormonal, chemotherapy, targeted therapy, and supportive care options. These treatments span the spectrum from neoadjuvant (preoperative or primary) chemotherapy to adjuvant therapy (following primary surgical resection) to the treatment of metastatic disease.

* Correspondence concerning this article should be addressed to Dr. Sukhbinder Dhesy-Thind, Division of Medical Oncology, Juravinski Cancer Centre, 699 Concession Street Hamilton, Ontario, Canada. L8V 5C2. Phone 905 387-9495 ext 64602; Fax: 905 575-6326; Email: bindi.dhesy@hrcc.on.ca.

1. Adjuvant Therapy

The decision to offer adjuvant systemic therapy is based on a number of prognostic variables that are used to determine a woman's risk of developing metastatic disease. These include the involvement of axillary lymph nodes, tumor size, tumor grade, the presence of lymphovascular invasion, estrogen (ER) and progesterone (PR) receptor status and the overexpression or amplification of the human epidermal growth factor receptor 2 (HER2/neu). Women with lymph-node positive disease or high-risk lymph-node negative disease are usually treated with adjuvant chemotherapy. The latter include women with large tumor size, high tumor grade (grade 3), lymphovascular invasion, ER negative or HER2/neu positive breast cancer. The use of decision aids has been beneficial in discussing adjuvant systemic therapy with patients, particularly those with node-negative breast cancer [4]. An on-line computer program is also available to help quantify a patient's risk of recurrence and the benefits of hormonal therapy and chemotherapy [5]. This program has been externally validated using the British Columbia Cancer agency's provincial registry [6]. Equally important to the decision making process is the side effect profile of the proposed agents and patient factors, including medical co-morbidities and patient preferences.

Adjuvant systemic therapy is given to most healthy women with breast cancer, the purpose being to treat occult metastatic disease (micrometastates). Women with axillary lymph node positive or high risk, lymph node-negative breast cancer are often treated with adjuvant chemotherapy. Patients with estrogen and/or progesterone positive disease are also treated with adjuvant hormonal therapy, the selection of which may be influenced by menopausal status. Premenopausal women may be treated with tamoxifen, ovarian ablation or ovarian ablation and an aromatase inhibitor. The latter is currently being investigated in the Breast Cancer International Research Group SOFT (Suppression of Ovarian Function Trial), TEXT (Tamoxifen/Exemestane Trial) and PERCHE (Premenopausal Endocrine Responsive Chemotherapy) studies.

1a. Adjuvant Hormonal Therapy

The importance of estrogen in breast carcinogenesis is well known with approximately 70% of breast cancers estrogen positive. This estrogen dependence is exploited through various therapeutic interventions [7]. Oophorectomy for palliation of advanced breast cancer in premenopausal women was first reported in 1896 by Beastson. [8]. A number of different drug therapies are also available for the treatment of hormone receptor positive breast cancer. Tamoxifen is a selective estrogen receptor modulator (SERM) competitively binding to the estrogen receptor where it may have antagonistic or agonistic estrogen effects depending on the target site. Its anti-estrogen effect in the breast led to its use in the treatment of hormone receptor positive breast cancer. In contrast, aromatase inhibitors block the peripheral conversion of androgens to estrogens, thus reducing estrogen levels in plasma [9]. The aromatase inhibitors are contraindicated in pre-menopausal women due to concerns of ovarian hyperstimulation and increased production of aromatase through endogenous feedback mechanisms.

Postmenopausal women with hormone receptor positive breast cancer may be treated with an aromatase inhibitor alone [10-12], tamoxifen alone, or a sequence of tamoxifen followed by an aromatase inhibitor [13-16]. For patients in whom adjuvant chemotherapy is planned, hormonal therapy should follow completion of chemotherapy as concurrent chemotherapy and tamoxifen has been associated with a worse outcome than sequential chemotherapy followed by tamoxifen [17]. Women whose tumors do not express ER or PR do not benefit from hormonal treatments [18,19].

In patients with hormone receptor positive breast cancer, five years of adjuvant tamoxifen therapy reduces the risk of breast-cancer recurrence by 47 percent and the risk of death by 26 percent [18,19]. This translates into a 10-year gain in breast cancer mortality compared to placebo for both node-positive (10.9% absolute gain) and node-negative patients (5.6%). Tamoxifen also reduces the risk of contralateral breast cancer risk by 40-50%. Benefits are seen in both pre- and post-menopausal women. The optimal duration of tamoxifen therapy appears to be five years.

The agonist action of tamoxifen on the endometrium are responsible for a 0.6% risk of developing endometrial cancer with an absolute excess of deaths from endometrial cancer of 1-2 per 1000. Tamoxifen is bone sparing in post-menopausal women and cardiac neutral [18,19].

Aromatase inhibitors block the peripheral conversion of androgens to estrogens, thus reducing estrogen levels in plasma. They include the non-steroidal agents anastrozole and letrozole and the steroidal agent exemestane. Two randomized, double-blind multicentre trials have compared initial aromatase inhibitors to tamoxifen [10-12]. The ATAC study (Arimidex, Tamoxifen, Alone or in Combination) randomized over 9000 patients to either 5 years of anastrozole alone, tamoxifen alone or a combination of the two [10,12]. The combination arm was discontinued after an interim analysis showed it to be no more effective than tamoxifen alone and inferior to anastrozole alone. The 68 month analysis showed an improved disease free survival (Hazard Ratio 0.87, (95% CI 0.78 to 0.97), p=0.013), translating into an absolute difference of 3.7%. Time to recurrence was also improved (p=0.005) and contralateral breast cancer incidence (p=0.014), but not overall survival or breast cancer deaths. There were also more non-breast cancer deaths in the anastrozole arm (6.2%) compared with tamoxifen (5.5%). There were significantly fewer side effects with anastrozole compared to tamoxifen with minimal effects on quality of life measures. Anastrozole was associated with fewer hot flashes, vaginal symptoms including endometrial cancer and venous thromboembolism 2.8% vs. 4.5%) than tamoxifen treated patients. Tamoxifen treated patients had fewer fractures and arthralgias than those receiving anastrozole.

The Breast International Group reported preliminary results of their four-arm study comparing 5 years of adjuvant letrozole to 5 years of adjuvant tamoxifen. Sequential treatment arms compare tamoxifen for 2 years followed by letrozole for 3 years to upfront letrozole with a switch to tamoxifen at 2 years [11]. Over 8000 post-menopausal women with hormone receptor-positive early stage breast cancer were randomized in this study. After a median follow-up of 25.8 months, letrozole resulted in a 19% reduction in disease-free survival compared to tamoxifen (HR 0.81, 95% CI 0.70-0.93, p=0.003). There was an absolute benefit of 2.6% at five years (p=0.0002) in breast cancer relapse rate and a significant improvement in time to development of distant metastases (HR 0.73, 95% CI) in the letrozole treated group. Women receiving letrozole had a higher incidence of skeletal and cardiac events and of hypercholesterolemia (43.5% vs. 19.1%) and lower rates of thromboembolism (0.8% vs. 2.0%), endometrial cancer and vaginal bleeding than those treated with tamoxifen.

Aromatase inhibitors have also been shown to be effective when used in sequence after 2 to 3 years of adjuvant tamoxifen. Anastrozole and exemestane have both been studied and found to be superior to five years of adjuvant tamoxifen. The Intergroup Exemestane Study (IES) randomized over 4500 post-menopausal women with hormone receptor positive breast cancer to switching to exemestane following 2 to 3 years of adjuvant tamoxifen or continuing with tamoxifen for a total of 5 years of treatment [13]. Disease-free survival was significantly improved in those women receiving exemestane (HR 0.73 95% CI 0.62 to 0.86, $p=0.0001$), absolute benefit of 4.7% at 3 years. There was a 30% relative risk reduction of local and distant recurrences ($p=0.0001$) and a 54% reduction of contralateral breast cancer ($p=0.04$). The side effect profile was similar to that of the other aromatase inhibitor studies. Significantly fewer gynecological symptoms ($p=0.002$) and thromboembolic events ($p<0.001$) and higher incidence of arthralgia ($p<0.001$) and myocardial infarction ($p=0.02$) were seen with exemestane treated patients. Sub-studies investigating the bone and gynecologic effects of exemestane are ongoing.

While the extension of tamoxifen beyond five years is of limited benefit, extended adjuvant hormonal therapy with aromatase inhibitors following 5 years of tamoxifen has been associated with an overall survival benefit in node-positive post-menopausal women [14]. This study of over 5000 post-menopausal women with hormone-receptor positive breast cancer showed a predicted 6% absolute improvement in risk of breast cancer recurrence at four years post randomization. This pivotal study highlights the late recurrences that may occur in ER positive women.

The collective studies discussed above show that aromatase inhibitors significantly improve breast cancer recurrence and rate of contralateral breast cancer compared to tamoxifen and compared to placebo following five years of tamoxifen. The aromatase inhibitors are associated with an increased incidence of fractures and osteoporosis, but fewer hot flashes, vaginal symptoms, endometrial cancer and venous thromboembolism than tamoxifen. The long-term effects of aromatase inhibitors and chronic and complete estrogen deprivation particularly with regards to cardiac disease, lipid metabolism and cognitive function are unknown at this time and require further investigation.

The question of the optimal adjuvant hormonal therapy regimen for post-menopausal women remains unanswered at this time. The American Society of Clinical Oncology (ASCO) Technology Assessment Panel has developed guidelines regarding use of aromatase inhibitors [15]. ASCO guidelines recommend that adjuvant treatment should include an aromatase inhibitor, as initial therapy or after treatment with tamoxifen. The particular regimen used is dependant on a woman's individual clinical situation and preference based on the risks and benefits of all the options. These issues should be clarified in the future as a number of studies are ongoing including first-line studies comparing the different aromatase inhibitors as well as the optimal duration of treatment. The BIG I-98 study also will address the question of whether upfront treatment with an aromatase inhibitor is preferable to a sequence of tamoxifen for two years followed by an aromatase inhibitor.

Ovarian ablation either through surgery (oophorectomy), radiation therapy or using gonadotrophin releasing hormone analogues (GnRH) may be an option for premenopausal women with hormone receptor positive breast cancer. The Oxford Overview found oophorectomy to be as effective as cyclophosphamide, methotrexate, and 5-fluorouracil (CMF) chemotherapy [18] but this strategy has not been compared to newer chemotherapy regimens. Studies are ongoing to evaluate the role of ovarian ablation in premenopausal women.

1b. Adjuvant Chemotherapy

Adjuvant chemotherapy is usually recommended for women with lymph node positive or high-risk lymph node negative breast cancer, including those with estrogen negative breast cancer. A number of chemotherapeutic options are available for healthy women. These include both anthracycline and non-anthracycline containing regimens and taxanes. The regimens vary in the number of chemotherapy drugs, frequency and route of administration and treatment duration. Direct comparison of the new treatment options is difficult, as randomized controlled trials have not been completed. This has resulted in significant variations in practice across countries and continents.

The selection of the chemotherapeutic regimen is dependent on tumor and patient characteristics and the degree of added benefit of more aggressive regimens (i.e. dose dense therapies) needs to be balanced against the extra toxicities. The Early Breast Cancer Trialists' overview [19] demonstrates the benefits of adjuvant chemotherapy to be most evident in women under 50 years of age, with less benefit in older patients. This meta-analysis of over 194 randomized controlled trials found that 6 months of anthracycline-based poly-chemotherapy (e.g. Fluorouracil, doxorubicin, cyclophosphamide (CAF), fluorouracil, epirubicin, cylcophosphamide (FEC)) reduces the annual breast cancer death rate by about 38% for women younger than 50 years and by 20% for women aged 50-69. This was irrespective of use of tamoxifen, ER status, nodal status or other tumor characteristics. The anthracycline-based regimens were significantly better than CMF chemotherapy ($p<0.00001$ for breast cancer mortality). This overview evaluates predominantly older chemotherapy regimens and the expectation is of greater improvements in long-term survival with the use of newer chemotherapy regimens which were not evaluated in the meta-analysis.

The most commonly used regimens are highlighted in Table 1. These include combinations that contain anthracyclines (adriamycin 50-60 mg/m^2 or epirubicin 100–120 mg/m^2 per cycle), taxanes (paclitaxel 175 mg/m^2) and accelerated or dose-dense regimens (given every two weeks with cell growth factor support).

Anthracycline containing regimens (doxorubicin and epirubicin) show greater efficacy in survival compared to cyclophosphamide, methotrexate and 5-flourouracil (CMF) but are associated with higher rates of alopecia, febrile neutropenia, and cardiotoxicity [20]. The exception is four cycles of doxorubicin (Adriamycin) and cyclophosphamide (AC) which was found to be equivalent to 6 cycles of CMF in relatively low-risk patients [21]. In patients with node positive breast cancer the addition of a taxane following anthracycline chemotherapy has shown a statistically significant improvement in disease free survival [22,23]. One of these studies showed an improvement in overall survival [22]. Both of these studies compared four cycles of adriamycin and cyclophosphamide (AC) with AC followed by paclitaxel (AC-T) for four cycles. The Breast Cancer International Research Group (BCIRG) 001 trial compared an anthracycline-taxane combination (TAC) with six cycles of an anthracycline-based regimen (FAC).

Table 1. Commonly used adjuvant chemotherapy regimens for Axillary Node Positive or High Risk Lymph Node Negative Breast Cancer

Regimen	Chemotherapy Drugs	Study Population	Disease Free Survival	Overall Survival
Non-anthracycline				
CMF-po	Cyclophosphamide Methotrexate Fluorouracil	Node positive	3 yr- 63% 5 yr- 53%	3 yr - 82% 5 yr – 70%
CMF –iv	Cyclophosphamide Methotrexate Fluorouracil	Node negative (N-) Node positive (N+)	5 yr – 67% (N-) 43% (N+)	5 yr – 81%(N-) 60% (N+)
Anthracycline				
AC	Doxorubicin Cyclophosphamide	Node positive	3 yr-62%	3 yr- 83%
FAC	Fluorouracil Doxorubicin Cyclophosphamide	Node positive	5 yr- 68%	5 yr- 81%
CEF	Cyclophosphamide Epirubicin Fluorouracil	Node positive	5 yr – 63% 10 yr- 52%	5 yr –77% 10 yr – 62%
FEC100	Fluorouracil Epirubicin Cyclophosphamide	Node positive	5 yr – 66.3%	5 yr – 77.4%
Taxane				
AC – T	Doxorubicin Cyclophosphamide Paclitaxel	Node positive	5 yr- 66%	5 yr- 79%
TAC	Docetaxel Doxorubicin Cyclophosphamide	Node positive	5 yr –75%	5 yr –87%
FEC - D	Fluorouracil Epirubicin Cyclophosphamide Docetaxel	Node positive	5 yr - 78.4%	5 yr – 90.7%
Dose-dense				
AC-T	Doxorubicin Cyclophosphamide Paclitaxel	Node positive	4 yr – 82%	3 yr – 92%

Table 2. Adjuvant Therapy with Trastuzumab

Study Treatment Arm	Median Follow-up (years)	DFS (%)	Disease-Free Survival Hazard Ratio (95% CI); p value	Overall Survival (%)	Overall Survival Hazard Ratio (95% CI); p value
NSABP-B31/NCCTG N9831 Combined Analysis	2	3yr DFS:		3 yr OS:	
AC→TH		87.1	0.48 (0.39 to 0.59);	94.3	0.67 (0.48 to 0.93);
AC→T		75.4	p<0.0001	91.7	p=0.015
HERA Trial	1	2 yr DFS:		2 yr OS:	
1° therapy→H		85.8	0.54	96	0.76
1° therapy → observation		77.4	(0.43-0.67); p<0.0001	95.1	(0.47 to 1.23); p=0.26
BCIRG 006 study	1.9	3 yr DFS			
AC→DH		80	0.49[1] (0.37 to 0.65); p<0.0001	n/a	n/a
DCbH		86	0.61[2] (0.47 to 0.79); p=0.0002	n/a	n/a
AC→D		77		n/a	n/a
FinHer Trial	3.2	3 yr DFS		3 yr OS	
DH / VinH→FEC		89.3	0.46;	96.3	0.43;
D or Vin →FEC		77.6	p=0.0078	89.7	p=0.08

1. for the comparison of AC →DH vs AC →D.
2. for the comparison of DCbH vs AC →D.

Abbreviations: AC = anthracycline + cyclophosphamide; BCIRG = Breast Cancer International Research Group; CI = confidence interval; D = docetaxel; DH = docetaxel+trastuzumab; DCbH = docetaxel + carboplatin + trastuzumab; FEC = 5-fluorouracil + epirubicin + cyclophosphamide; H = trastuzumab; HERA = Herceptin Adjuvant; HR = hazard ratio; n/a = not available; NCCTG = North Central Cancer Treatment Group; NSABP = National Surgical Adjuvant Breast and Bowel Project; T = paclitaxel; TH = paclitaxel + trastuzumab; Vin = vinorelbine; VinH = vinorelbine + trastuzumab.

This study found an improved overall survival and disease free survival benefit at 5 years but had significantly higher rate of febrile neutropenia [24].

The CALGB 9741 (Cancer and Leukemia group) of dose dense chemotherapy in node-positive breast cancer evaluated AC-T chemotherapy given every two weeks with growth factor support (Granulocyte colony stimulating factor or G-CSF) with the same standard three weekly treatment [25]. Both treatments were given for a total of 8 cycles and the more frequent treatment was associated with an improved disease free survival and overall survival. Four year disease free survival was 82% for the dose dense chemotherapy and 75% for the three weekly treatment. Fewer episodes of febrile neutropenia were seen with the dose dense group. The shorter duration of this dose dense treatment and reduced risk of infection may be preferable for many patients and clinicians.

A number of international groups have developed consensus guidelines for the treatment of early breast cancer [26-28]. Traditionally, treatment recommendations have focused on axillary nodal status (positive vs. negative) in selecting patients for whom chemotherapy may be appropriate. Women with lymph node positive disease have traditionally been felt to have a high risk of systemic recurrence and are offered adjuvant chemotherapy. However, the recommendations from the 2005 St. Gallen Breast Cancer meeting emphasizes endocrine responsiveness in choosing treatment [28], suggesting that some women with 1-3 positive axillary lymph nodes may not necessarily be at high risk for recurrence if they are also HER2/neu negative and ER positive. These women may be candidates for endocrine therapy alone or chemotherapy followed by endocrine therapy.

1c. Adjuvant Trastuzumab Therapy

Approximately 20-25% of breast cancers overexpress the HER2neu protein. This is associated with an adverse prognosis [29]. Trastuzumab is a humanized monoclonal antibody targeting the extracellular domain of the HER2neu protein. Five studies of adjuvant Trastuzumab have been reported showing a survival advantage with the addition of this monoclonal antibody to the HER2neu protein to chemotherapy [30-33] (Table 2). These studies are summarized in table 2. The HERA trial showed a significant improvement in disease free survival (hazard ratio 0.54). A pooled analysis of the NSABP and NCCTG trials also showed improvements in disease free survival (hazard ratio 0.48) and a significantly improved overall survival (hazard ratio 0.67). Long-term follow up is required particularly with regards to concerns about cardiotoxicity, especially in patients who have also received adjuvant anthracycline chemotherapy. Studies exploring the optimal duration of trastuzumab are ongoing.

1d. Adjuvant Bisphosphonates

Bisphosphonates inhibit osteoclast mediated bone resorption induced by tumor cells. Powles and colleagues randomly allocated 1069 women with operable breast cancer to 2 years of adjuvant clodronate or placebo [34]. There was a significant reduction in the development of skeletal metastases during the 2-year medication period and the 5-year follow-up. A statistically significant improvement in overall survival was found in patients treated with oral clodronate. Saarto and associates also reported a randomized controlled trial of adjuvant clodronate [36]. Two hundred and ninety-nine women with node-positive breast cancer received 3 years of adjuvant clodronate or no bisphosphonate therapy. At 10 years, there was no difference in bone metastases in the 2 groups. There was a statistically significant difference in disease-free survival in patients who received clodronate. However, this may have been due to an imbalance in prognostics factors between groups. A third study randomly allocated 302 women with primary breast cancer and micrometastatic cells in the bone marrow to 2 years of clodronate or standard therapy [38,39]. At a median follow-up of 103 months, there was no difference in the frequency of bone, visceral or distant metastases. Previous reports had demonstrated improved 3- and 5-year disease-free survival and overall survival in patients treated with clodronate. In the updated study, overall survival was improved; however, the improved disease-free survival was no longer evident. Given the differences in trial design and patient populations in these studies, it is premature to make recommendations regarding the use of bisphosphonates for the prevention of skeletal metastases.

Bisphosphonates have also been investigated as a means of counteracting the bone loss seen with aromatase inhibitors. The Z-FAST study found that women who received up-front zoledronate had reduced rates of osteoporosis as determined by dual energy xray absoptiometry scan (BMD scans) and also reduced rates of bone turnover measured by urine and serum bone markers. [40]

2. Metastatic Breast Cancer

Despite substantial improvements in screening and adjuvant treatments a significant number of women will develop metastatic disease. Studies do not show that routine screening in asymptomatic patients impact on survival [41-43]. Once metastatic disease develops it cannot be cured. The median survival for women with metastatic breast cancer is 18 to 24 months with few patients achieving complete remission. Factors predicting for longer survival include younger age, good performance status, long disease free interval, ER positive cancer, single site of metastases and lack of visceral metastases. The goals of treatment are palliation of symptoms, maintain or improve quality of life and possible prolongation of survival. The choice of systemic therapy will be dependant on patient and tumor factors including previous adjuvant therapy, performance status, co-morbid conditions, presence of visceral metastases, estrogen receptor status, HER2/neu status and patient preference.

Women with estrogen receptor positive disease and low volume metastatic disease or metastases limited to bone may be candidates for hormonal therapy including aromatase inhibitors or tamoxifen. Response rates to initial hormonal therapy range typically range from 20 to 35% with median overall survival of 30 to 40 months. Aromatase inhibitors have been shown to be superior to tamoxifen for the first-line treatment of metastatic breast cancer in postmenopausal women, with significantly higher response rates, time to treatment progression and significant improvements in one and two year survival rates compared to women who received tamoxifen [44].

Women with significant visceral metastases or rapidly progressive disease are often treated with chemotherapy. A number of combination chemotherapy regimens and single agents have been investigated. The benefit of combination chemotherapy as compared to sequential use of single chemotherapy agents is unknown. Combination regimens tested in randomized controlled studies include capecitabine and docetaxel as well as gemcitabine and paclitaxel. These regimens show significantly improved response rates and longer time to treatment progression than single agents but also have considerable toxicity, particularly febrile neutropenia. Capecitabine and docetaxel has an overall survival advantage of 14.5 months versus 11.5 months with single agent docetaxel. However, only 27% of patients on the single agent chemotherapy crossed over to receive capecitabine on disease progression [45]. A meta-analysis of single-agent versus combination chemotherapy showed a 9% absolute 1-year survival benefit for combination therapy [46]. This meta-analysis comprised small studies of non-taxane regimens and did not address the issue of sequential single agent therapy compared to combination therapy. Given the significant toxicities of combination therapy, it is usually recommended for those women with rapidly progressive or life-threatening metastases in whom combination therapy may be more likely to elicit a quick response.

Single agent chemotherapy response rates range from 20 to 65% with a median time to treatment progression of 6 months. Commonly used agents include anthracyclines (doxorubicin, epirubicin), alkylating agents (cyclophosphamide), taxanes (paclitaxel, docetaxel), vinca alkaloids (vinorelbine), capecitabine, and gemcitabine.

For women with HER2/neu positive breast cancer, trastuzumab (Herceptin) has been shown to improve median overall survival (25.1 months vs. 20.3 months) when combined with chemotherapy as compared to chemotherapy alone [47]. Response rates to single agent trastuzumab of 15% in heavily pretreated patients [48] to 35% in chemotherapy naïve patients [49]. The major toxicity of trastuzumab is cardiotoxicity, particularly in patients who previously received anthracycline chemotherapy.

Bevacizumab, a monoclonal antibody to the vascular endothelial growth factor (VEGF) receptor has also shown promise in combination with paclitaxel chemotherapy for the treatment of metastatic breast cancer [50].

Bisphosphonates should be considered for patients with skeletal metastases as randomized controlled studies have shown a reduction in skeletal related events including time to fracture, need for radiation therapy, and analgesic use [51]. ASCO practice guidelines recommend bisphosphonates for patients with lytic metastases on plain x-rays [52].

3. Locally Advanced Breast Cancer/ Inflammatory Breast Cancer

Locally advanced breast cancer refers to Stage III cancer which includes tumors of large size (>5 cm), associated with skin or chest wall involvement or fixed axillary lymph nodes, disease spread to the ipsilateral internal mammary or supraclavicualr lymph nodes or inflammatory breast cancer (a rapidly progressive breast cancer with skin involvement which may be seen as histological involvement of the dermal lymphatic system) [53]. Multimodality therapy consisting of neoadjuvant (preoperative or primary) chemotherapy, surgical resection and radiation therapy is the preferred treatment. The majority of studies of preoperative or neoadjuvant chemotherapy involve women with operable breast cancer, often with tumors of less than 3 cm. These studies have been extrapolated to patients with inoperable stage III disease.

The goals of neoadjuvant chemotherapy are to decrease the size of the primary breast cancer, which may result in optimization of the surgical resection and to reduce the risk of distant metastases. Neoadjuvant chemotherapy also permits the administration of drugs through intact vasculature and may provide insight into the responsiveness of the tumor to chemotherapy, providing a direct measurement of the sensitivity of the tumor to chemotherapy. This may also allow for the evaluation of biological markers in predicting tumor response to chemotherapy. The early detection of drug resistance may also lead to the discontinuation of an ineffective therapy.

The finding of a pathological complete response (absence of residual invasive or in situ disease following chemotherapy and surgery) is associated with a significant survival benefit and is a strong prognostic marker for both disease-free and overall survival [54].

Neoadjuvant hormonal therapy has also been extensively investigated and may be considered for patients who are medically unfit for or decline chemotherapy. Neoadjuvant therapy with an aromatase inhibitor has been shown to be superior to tamoxifen therapy, particularly in those women with HER2/neu positive breast cancer [55,56].

For patients with locally advanced operable breast cancer, neoadjuvant chemotherapy is associated with an increase in the overall rate of breast conservation surgery compared to mastectomy (22% with neoadjuvant chemotherapy vs. 8% without) [57]. Neoadjuvant chemotherapy regimens are often similar to those used in the adjuvant setting and usually comprise of an anthracycline-based regimen or a combination of an anthracycline and taxane. The NSABP-B 27 study randomized over 2000 women with operable breast cancer to either neoadjuvant doxorubicin and cyclophosphamide (AC) or AC followed by docetaxel (T) followed by surgery, or AC followed by surgery followed by postoperative adjuvant docetaxel. Neoadjuvant AC-T was shown to have a higher clinical complete response and higher pathological complete response (13.7% vs. 26.1%, $p<0.001$) [58]. A UK study also evaluated docetaxel in the neoadjuvant setting in patients with large operable and locally advanced breast cancer. Women who received docetaxel had higher pathological CR rates and longer relapse –free and overall survival [59].

In patients with inoperable locally advanced breast cancer, systemic chemotherapy is similar to that of operable locally advanced disease. The 5-year overall survival rate with neoadjuvant chemotherapy for these women ranges from 44 to 88%.

Inflammatory breast cancer typically presents with breast erythema and skin changes including a peau d'orange appearance. A palpable breast mass may or may not be evident. Inflammatory breast cancer has a poor prognosis and requires aggressive multimodality management. Treatment is as per inoperable locally advanced breast cancer.

In patients with HER2/neu overexpressing stage II to IIIA breast cancer, the addition of neoadjuvant trastuzumab (Herceptin) to chemotherapy is associated with a significantly higher pathological complete response rate (66.7% vs. 25% for chemotherapy alone, $p=0.02$) [60].

REFERENCES

[1] Levia, Fabio; Boxettic, Cristina; Lucchinib, Franca; Negric, Eva; La Veccgua, Carlo. Monitoring the decrease in breast cancer mortality in Europe. *European Journal of Cancer Prevention*, 2005 14, 497–502.

[2] International Agency for Research on Cancer. *Cancer incidence in five continents, volume VIII*. Lyon: IARC, 2002.

[3] Canadian Cancer Society/National Cancer Institute of Canada: Canadian Cancer Statistics 2005, Toronto, Canada, 2005.

[4] Whelan, T; Sawka, C; Levine, M; et al. Helping patients make informed choices: a randomized trial of a decision aid for adjuvant chemotherapy in lymph node-negative breast cancer. *J Natl Cancer Inst*, 2003 95, 581.

[5] Ravdin, PM; Siminoff, LA; Davos, GJ; et al. Computer program to assist in making decisions about adjuvant therapy for women with early breast cancer. *J Clin Oncol*, 2001 19, 980-991. www.adjuvantonline.com

[6] Olivotto, IA; Bajdik, CD; Ravdin, PM; et al. Population-based validation of the prognostic model ADJUVANT! for early breast cancer. *J Clin Oncol*, 2005 23, 2716-25.

[7] Yager, JD; Davidson, NE. Estrogen carcinogenesis in breast cancer. *N Engl J Med*, 2006 354, 270-82.

[8] Beastson, G. On the treatment of inoperable cases of carcinoma of the mamma: suggestions for a new method of treatment. *Lancet*, 1896 2, 104-7.

[9] Smith, IE; Dowsett, M. Aromatase inhibitors in breast cancer. *N Engl J Med* 2003 348, 2431-42.

[10] ATAC Trialists' Group. Results of the ATAC (Arimidex, Tamoxifen, Alone or in Combination) trial after completion of 5 years' adjuvant treatment for breast cancer. *Lancet*, 2005 365(9453), 60-2.

[11] BIG I-98 Collaborative Group. A comparison of letrozole and tamoxifen in postmenopausal women with early breast cancer. *N Engl J Med*, 2005 353, 2747-57.

[12] JCO, 2004, 22(21):4261-4271, Cella D, Fallowfield L, ATAC Trialist's Group. Five-year quality of life (QOL) follow-up of adjuvant endocrine therapy for post-menopausal women in the Arimidex, Tamoxifen, Alone or in Combination Trial. *Proc ASCO*, abstract 577, 2005

[13] Coombes, C; Hall, E; Gibson, L; et al. A randomized trial of exemestane after two to three years of tamoxifen therapy in post-menopausal women with primary breast cancer. *N Engl J Med*, 2004 350, 1081-92.

[14] Goss, PE; Ingle, JN; Martino, S; et al. A randomized trial of letrozole in postmenopausal women after five years of tamoxifen therapy for early-stage breast cancer. *N Engl J Med*, 2003 349, 1793-802.

[15] Winer, EP; Hudis, C; Burstein, HJ. American Society of Clinical Oncology Technology Assessment on the Use of Aromatase Inhibitors As Adjuvant Therapy for Postmenopausal Women With Hormone Receptor–Positive Breast Cancer: Status Report 2004. *J Clin Oncol*, 2005 23(3), 619-629.

[16] JCO, 2004, 22(21):4261-4271, Cella, D; Fallowfield, L, ATAC Trialist's Group. Five-year quality of life (QOL) follow-up of adjuvant endocrine therapy for post-menopausl women in the Arimidex, Tamoxifen, Alone or in Combination Trial. *Proc ASCO*, 2005, abstract 577

[17] Albain KS, Green SJ, Ravdin PM et al. Adjuvant chemohormonal therapy for primary breast cancer should be sequential instead of concurrent: initial results from intergroup trial 0100 (SWOG-8814). *Proc Am Soc Clin Oncol* 2002;21:37a (abstr 143)

[18] Early Breast Cancer Trialists' Collaborative Group. Ovarian ablation in early breast cancer: overview of the randomized trials. *Lancet*, 1996 348, 1189-1196.

[19] Early Breast Cancer Trialists' Collaborative Group. Effects of chemotherapy and hormonal therapy for early breast cancer on recurrence and 15-year survival: overview of the randomized trials. *Lancet*, 2005 365, 1687-1717.

[20] Levine, MN; Pritchard, KI; Bramwell, VH; et al. Randomized trial comparing cyclophosphamide, epirubicin, and fluorouracil with cyclophosphamide, methotrexate, and fluorouracil in premenopasual women with node- positive breast cancer: update of National Cancer Institute of Canada Clinical Trials Group Trial MA5. *J Clin Oncol*, 2005 23, 5166-70.

[21] Fisher, B; Brown, AM; Dimitrov, NV; et al. Two months of doxorubicin-cyclophosphamide with and without interval reinduction therapy compared with 6 months of cyclophosphamide, methotrexate, and fluorouracil in positive-node breast cancer patients with tamoxifen non responsive tumours: results from the National Surgical Adjuvant Breast and Bowel Project B-15. *J Clin Oncol*, 1990 8, 1483-96.

[22] Henderson, IC; Berry, DA; Demetri, GD; et al. Improved outcomes from adding sequential paclitaxel but not from escalating doxorubicin dose in an adjuvant chemotherapy regimen for patients with node-positive primary breast cancer. *J Clin Oncol*, 2003 21, 976-83.

[23] Amounas, EP; Bryant, J; Lembersky, B; et al. Paclitaxel after doxorubicin plus cyclophosphamide as adjuvant chemotherapy for node-positive breast cancer: results from NSABP B-28. *J Clin Oncol*, 2005 23, 3686-96.

[24] Martin, M; Pienkowski, T; Mackey, J; et al. Adjuvant Docetaxel for Node-Positive Breast Cancer, *N Engl J Med*, 2005 Volume 352, 2302-2313.

[25] Citron, MK; Verry, Da; Cirrincione, C; et al. Randomized trial of dose-dense versus conventially scheduled and sequential versus concurrent combination chemotherapy as ostoperative adjuvant treatment of node-positive primary breast cancer: first report of Intergroup Trial C9741/Cancer and Leukemia Group B Trial 9741. *J Clin Oncol*, 2003 21, 1431-1439.

[26] National Comprehensive Cancer Network Clinical Practice Guidelines: Breast Cancer Version 2, 2006.

[27] Adjuvant Therapy for Breast Cancer. NIH Consensus Statement Online. 2000 November 1-3, 2006 Mar 13, 17(4), 1-23.

[28] Goldhirsch, A; Glick, JH; Gelber, RD; et al. Meeting Highlights: International Expert Consensus on the Primary Therapy of Early Breast Cancer 2005. *Annals of Oncology*, 2005 16, 1569–1583.

[29] Slamon, DJ; Godolphin, W; Jones, LA; Holt, JA; Wong, SG; Keith, DE; et al. Studies of the HER-2/neu proto-oncogene in human breast and ovarian cancer. *Science*, 1989 244(4905), 707-12.

[30] Romond, H; Perez, EA; Bryant, J; et al. Trastuzzmab plus adjuvant chemotherapy for operable Her2 positive breast cancer. *N Engl J Med*, 2005 353, 1673-1684.

[31] Piccart-Gebhart, M; Procter, M; Leyland-Jones, B; et al. Trastuzumab after Adjuvant Chemotherapy in HER2-Positive Breast Cancer. *N Engl J Med*, 2005 353, 1659-1672.

[32] Slamon, D; Eiermann, W; Robert, N; et al. Phase III randomized trial comparing doxorubicin and cyclophosphamide followed by docetaxel (AC→T) with doxorubicin and cyclophosphamide followed by docetaxel and trastuzumab (AC→TH) with docetaxel, carboplatin and trastuzumab (TCH) in HER2 positive early breast cancer patients: BCIRG 006 study. *Breast Cancer Research and Treatment*, 2005 94(Suppl 1): abstract 1, S5.

[33] Joensuu, H; Kellokumpu-Lehtinen, PL; Bono, P; et al. Adjuvant Docetaxel or Vinorelbine with or without Trastuzumab for Breast Cancer. *N Engl J Med*, 2006 354, 809-820.

[34] Powles, T; Paterson, S; Kanis, JA; McCloskey, E; Ashley, S; Tidy, A; et.al. Randomized, placebo-controlled trial of clodronate in patients with primary operable breast cancer. *J Clin Oncol*, 2002, 20, 3219-24.

[35] Powles, T; Paterson, A; McCloskey, E; Kurkilahti, M; Kanis, J. Oral clodronate for adjuvant treatment of operable breast cancer: results of a randomized, double-blind, placebo-controlled multicenter trial [abstract]. *Proc Am Soc Clin Oncol*, 2004 23, 9.

[36] Saarto, T; Blomqvist, C; Virkkunen, P; Elomaa, I. Adjuvant clodronate treatment does not reduce the frequency of skeletal metastases in node-positive breast cancer patients: 5-year results of a randomized controlled trial. *J Clin Oncol*, 2001 19, 10-7.

[37] Saarto, T; Vehmanen, L; Blomqvist, C; Elomaa, I. Ten-year follow-up of a randomized controlled trial of adjuvant clodronate treatment in node-positive breast cancer patients [abstract]. *Proc Am Soc Clin Oncol*, 2004 23, 8.

[38] Diel, IJ; Solomayer, E; Gollan, C; Schutz, F; Bastert. Bisphosphonates in the reduction of metastases in breast cancer: results of the extended follow-up of the first study population [abstract]. *Proc Am Soc Clin Oncol*, 2000 19, 82a.

[39] Jaschke, A; Bastert, G; Solomayer, EF; Costa, S; Schuetz, F; Diel, IJ. Adjuvant clodronate treatment improves the overall survival of primary breast cancer patients with micrometastases to bone marrow - a longtime follow-up. *Proc Am Soc Clin Oncol*, 2004 23, 9.

[40] Brusfsy A, Harker W, Beck J, et al, The Z-FAST Study Group. Zoledronic acid (ZA) effectively inhibits cancer treatment-induced bone loss (CTIBL) in postmenopausal women (PMW) with early breast cancer (BCa) receiving adjuvant Letrozole (Let): 12 mos BMD results of the Z-FAST trial. *Journal of Clinical Oncology*, 2005 ASCO Annual Meeting Proceedings. Vol 23, No. 16S, Part I of II (June 1 Supplement), 2005: 533

[41] Rojas, MP; Telaro, E; Russo, A; et al. Follow-up strategies for women treated for early breast cancer. *The Cochrane Database of Systematic Reviews* 2005 Issue 1. Art. No.: CD001768.pub2. DOI:10.1002/14651858.CD001768.pub2.

[42] The Givio Investigators. Impact of follow-up testing on survival and health-related quality of life in breast cancer patients. A multi-center randomized controlled trial. *J Amer Medical Assoc*, 1994 271(20), 1587-92.

[43] Palli, D; Russo, A; Saieva, C; et al. Intensive vs clinical follow-up after treatment of primary breast cancer: 10-year update of a randomized trial. *J Amer Medical Assoc*, 1999 281(17), 1586.

[44] Mouridsen, H; Gershanovich, M; Sun, Y; et al. Phase III study of letrozole versus tamoxifen as first-line therapy of advanced breast cancer in postmenopausal women: analysis of survival and update of efficacy from the International Letrozole Breast Cancer Group. *J Clin Oncol*, 2003 21, 2101-9.

[45] O'Shaughnessy, J; Miles, D; Vukelja, S; et al. Superior survival with capecitabine plus docetaxel combination therapy in anthracycline –pretreated patients with advancer breast cancer: phase III trial results. *J Clin Oncol*, 2002 20, 2812

[46] Fossati, R; Confalonieri, C; Torri, V; et al. Cytotoxic and hormonal treatment for metastatic breast cancer: a systematic review of published randomized trials involving 31,510 women. *J Clin Oncol*, 1998 16, 3439-3460.

[47] Slamon, DJ; Leyland-Jones, V; Shak, S; et al. Use of chemotherapy plus a monoclonal antibody against HER2 for metastatic breast cancer that overexpresses HER2. *N Engl J Med*, 2001 344:783.

[48] Cobleigh, MA; Vogel, CL; Tripathy, D; et al. Multinational study of the efficacy and safety of humanized anti-HER2 monoclonal antibody in women who have HER2-overexpressing metastatic breast cancer that has progressed after chemotherapy for metastatic disease. *J Clin Oncol*, 1999 17, 2639.

[49] Vogel, CL; Cobleigh, MA; Tipathy, D; et al. Efficacy and safety of trastuzumab as a single agent in first-line treatment of HER2-overexpressing metastatic breast cancer. *J Clin Oncol*, 2002 20, 719.

[50] Miller KD, Wang M, Gralow J, et al. E2100: a randomized phase III trial of paclitaxel versus paclitaxel plus bevacizumab as first-line therapy for locally recurrent or metastatic breast cancer. *Proc Am Soc Clin Oncol*. 2005. Late-breaking session. Abstract

[51] Hortobagyi, GN; Theriault, RL; Porter, L; et al. Efficacy of pamidronate in reducing skeletal complications in patients with breast cancer and lytic bone metastases. Protocol 19 Aredia Breast Cancer Study Group. *N Engl J Med*, 1996 335, 1785.

[52] ASCO practice guidelines recommend bisphosphonates for patients with lytic metastases on plain x-rays. EXPAND (Hillner BE, Ingle JN, Chlebowski RT et al. American Society of Clinical Oncology 2003 update on the role of bisphosphonates and bone health issues in women with breast cancer. *J Clin Oncol*, 2003 21, 4042.

[53] Singletary, SE; Allred, C; Ashley, P; et al.: Revision of the American Joint Committee on Cancer staging system for breast cancer. *J Clin Oncol*, 2002 20(17), 3628-36.

[54] Wolmark, N; Wang, J; Mamounas, E; et al. Preoperative chemotherapy in patients with operable breast cancer: nine year results from the National Surgical Adjuvant Breast and Bowel Project B-18. *J Natl Cancer Inst Monogr*, 2001 30, 96-102.

[55] Ellis, MJ; Coop, A; Singh, B; et al. Letrozole is more effective neoadjuvant endocrine therapy than tamoxifen for ErbB-1- and/or ErbB-2-positive, estrogen receptor-positive

primary breast cancer: evidence from a phase III randomized trial. *J Clin Oncol*, 2001 19(18), 3808-16.

[56] Smith, I; Dowsett, M on behalf of the IMPACT Trialists. Comparison of anastrozole vs tamoxifen alone and in combination as neoadjuvant treatment of estrogen receptor-positive (ER+) operable breast cancer in postmenopausal women: The IMPACT trial. *Breast Cancer Res Treat* 2003, 82(Suppl 1):S6. Abstract 1.

[57] Fisher, B; Brown, A; Mamounas, E; et al. Effect or preoperative chemotherapy on local-regional disease in women with operable breast cancer: findings from the National Surgical Adjuvant Breast and Bowel Project B-18. *J Clin Oncol*, 1997 15, 2483.

[58] Bear, HD; Anderson, S; Brown, A; et al. The Effect on Tumor Response of Adding Sequential Preoperative Docetaxel to Preoperative Doxorubicin and Cyclophosphamide: Preliminary Results From National Surgical Adjuvant Breast and Bowel Project Protocol B-27. *J Clin Oncol*, 2003 2, 4165-4174.

[59] Smith, I; Heys, S; Hutcheon, A et al. Neoadjuvant chemotherapy in breast caners: Significantly enhanced response with docetaxel. *J Clin Oncol*, 2002 20, 1456-1466.

[60] Buzdar, AU; Ibrahim, NK; Francis, D; et al. Significantly higher pathologic complete remission rate after neoadjuvant therapy with trastuzumab, paclitaxel, and epirubicin chemotherapy: results of a randomized trial in human epidermal growth factor receptor 2-positive operable breast cancer. *J Clln Oncol*, 2005 23, 3676-3685.

In: Women and Cancer
Editor: Laurie Elit, pp. 75-83
ISBN: 978-1-60021-494-3

Chapter III

RADIATION THERAPY FOR BREAST CANCER

Jonathan Sussman*
Juravinski Cancer Centre, Hamilton, Ontario and Department of Oncology McMaster, University, Hamilton, Canada.

ABSTRACT

Radiation therapy is an important modality of treatment for breast cancers in the early as well as later stages of disease. Ongoing trials will help answer the questions of whether additional radiation to regional nodal areas is of benefit in node positive breast cancers as well as determine whether accelerated partial breast radiation is equivalent to whole breast radiation in early stage (node negative) disease. The use of new imaging and treatment modalities holds the promise of maintaining excellent control rates while further improving convenience and possibly further reducing morbidity.

INTRODUCTION

Radiation therapy is an important modality of treatment for breast cancers in the early as well as later stages of disease. Advances through randomized clinical trials have lead to significant improvements in outcomes both in terms of disease control and morbidity. Recent advances in planning and treatment technologies have the potential to further improve outcomes. In this chapter the role of radiation therapy for breast cancer will be reviewed and the current issues regarding the evolution of radiation therapy will be presented.

* Correspondence concerning this article should be addressed to Dr. J. Sussman Division Radiation Oncology, Juravinski Cancer Centre 699 Concession Street, Hamilton, Ontario, L8V 5C2, Canada. Phone 905 389-9495.

Ductal Carcinoma in Situ

The results of the NSABP B17 randomized trial [1] were pivotal in changing the standard approach to the treament of DCIS from mastectomy to breast conserving therapy (BCT) that involved segmental resection and adjuvant radiation therapy. Currently, this is considered the standard of care for DCIS for the majority of presentations. In the B17 study, women were randomized to segmental resection alone or segmental resection with adjuvant radiation therapy of 5000 cGy in 25 fractions. Survival was equivalent between groups but recurrence rates (that included both DCIS and invasive breast cancer) were significantly reduced with the addition of radiation therapy at 8 years of follow up. (overall recurrence rates 26.8% vs. 12.1% $p<0.000005$). Similar results were achieved in the UKCCR and EORTC trials [2,3]. In a subsequent study, the NSABP B 24, the standard of BCT (segmental resection and adjuvant radiation) to BCT and tamoxifen was evaluated [4]. The study demonstrated a lower breast cancer event rate in the tamoxifen group (8.2% vs 13.4%) but no difference in overall survival. The study did include women with involved and undetermined margin status, who had a much higher recurrence rate than those with negative margins and significantly higher benefit with the addition of tamoxifen. Given the additional morbidity of tamoxifen therapy, the results of this study in the group of women with clear surgical margins remain controversial. The Van Nuys group in California has published on their experience with DCIS and have proposed a risk stratification schema with the implication that very low risk women may not require adjuvant radiation therapy [5]. There was an attempt to study this further in a randomized trial lead by the RTOG that has been recently closed due to poor accrual [6]. The question of whether a very low risk subgroup of patients who are unlikely to benefit from adjuvant radiation currently remains unanswered.

Node Negative Breast Cancer

The benefit of radiation therapy as local adjuvant treatment to support breast conservation therapy (BCT) has been established through a number of randomized trials conducted over the last 20 years [7,8,9,10]. These trials have been further analyzed by the Early Breast Trialists Collaborative group with a series of meta analysesdemonstrating that local control rates of upwards of 90% can be achieved with the addition of adjuvant radiation to segmental resection [11]. Although individual trials have not demonstrated a survival advantage, a recent analysis of long term data suggests that cause specific survival is also improved with the addition of radiation therapy and perhaps more importantly that radiation therapy to the breast after surgery is not associated with late morbidities that can affect survival [12]. A number of studies have evaluated different fractionation schemes to determine the optimal dose and number of treatments. A Canadian study compared a 5 week (5000 cGy in 25 fractions) to a biologically equivalent but accelerated 3 week course (4250 cGy in 16 fractions) and found no differences in recurrence, morbidity or survival supporting an accelerated treatment approach that is more convenient for patients [13]. This treatment regime has been adopted in a number of jurisdictions primarily in Canada and Europe as the current standard of treatment for early stage disease.

It is well established that within the group of early breast cancers, subgroups of lower and higher risk of local recurrence exist. The factors associated with higher risk of recurrence include age, tumour grade and margin status [25]. This observation has lead to the question of whether a subgroup of very low risk patients exists who can be safely treated without adjuvant radiation therapy after segmental resection. This question was addressed in two recently published randomized controlled studies in post menopausal women with small (less than or equal to 2 cm) early stage, node negative breast cancers who were Estrogen and/or Progesterone receptor positive. In the study conducted by the NSABP [14], patients were randomized to: tamoxifen alone, radiation alone or combination tamoxifen and radiation therapy after surgical excision. The recurrence rates were 16.5%, 9.3% and 2.8% respectively. In the study by Fyles et al [15], patients were randomized between tamoxifen alone or with radiation therapy. The recurrence rates in this trial were 7.7% and 0.6% respectively. Subgroup analysis has not demonstrated any risk group that does not benefit from radiation therapy and thus the current recommendations of offering adjuvant whole breast radiation to all women with early stage breast cancer regardless of tumour or patient profile or use of adjuvant systemic therapy are considered standard of care.

Node Positive Breast Cancer

Current clinical questions include whether there is additional benefit of nodal radiation in node positive patients (who do not have advanced disease) which is being examined in 2 randomized trials [16,17]. The results of these studies will not be available for a number of years and the current standard of care should not include nodal irradiation for node positive patients who do not have advanced disease (T1 or T2 disease with 4 or fewer lymph nodes positive). Despite the fact that nodal radiation comes at a cost of increases in morbidity from irradiation of larger volumes of lung as well as the axillary bed, many radiation oncologists advocate for routine nodal irradiation in patients with heavy node positive disease (=> 4 nodes positive) [18]. Recent studies of failure patterns have suggested that relapse rates with level I and II axillary dissection and appropriate systemic therapy are not high and are unlikely to improve with addition of nodal radiation [19]. This will likely remain an area of controversy for some time to come. At the present time, patients who have undergone breast conserving surgery and have had a level I and II nodal dissection and who are not found to have locally advanced disease should receive radiation to the breast alone.

Boost Radiation Therapy to the Tumour Bed

The addition of a "boost" of radiation therapy to give a higher dose to the tumour bed and reduce the risk of local recurrence is considered in a number of situations. Typically, 5 to 8 treatments directed at the tumour bed are given to patients with high risk features for local recurrence such as close or positive margins for which further resection is not to be undertaken and young age [25]. A large randomized study conducted by the EORTC [20] demonstrated a significant reduction in local recurrence rates with addition of boost radiation to standard whole breast radiation therapy in patients with early stage breast cancer and pathologically negative margins (6.8 % vs 4.5%, p<0.0001) Critics of this study have suggested that the recurrence rates in the no boost group where much higher than in other randomized studies of radiotherapy. Most agree though that the subgroup of younger patients clearly had a high rate of recurrence in the standard treatment arm and had a clinically meaningful reduction in local recurrence with the addition of boost radiation therapy. Thus, although a boost will further reduce the risk of local recurrence, this must be balanced against the increased cosmetic morbidity of additional radiation treatment. Currently, there are no widely disseminated guidelines regarding the use of boost and thus significant variation in its use exists.

Post Mastectomy Radiation Therapy

The benefits of radiation therapy after mastectomy have been defined through a series of clinical trials and a recent meta analyses demonstrating benefits in terms of locoregional control and survival for women who have either advanced local disease (T3 or T4 or advanced nodal disease i.e > 4 nodes positive in the axilla) or incomplete resection due to positive margins despite mastectomy [21]. The intention is to treat subclinical or residual disease in the chest wall and regional nodal basins. In this population, the estimated risk of local regional recurrences without radiation is approximately 30-40 %, which is reduced to 10-15% with radiation. Failure pattern studies in patients who did not receive up front radiation treatment have shown that 1/3 of recurrences are in the nodal regions (with or without chest wall recurrence) with 2/3 being isolated chest wall recurrences [22,23]. Standard loco regional radiation therapy is delivered to the chest wall and regional lymph nodes over a 5-week course. The most recent meta analysis of post mastectomy radiation therapy by Whelan et al. has identified that there is likely a small survival benefit conferred with the addition of loco regional to radiation therapy to systemic therapy after mastectomy in women with high risk disease (T3 or T4 with 4 or more axillary nodes involved) although some argue that these studies were conducted with less effective chemotherapy agents and that these results must be balanced against the toxicities of radiation therapy, especially to the axilla and supraclavicular regions. One ongoing area of controversy is the need to irradiate the internal mammary lymph nodes as this is known to be increase normal tissue irradiation (lung and on the left side, the heart) and possibly increase the risk of late toxicities [24].

Pallative Radiation Therapy

Radiation is an effective modality of treatment in the palliative setting with the intention of treatment being the minimization of symptoms related to metastatic sites and improvements in quality of life. Bone metastases respond well to short courses (between 1 and 10 treatments) of radiation therapy with response rates of pain reduction as well as reduction in use of analgesic medications of 50-80%.[32] In general, palliative radiotherapy is well tolerated with minimal side effects and long term follow studies have reported that the rate of pathological fractures attributable to radiation treatment itself is low. The use of radiation therapy to prophylactically treat a site of bone metastases that is considered at risk for pathological fracture is controversial with no prospective data to demonstrate that this is an expected benefit of therapy although when associated with spinal cord compression, palliative radiation therapy is often used either alone or in conjuction with surgical decompression as early as possible to help maintain ambulation and prevent neurological deterioration. In the setting of brain metastases, radiation therapy to the whole brain[33] can be effective in palliation of symptoms and stabilization of neurological function although prognosis is generally poor with survival measured in months. Recently, studies have demonstrated that in the subgroup of patients with few metastases (between 1 and 3) and controlled visceral disease, more aggressive approaches with surgery or higher doses of radiation targeted to the metastases may improve neurological outcomes [34] .

Contraindications to Radiation Therapy

There are few absolute contra indications to radiation therapy for breast cancer. Those factors that are generally felt to be contraindiations include:

1. Women with two or more primary tumours in separate quadrants of the breast or with diffuse malignant appearing microcalcifications (not candidates for BCT)
2. A history of previous irradiation to the breast region
3. Pregnancy as there is a risk to the fetus from scattered radiation.

Relative contraindications include the following:

1. A history of active lupus erythematosus or scleroderma as there is published data suggesting poor tolerance of radiation, especially in the latter disorder
2. A probable poor cosmetic resulting from BCT due to tumour or patient factors (ie a large tumour in a small breast) is relative contra indication as in these situations women should be offered the choice of mastectomy with reconstruction.

These issues need to be considered at the time of surgery and if there is concern, consultation between the surgeon and radiation oncologist is needed to ensure appropriate multidisciplinary planning.

Side Effects of Radiation Therapy

Side effects associated with radiation therapy include those that occur acutely (during and for the few weeks after treatment), in an intermediate period (4 to 12 weeks after treatment) and those that occur late, generally accepted to be 6 months or more after treatment. As a local therapy, radiation does not have systemic side effects (i.e. effects outside of the area treated) although a number of women report fatigue during therapy. The cause for this is not known. This fatigue is self limited, generally resolving within 4-8 weeks of completion of therapy.

Other acute effects are generally inflammatory which manifest as erythema and swelling in the breast and chest wall tissues with occasional associated pain. There may be desquamation of the skin especially in areas of folds and around the nipple areolar complex. Treatment is conservative and includes skin care (avoidance of abrasive clothing), gentle washing and use of water based moisturizing agents. Significant moist desquamation of the skin is rare with modern techniques but in the few cases where it occurs, aggressive skin care management is required.

Clinically significant intermediate side effects are rare and include radiation pneumonitis and very rarely pericarditis when treating the left side due to exposure of thelung and heart respectivelyto radiation treatment. These side effects are dose and volume sensitive (ie the amount of organ exposed and dosage received) and should only be suspected if clinical and radiological manifestation correspond with areas within the treatment fields. Use of modern planning techniques including advanced imaging with CT result in shielding of these areas and subsequently, much lower risks (<5%) than reported in historical cohorts.

The most common late effects of radiation to the breast and chest wall include the risks of soft tissue fibrotic change that can manifest as cosmetic change in the breast (telangiectasias of the skin and generalized firmness of the breast tissue). Long term follow up studies have demonstrated that these effects are clinically significant in fewer than 15% of women in the years after treatment.A few long term follow up cohort studieshave reported increased rib fragility on the treated side, clinically significant fibrosis of the small volumes of lung exposed to radiation on the treated side, radiation induced heart disease in patient treated on the left hand side and very rarely, secondary malignancies. These rare late effects are likely manifestations of older techniques which are no longer used and it is felt that they are now very unlikely to occur with modern treatment [25]. Modern radiation treatment ofthe regional lymph nodes is associated with small increased risk of pneumonitis, lymphedema and brachial plexopathy.

Future Directions

The dogma of adjuvant breast radiation treatment in early stage disease has been founded on the belief that the whole breast was at risk of recurrence following BCS. This was consistent with the rationale behind the use of mastectomy. Pathologic data of mastectomy specimens suggested that for large tumours microscopic disease was likely to extend within the breast 2-4 cm beyond the primary tumour site [29]. Thus radiation is normally delivered to the whole breast following BCS. However, subsequent trials evaluating the role of breast irradiation following BCS suggest that if local recurrences recur, they are most likely (70-80% of cases) to occur at the site of the primary tumour with or without radiation therapy. The risk of recurrence in the breast away from the primary tumour site is only 1.5-3.5%, and is consistent with the rate of developing a contralateral breast cancer. These data support that the primary role of whole breast irradiation is to reduce the risk of recurrence at the primary tumour site. Recent pathological studies also suggest that with smaller or mammographically-screened cancers, the risk of microscopic extension of tumour within the surrounding breast is rare [30]. The importance of these observations is that radiation therapy may be limited to the primary tumour site (called partial breast irradiation) rather than the whole breast resulting potentially in less morbidity and shorter overall treatments [27]. Radiation morbidity is directly related to the volume of tissue irradiated and radiation therapy dose per fraction [31]. By limiting the volume treated, larger doses of radiation can be delivered in even shorter periods of time (up to one week) with the expectation that there will be limited morbidity [28]. Currently, there are 2 phase 3 clinical trials underway in North America to evaluate acclerated partial breast radiation therapy for early stage disease. If these studies find that outcomes are equivalent to whole breast radiation therapy with similar or improved morbidities, these regimens will become the new standard of care.

Conclusion

Over the past 30 years, clinical trials with long term follow up have demonstrated the important role that radiation therapy plays as part of breast conservation. Ongoing trials will help answer the questions of whether additional radiation to regional nodal areas is of benefit in node positive breast cancers as well as determine whether acclerated partial breast radiation is equivalent to whole breast radiation in early stage (node negative) disease. In locally advanced disease, the addition of radiation contributes to local control and survival. The use of new imaging and treatment modalities holds the promise of maintaining excellent control rates while further improving convenience and possibly further reducing morbidity.

References

[1] Fisher B, Dignam J, Wolmark N, Mamounas E, Costantino J, Poller W, Fisher ER, Wickerham DL, Deutsch M, Margolese R, Dimitrov N, Kavanah M.Lumpectomy and radiation therapy for the treatment of intraductal breast cancer: findings from National Surgical Adjuvant Breast and Bowel Project B-17. *J Clin Oncol.* 1998 Feb;16(2):441-52.

[2] Houghton J, George WD, Cuzik J, Duggan C, Fentiman IS, Spittle M. Radiotherapy and tamoxifen in women with completely excised ductal carcinoma in situ of the breast in the UK, Australia, and New Zealand: randomised controlled trial. *Lancet.* 2003 Jul 12;362(9378):95-102

[3] Bijker N, Peterse JL, Duchateau L, Julien JP, Fentiman IS, Duval C, Di Palma S, Simony-Lafontaine J et al. Risk factors for recurrence and metastasis after breast-conserving therapy for ductal carcinoma-in-situ: analysis of European Organization for Research and Treatment of Cancer Trial 10853. *J Clin Oncol.* 2001 Apr 15;19(8):2263-71

[4] Fisher B, Dignam J, Wolmark N, Wickerham DL, Fisher EL, Mamounas E, Smith R, Begovic M, Dimitrov NV, Margolese RG, Kardinal CG, Kavanah MT et al. Tamoxifen in treatment of intraductal breast cancer: National Surgical Adjuvant Breast and Bowel Project B-24 randomised controlled trial. *Lancet.* 1999 Jun 12;353(9169):1993-2000.

[5] Silverstein MJ, Lagois MD, Craig PH, Waisman JR, Lewinsky BS et al. A prognostic index for ductal carcinoma in situ of the breast. *Cancer.* 1996 Jun 1;77(11):2267-74.

[6] http://www.rtog.org/qa/98-04/9804broadcast.html

[7] Fisher B, Anderson S, Redmond R, et al. Re-analysis and results after 12 years of follow-up in a randomized clinical trial comparing total mastectomy with lumpectomy

with or without irradiation in the treatment of breast cancer. *N Engl J Med* 1995;333:1456-61.

[8] Clark RM, Whelan T, Levine M, et al. Randomized clinical trial of breast irradiation following lumpectomy and axillary dissection for node-negative breast cancer. An update. *J Natl Cancer Inst* 1996;88:1659-64.

[9] Liljegren G, Holmberg , L. Bergh, J. Lindgren, A. Tabar, L. Nordgen, H Adami, H.O. and the Uppsala-Orebro Breast Cancer Study Group. 10-Year results after sector resection with or without postoperative radiotherapy for stage 1 breast cancer: A randomized trial. *J Clin Oncol* 1999; 17: 2326-33.

[10] Veronesi U, Luini A, Del Vecchio M, et al. Radiotherapy after breast-conserving surgery in women with localized cancer of the breast. *N Engl J Med* 1993;328:1633-34.

[11] Early Breast Cancer Trialists' Collaborative Group. Favourable and unfavourable effects on long-term survival of radiotherapy for earlybreast cancer: an overview of the randomized trials. *Lancet* 2000;355:1757-69

[12] Van de Steen J, Soete G, Storm G. Adjuvant radiotherapy for breast cancer significantly improves overall survival: the missing link. *Radiother Oncol.* 2000 Jun;55(3):263-72.

[13] Whelan T, Mackenzie R, Julian J, et al. Randomized trial of breast irradiation schedules after lumpectomy with lymph node-negative breast cancer. *J Natl Cancer Inst* 94:1143-50, 2002

[14] Fisher B, Bryant J, Dignam JJ, Wickerham Dl et al. Tamoxifen, radiation therapy, or both for prevention of ipsilateral breast tumor recurrence after lumpectomy in women with invasive breast cancers of one centimeter or less. *J Clin Oncol.* 2002 Oct 15;20(20):4141-9

[15] Fyles AW, McCready DR, Manchul LA, Trudeau ME, Merante P, Pintilie M, Weir LM, Olivotto IATamoxifen with or without breast irradiation in women 50 years of age or older with early breast cancer. *N Engl J Med.* 2004 Sep 2;351(10):963-70.

[16] Olivotto IA, Chua B, Elliot EA, Parda DS, Pierce LJ, Shepherd L, Vallow LA, White JR, Whelan TJA clinical trial of breast radiation therapy versus breast plus regional radiation therapy in early-stage breast cancer: the MA20 trial. *Clin Breast Cancer.* 2003 Dec;4(5):361-3

[17] http://www.eortc.be/protoc/details.asp?protocol=22922

[18] Fowble B. Radiotherapeutic considerations in the treatment of primary breast cancer. *J Natl Cancer Inst Monogr.* 1992;(11):49-58.

[19] Fortin A, Dagnault A, Blondeau L, Vu TT, Larochelle M. The impact of the number of excised axillary nodes and of the percentage of involved nodes on regional nodal failure in patients treated by breast-conserving surgery with or without regional irradiation. *Int J Radiat Oncol Biol Phys.* 2006 May 1;65(1):33-9

[20] Bartelink H, Horiot JC, Poortmans P, Struikmans H, Van den Bogaert W, Barillot I, Fourquet A, Borger J, Jager J, Hoogenraad W, Collette L, Pierart M.Recurrence rates after treatment of breast cancer with standard radiotherapy with or without additional radiation. *N Engl J Med.* 2001 Nov 8;345(19):1378-87.

[21] Whelan TJ, Julian J, Wright J, Jadad AR, Levine ML.Does locoregional radiation therapy improve survival in breast cancer? A meta-analysis. *J Clin Oncol.* 2000 Mar;18(6):1220-9.

[22] Shenkier T, Weir L, Levine M, Olivotto I, Whelan T, Reyno L. Clinical practice guidelines for the care and treatment of breast cancer: 15. Treatment for women with stage III or locally advanced breast cancer. *CMAJ.* 2004 Mar 16;170(6):983-94

[23] Recht A, Edge SB Evidence-based indications for postmastectomy irradiation. *Surg Clin North Am.* 2003 Aug;83(4):995-1013

[24] Whelan T. Treatment of the internal mammary nodes in early breast cancer: back to the future. *Clin Oncol (R Coll Radiol).* 2003 Feb;15(1):14-6

[25] *Diseases of The Breast*: Harris J, Lippman M, Morrow M, Osborne K eds. Lippincott Williams and Wilkins, Philadelphia. 2000.

[26] Fowler JF. The linear-quadratic formula and progress in fractionated radiotherapy. *Br J Radiol 62*:679-694, 1989

[27] Vicini FA, Baglan KL, Kestin LL, Mitchell C, Chen PY, et al. Accelerated treatment of breast cancer. *J Clin Oncol.* 2001;19(7):1993-2001

[28] Arthur D, ViciniF, Kuske RR et al. Accelerated Partial Breast Irradiation: An updated report from the American Brachytherapy Society. *Brachytherapy* 2002;1(4): 184-190

[29] Holland R, Veling SH, Mravunac M, Hendricks JH. Histologic Multifocality of Tis, T1-2 breast carcinoma. Implications for clinical trials of breast conserving surgery. *Cancer* 1985;56(5):979-990.

[30] Imamura H, Haga S, Shimizu T et al. Relationship between the morphological and biological characteristics of intraductal components accompanying invasive ductal breast carcinoma and patient age. *Breast Cancer Res Treat* 2000;62:177-184.

[31] Lymon JT. Complication probability as assessed from the dose-volume histograms. *Radiat Res Suppl.* 1985;8(S1)3-9

[32] Wu JS, Wong R, Johnson M et al. Meta-analysis of dose-fractionation radiotherapy trials for palliation of painful bone metastases. *Int J Radiat Oncol Phys.* 2003 Mar 1;55(3):594-605

[33] Khuntia D, Brown P, Li J, Mehta MP. Whole brain radiotherapy in the management of brain metastases. *J Clin Oncol.* 2006 Mar. 10;24(8):295-304.

[34] Mehta MP, Tsao MN, Whelan TJ et al. The American Society for Therapeutic Radiology and Oncology (ASTRO) evidence-based review of the role of radiosurgery for brain metastases. *Int J Radiat Oncol Biol Phys.* 2005 Sep 1;63 (1): 37-46.

In: Women and Cancer
Editor: Laurie Elit, pp. 85-106
ISBN: 978-1-60021-494-3

Chapter IV

Breast Reconstructive Surgery: A Female Surgeon's Perspective

*Arianna Dal Cin**
McMaster University, Hamilton Health Sciences and Juravinski Cancer Centre Hamilton, Ontario, Canada.

Abstract

Breast reconstruction after breast cancer surgery is gaining popularity. The reported frequency has increased 3.5 fold to 35 percent from 8 to 10 percent a few years ago. This is anticipated to increase further with patient education and earlier detection.

Herein is provided a surgical algorithm for the approach to breast reconstruction that incorporates patient factors and surgical options. Patient factors include stage of disease, comorbidities and body habitus. Surgical options include consideration of timing of reconstruction, use of prosthesis versus autologous tissue and reconstruction of the nipple-areolar complex.

Finally a woman's perspective towards breast reconstruction is discussed

Introduction

Breast reconstruction is the creation of a soft supple breast mound with an overlying visually realistic nipple areolar complex following mastectomy. The goal is to provide symmetry to the anterior chest wall such that the patient is less reminded on a daily basis of her breast cancer diagnosis. It is to facilitate the patient's daily dressing. Often patients find the external prosthesis heavy, hot and cumbersome, frequently reporting that the external prosthesis falls out of any garments they wear during sports activities such as swimming.

* Correspondence concerning this article should be addressed to Arianna Dal Cin MD, 504-304 Victoria Ave North Hamilton, Ontario, Canada L8L 5G4. Phone: 905 526-0811; Fax: 905 526-0890.

Another goal of reconstruction is to enhance the patient's mood and decrease her anxiety, not only with her diagnosis of breast cancer but to enhance her activities of daily living, thereby enhancing her overall body image including sexuality.

The breast mound is to be created with minimal donor site morbidity and scarring in a timely fashion that expedites the patient's overall time to recovery with minimal to no interference with adjuvant treatment be it with chemotherapy or radiation therapy. Meeting all of these requirements is a challenge for the oncological surgeon and the plastic surgeon. Frequent, open dialogue between surgeons, as well as with the patient and various members of the healthcare team needs to be performed regularly in order to expedite the patient's recovery with restoration to health in a timely fashion. These goals are enormous.

Herein will be provided a discussion and layout of reconstructive options and an algorithm that must be individualized to each patient in order to achieve success and satisfaction from both the patient and surgeon's perspective.

Rates of Breast Reconstruction

The approach to breast resection and reconstruction for invasive breast carcincoma has undergone a revolution in the past twenty-five years. Mastectomy rates declined by approximately 60% between 1981 and 2000 in Canada to an average national mastectomy rate of 37.9/100,000 [1]. Following the publication in particular of the NSABP B-06 clinical trial, there has been a surge in the number of lumpectomies over mastectomies which remains consistent [1,2]. Lumpectomies now outnumber mastectomies by a 5:1 ratio [2]. The rate of prophylactic mastectomy has risen as we have come to understand the genetics of breast cancer with the discovery of the BRCA 1 and 2 genes. Prophylactic mastectomy is offered as an alternative to preventive chemotherapy and surveillance. In a prospective observational study, approximately 27% [8] of the BRCA 1 or 2 carriers underwent prophylactic mastectomy during the one year follow-up period [6]. Thus, reconstruction is now considered after a variety of surgical approaches to breast cancer.

Reconstruction rates after mastectomy range from 8 to 10% in the Province of Ontario in Canada in 2005 [7]. Some American studies have shown reconstruction rates up to 30% [4] with a variability in practice ascribed to the patient's age, race, status of disease and geographic location [4].

Morrow et al [3] identified women younger than 79 years of age who were diagnosed with breast cancer between 2001 and January 2003 from the Surveillance Epidemiology and End Results (SEER) Registries of Detroit and Los Angeles. Of the approximate 2000 respondents, 35% of women had undergone mastectomy and 38% of these patients underwent breast reconstruction. Younger patient age, higher education level and earlier stage of disease were significant factors associated with breast reconstruction. Approximately 78% of the women reported that they had received information about reconstruction but only 11% correctly answered basic knowledge questions regarding the procedure, indicating that patients are receiving information about breast reconstruction but the information may be overwhelming, too enormous to absorb or as indicated by the patients not desiring of more surgery. Thus, the majority of women were aware of breast reconstruction but chose not to undergo the procedure. The most common reason for *not* undergoing reconstruction was the desire to avoid more surgery.

The frequency of reconstruction after lumpectomy or breast conserving surgery (BCS) is unknown. Patients undergoing BCS generally receive adjuvant therapy with radiation creating specific aesthetic problems due to breast and chest wall fibrosis and altered wound healing. Another factor is the volume of the lumpectomy which can produce significant distortion of the breast contour sufficient to warrant reconstruction. Veronesi in his original work described quadrantectomy of the breast which over the years has now evolved to a variable resection of breast volume. Bajaj et al [9] showed that all patients have some asymmetry after breast conserving surgery with significant asymmetry noted in 35%. However, it is interesting to note that 86% were satisfied with their aesthetic outcome and did not wish for further surgery.

An area of controversy in breast cancer surgery is the optimal approach to breast resection to produce the most esthetically pleasing result after reconstruction without compromising tumour control. Cocquyt [10] found that cosmetic results are superior after reconstruction for skin sparing mastectomy rather than breast cancer treatment. However, Gendy [11] found that BCS followed by mini-flap reconstruction was associated with fewer adverse effects than skin sparing mastectomy and myocutaneous flap reconstruction, without significant difference in cosmetic outcome. Thus some authors advocate skin sparing mastectomy [10], that is removal of all breast tissue, while others support lumpectomy or the removal of the least amount of tissue [11] and reconstruction. Caution is needed in interpreting these studies because they are usually retrospective case series, from an individual surgeon's practice and are subject to bias based on the preferences of the surgeon and issues of reimbursement. This is an important area requiring prospective, unbiased studies.

Timing of Reconstruction

Breast reconstruction may be immediate, early or late. Immediate reconstruction is defined as development or maintenance of the breast mound at the time of mastectomy [12]. A variant described by Kronowitz [5] is termed delayed immediate reconstruction in which the breast mound is supported at the time of mastectomy with a tissue expander with definitive breast reconstruction being completed once the final pathology report has indicated that adjuvant radiation therapy is *not* required. This usually occurs within two weeks from time of mastectomy. Early delayed reconstruction [4] occurs within three to four months of mastectomy and late delayed reconstruction usually occurs more than three months post-mastectomy.

Timing of breast reconstruction is predicated on a number of factors, including the stage of disease, the need for adjuvant chemo or radiation therapy and the risk of recurrence as well as patient preference. It is generally accepted that patients desiring prophylactic mastectomy or having early stage breast cancer, that is, in situ disease, stage 1 or stage 2A disease, are candidates for immediate reconstruction. A major concern with immediate reconstruction has been the risk of masking tumour recurrence. However, a number of studies have demonstrated that the risk of local recurrence is low [18,19] and long-term outcomes are no different between patients with or without reconstruction.

A second concern is the patient acceptance of the aesthetic outcome. The patient who has had a period of time without a breast mound is more likely to accept the newly created breast mound. A number of retrospective studies have noted that women who underwent immediate reconstruction compared with those who underwent delayed reconstruction reported lower post-operative psychological disturbance and improvement in self-image [56,58,59]. However, prospective studies have *not* been as universal in supporting the relative benefits of immediate reconstruction at the time of mastectomy. Dean noted [60] significant psychological benefits for immediate reconstruction at three months, but at one year no difference in psychological status or sexual functioning was observed between the groups. Harcourt [61] compared three groups of women; those who received mastectomy alone, mastectomy and immediate breast reconstruction or mastectomy with delayed reconstruction and observed that all three groups showed significant improvement in quality of life and psychological functioning within the first year after surgery equivalently [61]. Rowland [59] found a positive association between time of mastectomy and reconstruction and higher patient satisfaction with the surgical outcome. There is evidence that women, who seek immediate reconstruction compared with those who delay, are more distressed about the effects of mastectomy on their feelings of femininity and sexuality [44]. Prospective studies are supporting the old notion that delayed reconstruction may better identify women with pre-existing anxiety or depression and concerns with femininity and sexuality. These concerns decrease within the first year of following breast cancer treatment, particularly mastectomy [44]. From a psychological perspective it would seem that delayed reconstruction should be favoured.

Retrospective studies even today [6] reveal 92% of woman who carry the BRAC 1 or 2 gene and who desire prophylactic mastectomy, also desire immediate breast reconstruction. The major rate limiting factor from a surgeon's perspective was that of possibly masking tumour occurrence [18,19] while also allowing the patient time to adjust to her new body image without a breast [44].

In 1991, the skin sparing mastectomy was introduced by Toth and Lappert [13]. This change in mastectomy style allowed for softening and a more natural appearance to the reconstructed breast via preservation of the skin envelope and infra-mammary fold. Subsequent studies by Singletary at the MD Anderson Cancer Centre in 1996 [14] and Slavin and Goldwyn et al in 1993 and 1998 [15,17,19] demonstrated that the skin sparing mastectomy with immediate breast reconstruction studied retrospectively was safe and did not yield a local recurrence risk or metastatic disease risk different from the risk established and known by the modified radical mastectomy and delayed reconstruction group in early breast cancer. The fear of masking local recurrence in the setting of skin sparing mastectomy in immediate reconstruction has been dispelled in early breast cancer. However, it does not necessarily abate the fear of the individual cancer patient or surgeon. It is known that in patients with locally advanced disease (stage 2B or greater), that local recurrence in advanced breast disease usually manifests itself within two to two and a half years [19]. It is recommended by Langenstein et al [18] that breast reconstruction, for this patient group is delayed until this time period has elapsed and the patient remains disease-free.

Local recurrences after immediate breast reconstruction have been examined by at least six authors between 1997 and 2003. Mustonen [19] in 2005 reviewed these studies as well as their own data in 79 patients between 1998 and 2001. They examined the incidence and reason for local recurrence after immediate breast reconstruction in breast cancer patients. All recurrences appeared within the first two years after the initial therapy. The predominant risk factors were the patient's young age (41 years of age or younger) and increasing tumour size (21.6% recurrence in T2 or larger tumours) [19]. Therefore a patient 41 years or less with stage 2 tumour or higher breast carcinoma should wait two years for breast reconstruction.

Some studies [19,20,21,22,25] are suggesting patients with advanced disease can undergo immediate breast reconstruction, if one considers that the outcome depends on disease status, which is already predetermined at the time of diagnosis. Concern is legitimate that autologous reconstruction in particular can impede surveillance for local recurrence although studies such as that by Langenstein in 2003 [18] have shown that most local recurrences occur within the skin and subcutaneous fat of the chest wall skin. His study noted that 57% of the patients who developed skin and soft tissue recurrence, developed metastases within five years, whereas 91% of the patients who developed skeletal or muscle recurrences went on to metastases within five years. Perhaps an increase in the reconstruction rate for advanced breast disease will occur with the development of more sensitive tools for surveillance such as the wider availability of MRI [24] and with the PET/CT scanner combination which has the ability to detect microdisease in asymptomatic patients [23].

The American Society of Clinical Oncology recommends that reconstruction be delayed in patients expected to undergo radiation treatment post breast cancer resection [26,73]. Radiation therapy can adversely increase the complication rates in reconstructive patients with either autologous tissue and/or prostheses. With respect to the autologous reconstruction, there are significant increases reported in dehiscence, infection and fat necrosis (up to 40%) resulting in flap contractures (75%) [27] which can be difficult to correct even with additional flaps needed in up to 30% of patients [27,28,29].

Radiation of the chest wall in patients reconstructed with implants results in severe capsular contracture in over 50% of patients [26]. Capsular contractures can result in chest wall pain, implant rupture, implant exposure or superior migration of the implant often needing further surgical treatment. Isolated articles exist reporting good to excellent aesthetic outcomes with the use of autologous tissue in breast reconstruction prior to radiation therapy but the number of women studied retrospectively are small in number [30,31].

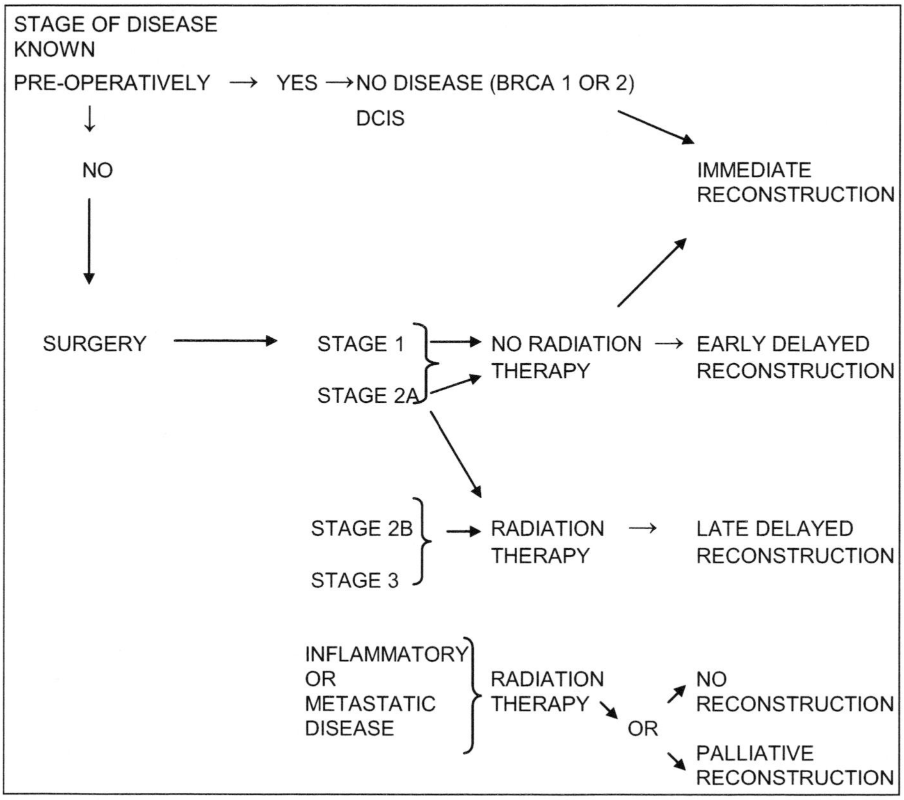

Figure 1. Algorithm to determine the timing of breast reconstruction.

Modalities of Breast Reconstruction

In 1906, Tanzini described an autoplastic flap from the back in its modified version of the latissimus dorsi myocutaneous flap for reconstruction of the anterior chest wall. This was further refined by Campbell in 1950 and with the advent of silicone gel prostheses as described in 1963 by Cronin and Gerow [75], two mainstream choices for reconstruction emerged and have continued to exist.

Autologous Tissue Reconstruction

The preferred modality of breast reconstruction by plastic surgeons and patients alike is that of reconstruction with autologous tissue, commonly transverse rectus abdominus myocutaneous (TRAM) flap, deep inferior epigastric perforator (DIEP) flap, latissimus dorsi (LD) myocutaneous flap. Though this modality of reconstruction requires specialized microsurgical expertise, is of greater complexity and is associated with increased operative time, as well as potentially increased post-operative recovery time, it has overall sustained patient and surgeon satisfaction in the immediate and long-term post-operative periods.

Table 1. Indications and Contraindications to Autologous Flap Reconstruction

INDICATIONS	CONTRAINDICATIONS
Modified Radical Mastectomy with - tight thin chest wall - failed previous reconstruction - irradiation of chest wall - large ptotic opposite breast - Congenital chest wall deformities - Failure of alternate methods of reconstruction	- moderate to severe respiratory disease - severe cardiovascular disease - uncontrolled hypertension - morbid obesity - IDDM - Abdominal scars associated with disruption of perforating vessel - Autoimmune disease affecting small vessels (ie.connective tissue disease eg. scleroderma) - severe social problems - adverse patient attitude, - i.e., unwilling, unable to invest time required for healing

Hartrampf [33] pp 33-35.

Indications for autologous soft tissue chest wall reconstruction were initially well-outlined by Hartrampf. See Table 1 [33]. Provided these co-morbidities are not present including significant transverse abdominal scars and back scars, reconstruction even in the radiated patient using this modality can be performed successfully. Table 2 A and B outline the choices of flaps available for reconstruction for the post-mastectomy or post-lumpectomy patient.

Local flaps may also be utilized for reconstruction, the most commonly described flaps are the thoraco-epigastric or lateral thoracic transposition flaps [67].

Flaps have been successfully performed in settings of abdominal scarring with lower and midline quadrant scars [37]. The abdominal scar from the Pfannenstiel incision has been proven microscopically and clinically to have no deleterious effects on successful reconstruction with a TRAM flap. Patients who have undergone an open abdominal hysterectomy should be judged on a case-by-case basis by the reconstructing surgeon. The scar from an open cholecystectomy places technical limits on the placement of the TRAM flap, but a laparoscopic cholecystectomy rarely has an impact on reconstruction. Similarly, laparoscopic hysterectomy is unlikely to interfere with the use of the TRAM flap. The TRAM flap should be avoided in the young pre-menopausal patient who may be entertaining future pregnancies following completion of treatment and a period of disease-free survival.

Table 2A. Common Flap Choices

Flap	**Author**	**Picture**	**Blood supply**	**Flap Specific Qualities/ Complications**
TRAM Transverse Rectus Abdominus muscle flap	Hartrampf Scheflan Black (1982)		deep inferior epigastric artery	10% abdominal incidence bulge/hernia
Types Unipedicled Bipedicled Supercharged Free		 1 2 3	 superior epigastric artery deep inferior epigastric artery	 36% vascular complications 5% vascular complications (venous occlusion most commonly) (30)
Deep Inferior Epigastric Perforator flap (variant of TRAM) DIEP Flap	Blondeel (1994)		deep inferior epigastric artery peforator derivative	0.7-5% incidence abdominal bulge
Latissimus Dorsi (LD)	Schneider Muhlbauer (1977)	4	thoracodorsal artery	- seroma and scar on back - need implant also for projection and volume usually - potential shoulder dysfunction

References: [38,63].

Table 2B. Less Common Flap Choices

Flap	Author	Picture	Blood supply	Flap Specific Qualities/ Complications
Gluteal Flap SGAP Flap	Fujino (1975) Koshima (1989)	5	Superior or Inferior Gluteal arteries Superior Gluteal Artery Perforator	- skin paddle width limited (13W x 10-30cm L) - short pedicle - Longer pedicle - Technically demanding
Superficial Inferior Epigastric or Superficial Circumflex Iliac Artery (SIEAA, SCIA) Flap	Taylor & Daniel (1975) 1st used Grotting (1991)	 6	superficial inferior epigastric artery	not present in 51% of patients - inconsistent vascular anatomy - short pedicle - small diameter
Lateral Thigh Flap		7	lateral femoral circumflex vessels	- need sufficient upper lateral thigh fullness - 6-8 cm pedicle
Reuben's Flap			deep circumflex Iliac arteries	- abdominal, groin hernia - inconsistent vessel anatomy
Local Flaps Thoraco-Epigastric Lateral-Thoracodorsal	 TD Cronin (1990) Holmstrom & Lossing (1986)	 8		 - transposition flap (mini flaps)

**The recipient vessels used are those of the thoracodorsal arcade in the axilla or the internal mammary vasculature, in the medial chest. Either artery is unusable in 20 – 26% of cases [26,38,64].

References: [38,39,67]

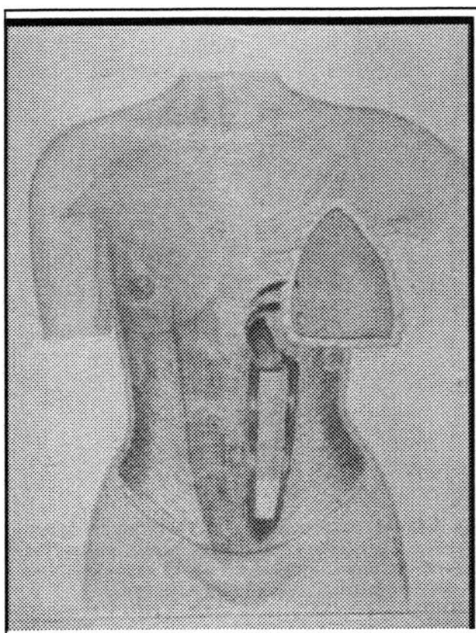

Picture 1

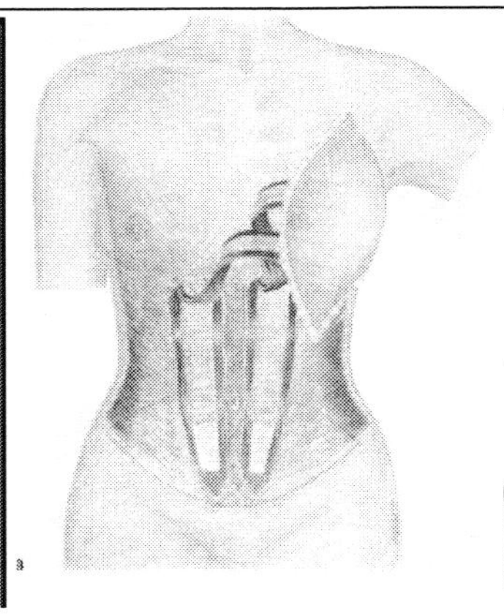

Picture 2

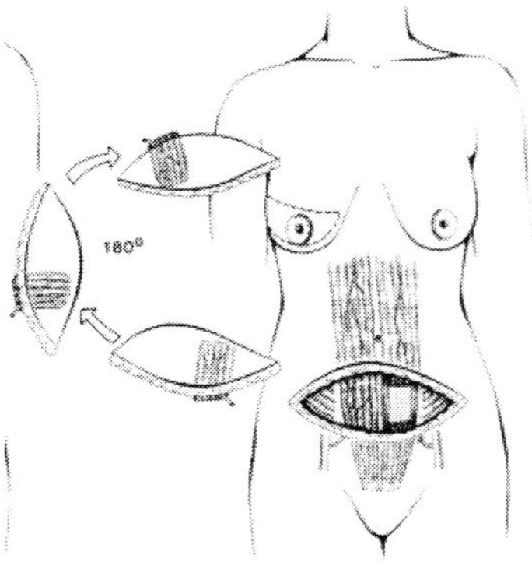

Picture 3

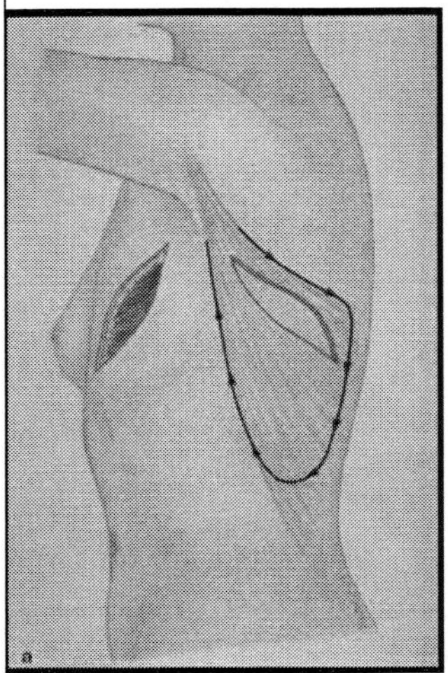

Picture 4

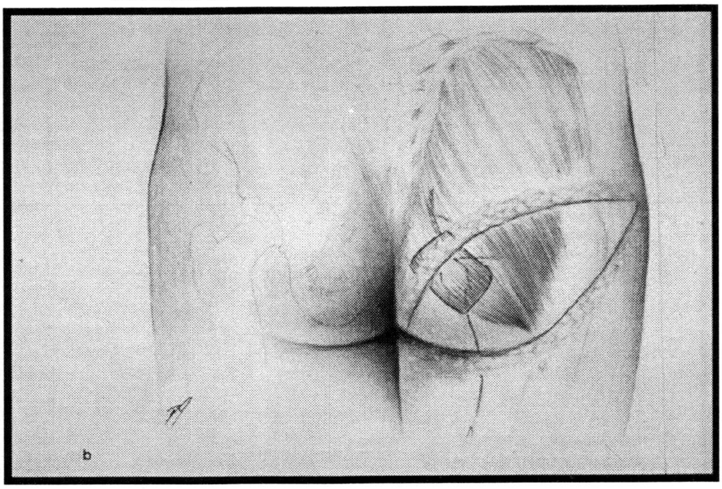

Picture 5

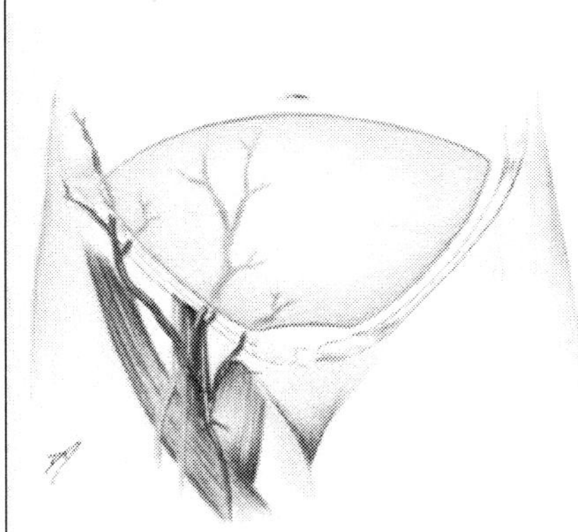

Picture 6

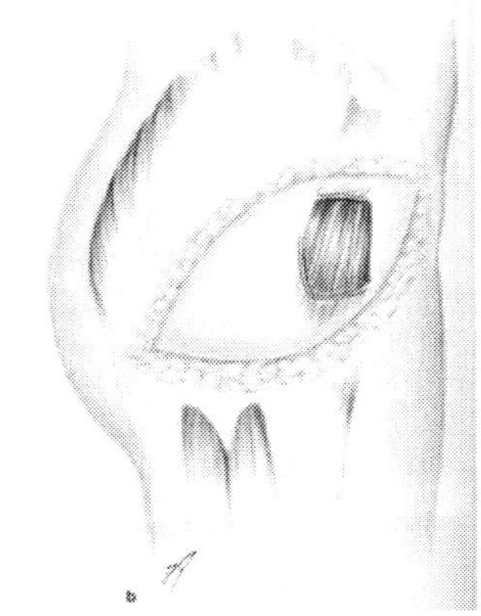

Picture 7

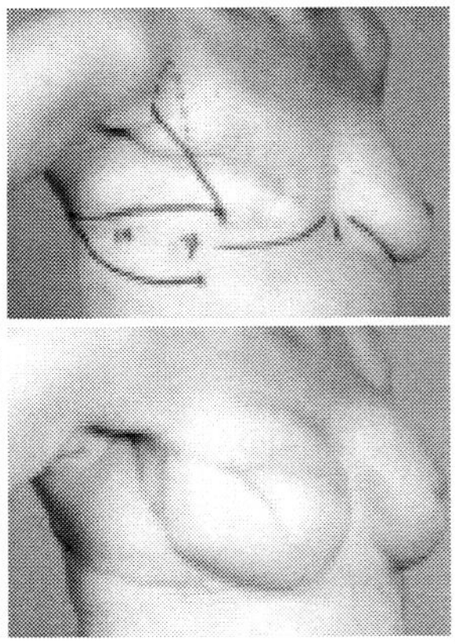

Picture 8

Pictures 1-8 (see Table 2A and 2B).

Complications of Autologous Reconstruction of the Breast

Table 3. TRAM Flap Complications

NON RADIATED TRAM	***Flap***	***Incidence***
	Infection	
	Seroma	
	Hematoma	
	Delayed Healing	
	Fat Necrosis	
	Partial Flap Necrosis	
	Total Flap Loss	
RADIATION BEFORE TRAM	***Flap***	***Incidence***
	Infection	4.8%
	Seroma	NR
	Hematoma	4.8%
	Delayed Healing	4.8%
	Fat Necrosis	23.8%
	Partial Flap Necrosis	9.5%
	Total Flap Loss	2.4%
RADIATION AFTER TRAM	***Flap***	***Incidence***
	Infection	5.3%
	Seroma	NR
	Hematoma	10.5%
	Delayed Healing	5.3%
	Fat Necrosis	23.7%
	Partial Flap Necrosis	0%
	Total Flap Loss	0%
	DONOR	***Incidence***
	Infection	2.6%
	Seroma	33%
	Delayed Healing	2.6%
	Hernia	2.6%

NR – Not Recorded

**With regards to flap complications, no statistical significance between 3 groups was found. Donor site complications occurred in approximately 30% of patients in all groups (Spear et al [16,73]).

Complications in autologous tissue reconstruction pertain not only to the transferred flap but also to the surrounding chest wall tissues, microvasculature and donor site (Table 3). In a recent review comparing the various flap modalities of breast reconstruction (TRAM, DIEP and SGAP), Nahabedian et al [35] found that venous occlusion and flap necrosis occurred in approximately 1 to 5% of cases regardless of the flap modality utilized, resulting in partial or total flap loss. Operative re-exploration of all flaps is needed in 5 to 10% of cases. With respect to the surrounding chest wall soft tissues, chest wall skin loss occurred in as many as 16% of patients reconstructed immediately with free TRAM flap but not in patients undergoing delayed reconstruction [42].

Other described complications of, in particular the TRAM flap reconstruction, is that of partial flap necrosis. In the contralateral pedicled TRAM flap, the incidence has been reported to be in the range of 5 to 44 percent; with the ipsilateral pedicled TRAM flap, Clugston et al [72] described a reduction of flap necrosis to 2 percent. In 2002 in free TRAM reconstruction, fat necrosis was noted in 5 to 10 percent of patients [42].

Obesity is a factor increasing postoperative complications following TRAM flap reconstruction [40] at times altering the placement of flap harvest such as the mid abdomen instead of lower abdomen [57]. Wang et al [68] retrospectively reviewed 107 patients who underwent delayed TRAM reconstruction and found that there was no significant difference in the fat necrosis rate (10 percent) regardless of whether the BMI was greater than or less than 30 kg/m^2. What was significant in this retrospective study was the incidence of deep vein thrombosis and pulmonary embolus which was significantly greater in the obese group (31.6 percent versus 8 percent in the non-obese group). Similarly Moran et al [69] and Ducic et al [70] found that there were no significant differences between the free and pedicled TRAM flap in the overall complication rates of obese patients however if obesity was linked with active smoking, the patients were likely to have two or more complications including infection as well as delayed healing. Obesity (BMI index greater than or equal to 30) was found to significantly increase risk for overall postoperative, both flap and donor site complications [40,70].

With respect to smoking it is a recognized accelerator of postoperative complications. In 2000, Chang et al [74] reviewed 718 patients who underwent the Free TRAM Flap reconstruction. Patients who were smokers and who underwent breast reconstruction had a 20 percent incidence of mastectomy skin flap necrosis and a 25 percent incidence of donor site complications. This was true in greater than 10 pack-year smokers thus patients who fall within this category are relative contraindicated undergoing a free TRAM flap reconstruction. It is recommended that reconstruction in this group of patients be delayed until the patient has stopped smoking for at least 4 weeks prior to the reconstructive surgery [74,70].

From a functional perspective, there is a 10% risk of abdominal wall bulge or hernia following harvest of the TRAM flap which is reduced to 0.7 – 5% with the DIEP modification [36,41]. Minimal functional disability is noted following harvest of the latissimus dorsi myocutaneous flap but lymphedema has been reported to be exacerbated [35]. The addition of scars can also be perceived as added disadvantage to this modality of reconstruction. However, studies overall support autologous reconstruction as it provides a more natural and aesthetic appearing breast especially in the patient with unilateral breast reconstruction.

Reconstruction with Prostheses

Choices in Prosthetic Reconstruction

Reconstruction usually commences with insertion of a tissue expander with either an internal or external port. This usually depends on the surgeon's preference and comfort with using either modality of tissue expander. Contraindications to the use of the tissue expander with the internal metallic magnetic port are presence of a pacemaker, patient's need for use of infusion pumps such as for delivery of chemotherapeutic agents, electrocardiogram equipment and use of the MRI for tumour surveillance while a tissue expander with internal metallic and magnetic port is in situ is contraindicated. The tissue expander may be slowly (60 cc per week) or rapidly expanded (120 cc per week) [43] depending on the quality of the patient's soft tissues, wound healing abilities and surgeon's preference. When fully expanded, the tissue expander is left in situ for a minimum of six to eight weeks but usually three to four months to allow the final contour and possible development of capsular contracture as well inframammary fold to evolve.

Patients can successfully undergo chemotherapy while also undergoing tissue expansion (6h) [65,66] though an increased incidence of wound complications such as hematoma, infection, and skin loss can occur.

Once tissue expansion has been completed, the expander is removed and replaced with a reconstructive implant filled either with saline solution or silicone. These prostheses may be round or tear-drop in shape and it is felt that in the breast reconstruction patient, the tear-drop shape is preferable to the round prosthesis. Each of these prostheses can have a smooth or textured surface. Textured implants are believed to reduce the risk of capsular contractures [54].

The reconstruction process utilizing this modality can take six to eight months to complete from time of expander insertion to insertion of final implant. With rapid tissue expansion [36], which is most possible in the non-radiated patient, this can be reduced to approximately three to four months. However, time is often needed for development of ptosis and development of an infra-mammary fold. Hence, there is longer time to completion of the reconstruction utilizing this modality. The advantages of reconstruction utilizing implants are: no additional donor site, can be performed on an out-patient basis, short operative time, often requested by patients with young families (example pre-menopausal group). Disadvantages of this modality of reconstruction include the need for a second surgical procedure, inability to undergo an MRI investigation if an expander with an internal magnetic port is utilized, pain immediately following each weekly expansion potentially limiting the activities of daily living temporarily following expansion, and the length of time to completion.

Of greater concern, however, are the potential risks associated with implant reconstruction which include implant rupture (1 to 7 percent) [44,45] and extrusion [26], contracture (10 to 32 percent) [32] and finally that of infection. The incidence of infection following reconstruction of the breast with expanders and implants ranges from 1 to 24 percent [45,46]. In a recent review by Pittet [47], the infectious complication rate of breast implants was as low as 2 to 2.5 percent in most case series. Nahabedian et al [47] examined a total of 168 implant reconstructions retrospectively and found a significant association between implant infection and radiation therapy. Implants exposed to radiation therapy were 4.8 times more likely to develop infection. The chance of implant infection increased to 6.29 times higher than normal in women who had undergone lymph node dissection than in patients who had not undergone axillary lymphadenectomy. In a recent prospective cohort study performed by Alderman et al [40] the statistically significant high rate of complications in radiated patients who underwent implant reconstructions was not found. This prospective study differs from previous retrospective studies. The cohort prospective study of Alderman does recognize, however, that they had a limited sample size which could contribute to the lack of statistical significance.

Goodwin et al [49] retrospectively reviewed complications following tissue expansion in over 500 patients and overall complications were 2.5 times more common in smokers compared with non-smokers.

A final option for breast reconstruction is the combination of modalities using both TRAM flaps and prosthesis on opposite sides of the chest wall or in combination (ipsilateral fashion) which are occurring with greater frequency. In a retrospective review by Spear, the greatest problem was seen in 19% of patients reconstructed with implants which became infected and required explantation, although the majority of the patients in this group had been radiated [48,73].

Reconstruction of the Radiated Patient

With the development and evolution of autologous tissue reconstruction, that is microsurgical transfer of free flaps and their perforator derivatives, the role of implants in breast reconstruction has come into question. This has further been highlighted by the recognized increased use of radiation therapy and breast conserving surgery as well as the concern regarding tumour control following mastectomy. Reconstruction of the radiated chest wall with prostheses have a recognized complication rate of 17 to 80 percent [26,71]. It is recognized that capsular contracture rates of up to 32% [32] can occur in patients undergoing breast reconstruction with prosthesis following radiation therapy. In one study, non-radiated patients reconstructed with implants had a 10% incidence of capsular contracture while 50% of the radiated population who developed capsular contracture rates then went on to flap salvage [32,34]. Other potential risks include wound dehiscence, infection, implant rupture and implant exposure [26,34]. This therefore has limited the use of the tissue expander and implant modality reconstruction to the non-radiated chest wall patient with small to moderate sized minimally ptotic breasts, and bilateral chest wall reconstruction as well as prophylactic mastectomy (see Table 4). In the radiated patient, reconstruction utilizing a tissue expander and implant is relatively contraindicated paralleling the non-radiated patient just described provided adequate soft tissue coverage of the chest wall is present. This can be determined by the pinch test as well as physical examination of the radiated chest wall ensuring the presence of minimal post-radiation skin changes. Findings of severe hyperpigmentation, fibrosis, thin or atrophic tissues, or prominent surface telangiectasia following radiation therapy to the chest wall are signs that damage from radiation is severe indicating that utilizing the tissue expander and implant modality is likely to result in failure. These physical findings are best treated with autologous breast reconstruction or no reconstruction at all. Breast reconstruction following radiation therapy can commence as early as three months up to one year following completion of adjuvant radiation therapy.

Breast reconstruction in the to-be radiated patient, should be performed in a delayed fashion. Reconstruction should also be delayed in the patient with locally advanced or aggressive breast cancer for a minimum of two years. Breast reconstruction following radiation therapy can commence as early as three months up to one year following completion of adjuvant radiation therapy. Though in the post-radiated patient, reconstruction via autologous tissue is preferred, reconstruction with a prosthetic device can be considered. Previous radiation therapy to the anterior chest wall is a relative contraindication to reconstruction with prostheses. If the skin changes secondary to radiation therapy are minimal in nature or essentially non-existent, and there is adequate soft tissue coverage of the anterior chest wall (pinch test), then reconstruction via prostheses can be entertained.

Table 4. Modalities of Reconstruction

MODALITY	PATIENT FACTORS
PROSTHESES	- prophylactic mastectomy - bilateral mastectomy - young patient - adequate soft tissue coverage (pinch test) - minimum to no radiation changes (preferably none) - small to moderate sized opposite breast - minimum to no ptosis on the remaining breast unless patient agrees to contralateral mastopexy or reduction - patient preference
AUTOLOGOUS TISSUE	- unilateral reconstruction - tight thin chest wall scar - contracted skin/soft tissues of chest wall - post-radiated patient - patient preference - no contraindicating scars on abdomen, back or other donor sites - older patient (≥40)

NIPPLE AREOLAR COMPLEX RECONSTRUCTION

Early studies indicated that approximately 50% of women who had undergone breast mound reconstruction then proceeded to nipple areolar complex reconstruction [53]; this figure is now believed to be close to 90% [51]. The most common method is fabrication of the nipple with a local flap and of the areola with skin graft or micropigmentation (tattooing) (or combination of the two).

In patients with adequate soft tissue coverage that has excellent vascularity, a variety of flaps have been described for reconstruction of this unit. In a recent study by M. Jabor et al [53], only 12% of patients in their study group chose not to undergo nipple areolar complex reconstruction. Sixty-four percent of their patients reported excellent to good satisfaction with the nipple areolar complex reconstruction and 14% reported a poor satisfaction with the reconstruction. Jabor et al examined nipple areolar reconstruction in a variety of settings including not only implants but also TRAM and latissimus dorsi flaps.

The greatest area of dissatisfaction for the patients was lack of projection followed by colour match and shape. Approximately 30% of patients studied required retattooing due to fading of the pigment, poor take of the pigment or revision of the shape of the pigment to the area. Greater satisfaction was also noted if patients underwent nipple areolar complex reconstruction within one year of completion of the breast mound [53]. Approximately 1/3 of the patients required two procedures, most of which (85%) were for retattooing, 15% of the secondary procedures were for revision of the nipple.

In patients reconstructed with TRAM or other flaps, caution is used in nipple reconstruction in patients who have been radiated and/or have thin soft tissues covering the implant. In one study [53] 11% of patients experienced nipple necrosis. Due to altered blood supply, there are increased risks of implant exposure and infection in reconstruction of the nipple in thin and/or radiated patients who have been reconstructed with implants. At times, micro-implantation alone or prosthetic addition of nipple is recommended.

Choosing not to Undergo Breast Reconstruction

Finally, a woman may choose to not undergo breast reconstruction if she feels it is not essential for her physical or emotional well-being, fears complications or prefers not to undergo additional surgery. In addition, patients may lack family support, be unable to undergo a specific type of reconstruction, or fear the perception by friends and family of the surgery as cosmetic in nature and some may fear being too old for the procedure [58]. Other factors include socioeconomic factors, geographic location [7,3] and not being able to take the time away from work for possible repeated office visits and finally advanced stage of disease may not allow for early breast reconstruction. A patient also may decline reconstruction if she does not wish any additional scars. For example, she may not wish to add scars to her flat toned abdominal wall. It is generally recommended that patients with stage IV disease not undergo reconstruction.

Satisfaction with Reconstruction

Given the variety of reconstructable patients and selection of modalities be they autologous tissue, implants or combination thereof, the final evaluation of the end result lies predominantly with the patient but also with the reconstructive surgeon. Several retrospective studies since 1992 have tried to better delineate patient esthetic satisfaction, with the various modalities of breast reconstruction with conflicting results. Several studies have shown a higher patient satisfaction with autologous reconstruction specifically the TRAM flap compared to the implant modality reconstruction [51]. Though several reports have shown that immediate reconstruction is less psychologically traumatizing for patients than in patients who undergo delayed reconstruction, other studies have found no differences between these two groups with respect to their body image [50]. Prospective cohort studies now are suggesting delayed reconstruction may in fact be better psychologically as women adjust to the cancer diagnosis and treatments especially if they have pre-existing anxiety with self-image and sexuality.

Andrade et al [50] found that patient dissatisfaction with reconstruction correlated with significant post-operative complications. Patient satisfaction with their reconstruction, regardless of method, rested more on the lack of post-operative complications rather than the form itself (implant vs flap). Shaikh-Naidu et al [51] in their retrospective satisfaction survey found that in patients who underwent bilateral reconstruction, the modality of reconstruction was not significant. In unilateral reconstruction, the flap modality was preferred, patients having rated higher their esthetic satisfaction with breast shape and symmetry as well as volume than did implant patients [51]. In their study, patients who had undergone post-operation radiation were most dissatisfied with their reconstructed breast and the most significant factor was the presence of nipple areolar reconstruction which yielded the highest satisfaction [51 pg 467] with breast reconstruction.

Patients should be informed of the possible number of secondary procedures following reconstruction regardless of the modality utilized. Losken et al [52] retrospectively determined that the average number of secondary procedures was approximately four in unilateral autologous reconstruction and almost six in number for bilateral autologous reconstruction mainly donor site revisions. Factors increasing the number of secondary procedures were noted to be delayed reconstruction, radiation therapy in patients who had suffered post-operative complications, significant patient co-morbidities and in patients who had undergone autologous tissue reconstruction. Patients who had undergone reconstruction with latissimus dorsi myocutaneous flap with or without implant were also studied and are included in the flap group. The number of secondary procedures was higher in the TRAM flap reconstruction group attributed to further refinement of the abdominal wall donor site. The study, however, examined the secondary procedures in the immediate post-operative period and did not examine long-term secondary procedures such as treatment of capsular contractures in the group reconstructed with breast implants.

CONCLUSION

Though ideally all breast cancer patients should be reconstructed at the time of mastectomy, staging of disease and co-morbid factors limit this possibility. In patients with advanced disease, most recurrences develop within the first two years following diagnosis, thus this group of patients is best reconstructed in delayed fashion. Post-operative cancer monitoring currently is limited and future growth lies with application of investigative tools currently used for monitoring of breast cancer patients who have not undergone reconstruction. A reconstructive patient must be an active participant in the decision making process with regards to breast reconstruction. Concerns pertaining to scars and lifestyle must be respected by the reconstructing surgeon. Post-operative complications must be fully delineated. An educated open dialogue must therefore occur amongst members of the multi-disciplinary team and between surgeon and patient who together decide on the ultimate timing and modality of breast reconstruction.

REFERENCES

[1] Gaudette, LA; Gao, RN; Spence, A; et al. Declining Use of Mastectomy for Invasive Breast Cancer in Canada, 1981-2000. *Can J Public Health*. 2004 Sept-Oct 5(5), 325-8.

[2] Thompson, TA; Pusic, A; Kerrigan, CL; et al. Surgeon Perspectives on Surgical Options for Early-Stage Breast Cancer. *Plast Reconstr Surg*, 2000 Mar 105(3), 910-8.

[3] Morrow, M; Mujahid, M; Lantz, P; et al. Correlates of Breast Reconstruction – Results from a Population-Based Study. *American Cancer Society*. 2005 Dec 104, 2340-6.

[4] Joslyn, S. Patterns of Care for Immediate and Early Delayed Breast Reconstruction Following Mastectomy. *Plast Reconstr Surg*, 2005 Apr 115(5), 1289-1296.

[5] Kronowitz, S; Hunt, KK; Kuerer, HM; et al. Delayed-Immediate Breast Reconstruction. *Plast Reconstr Surg*, 2004 May 113, 1617-28.

[6] *Eur J Surg Oncology*, 2002 Sept 28(6), 627-32.

[7] Baxter, N; Goel, V; Semple, J. Utilization and Regional Variation of Breast Reconstruction in Canada. *Plast Reconstr Surg*, 2005 Jan 115(1), 338-339.

[8] Metcalfe, KA; Snyder, C; Seidel, J; et al. The Use of Preventative Measures Among Healthy Women Who Carry a BRAC1 or BRCA2 Mutation. *Fam Cancer*, 2005 4(2), 97-103.

[9] Bajaj, AK; Kon, PS; Oberg, KC; et al. Aesthetic Outcomes in Patients Undergoing Breast Conservation Therapy for the Treatment of Localized Breast Cancer. *Plast Reconstr Surg*, 2004 Nov 114(6), 1442-9.

[10] Cocquyt, VF; Blondeel, PN; Depypere, HT; et al. Better Cosmetic Results and Comparable Quality of Life After Skin-Sparing Mastectomy and Immediate Autologous Breast Reconstruction Compared to Breast Conservative Treatment. *Br J Plast Surg*, 2003 July 56(5), 762-70.

[11] Gendy, RK; Able, JA; Rainsbury, RM. Impact of Skin-Sparing Mastectomy With Immediate Reconstruction and Breast-Sparing Reconstruction via Miniflaps on the Outcomes of Oncoplastic Breast Surgery. *BR J Surg*, 2003 Apr 90(4), 433-9.

[12] Mortenson, MM; Schneider, PD; Khatri, VP; et al. Immediate Breast Reconstruction After Mastectomy Increases Wound Complications. *Arch Surg*, 2004139, 988-91.

[13] Toth, BA; Lappert, P. Modified Skin Incisions for Mastectomy: The Need for Plastic Surgical Input in Preoperative Planning. *Plast Reconstr Surg*, 1991 87, 1048-1053.

[14] Singletary, SE. Skin-Sparing Mastectomy With Immediate Breast Reconstruction: The MD Anderson Cancer Center Experience. *Ann Surg Oncol*, 1996 3, 411-416.

[15] Slavin, SA; Schnitt, SJ; Duda, R; et al. Skin-Sparing Mastectomy and Immediate Reconstruction: Oncologic Risks and Aesthetic Results in Patients With Early Stage Breast Cancer. Plast Reconstr Surg, 1998 102, 49-62.

[16] Spear, SL; Carter, ME; Schwarz, K. Prophylactic Mastectomy: Indications, Options, and Reconstructive Alternatives. *Plast Reconstr Surg*, 2005 Mar 115(3), 891-909.

[17] Slavin, SA; Love, SM; Goldwyn, RM. Recurrent Breast Cancer Following Immediate Breast Reconstruction with Myocutaneous Flaps. *Plast Reconstr Surg*, 1994 May 93, 1191-1204.

[18] Langstein, HN; Cheng, MH; Singletary, SE; et al. Breast Cancer Recurrence After Immediate Reconstruction: Patterns and Significance. *Plast Reconstr Surg*, 2003 Feb 112(2), 712-720.

[19] Mustonen, P; Katja, V; Berg, M; et al. Recurrences After Immediate Reconstruction in Breast Cancer. *Scandinavian Journal of Surgery*, 2005 94, 21-24.

[20] Carlson, GW; Styblo, TM; Lyles, RH; et al. Local Recurrence After Skin-Sparing Mastectomy: Tumor Biology or Surgical Conservatism? *Annals of Surg. Onc*, 2003 10(2), 108-112.

[21] Fersis, N; Hoenig, A; Relakis, K; et al. Skin-Sparing Mastectomy and Immediate Breast Reconstruction: Incidence of Recurrence in Patients with Invasive Breast Cancer. *The Breast*, 2004 13, 488-493.

[22] Sandelin, K; Wickman. M; Billgren, AM. Oncological Outcome After Immediate Breast Reconstruction for Invasive Breast Cancer: A Long-Term Study. *The Breast*, 2004 13, 210-218.

[23] Juweid, ME; Cheson, BD. Positron-Emission Tomography and Assessment of Cancer Therapy. *N Engl J Med*, 2006 354, 496-507.

[24] Rieber, A; Schramm, K; Helms, G; et al. Breast-Conserving Surgery and Autogenous Tissue Reconstruction in Patients with Breast Cancer: Efficacy of MRI of Breast in the Detection of Recurrent Disease. *Eur. Radiol*, 2003 13, 780-787.

[25] Downes, KJ; Glatt, BS; Kanchwala, SK; et al. Skin-Sparing Mastectomy and Immediate Reconstruction Is an Acceptable Treatment Option for Patients with High-Risk Breast Carcinoma. *Cancer*, 2005 103, 906-13.

[26] Senkus-Konefka, E; Welnicka-Jaskiewicz, M; Kaskiewicz, J; et al. Radiotherapy for Breast Cancer in Patients Undergoing Breast Reconstruction or Augmentation. *Cancer Treatment Reviews*, 2004 30, 671-682.

[27] Tran, NV; Chang, DW; Gupta, A; et al. Comparison of Immediate and Delayed Free TRAM Flap Breast Reconstruction in Patients Receiving Postmastectomy Radiation Therapy. *Plast Reconstr Surg*, 2001 108, 78-82.

[28] Kronowitz, SJ; Robb, GL. Breast Recontruction with Postmastectomy Radiation Therapy: Current Issues. *Plast Reconstr Surg*; 2004 114, 950-960.

[29] Spear, SL; Ducic, I; Low, M; et al. The Effect of Radiation on Pedicled TRAM Flap Breast Reconstruction: Outcomes and Implications. *Plast Reconstr Surg*, 2005 115, 84-95.

[30] Halyard, M; McCombs, K; Wong, W; et al. Acute and Chronic Results of Adjuvant Radiotherapy After Mastectomy and Transverse Rectus Abdominis Myocutaneous

(TRAM) Flap Reconstruction for Breast Cancer. *Am J of Clin Oncol*, 2004 27, 389-394.

[31] Soong, IS; Yau, TK; Ho, CM; et al. Post-mastectomy Radiotherapy after Immediate Autologous Breast Reconstruction in Primary Treatment of Breast Cancers. *Clinical Oncology*, 2004 16, 283-289.

[32] Spear, SL; Onyewu, C. taged Breast Reconstruction with Saline-Filled Implants in the Irradiated Breast: Recent Trends and Therapeutic Implications. Plast Reconstr Surg, 2000 Mar 105(3), 930-942.

[33] Hartrampf, CR. *Breast Reconstruction with Living Tissue*. Edition 1991: 33-35.

[34] Karanas, YL; Leong, DS; Da Lio, A; et al. Surgical Treatment of Breast Cancer in Previously Augmented Patients. *Plast Reconstr Surg*, 2003 March 111(3), 1078-1083.

[35] Nahabedian, MY; Momen, B; Manson, PN. Factors Associated with Anastomotic Failure after Microvascular Reconstruction of the Breast. *Plast Reconstr Surg*, 2004 114, 74-82.

[36] Nahabedian, MY, FACS; Momen B. Lower Abdominal Bulge After Deep Inferior Epigastric Perforator Flap (DIEP) Breast Reconstruction. *Ann Plast Surg*, 2005 54, 124-129.

[37] Dayhim, F; Wilkins, EG. The Impact of Pfannestiel Scars on TRAM flap Complications. *Ann Plast Surg,* 2004 53, 432-435.

[38] Tachi, M; Yamada, A. Choice of Flaps for Breast Reconstruction. *Int J Clin Oncol*, 2005 10, 289-297.

[39] Blondeel, PN. The Sensate Free Superior Gluteal Artery Perforator (S-GAP) Flap: A Valuable Alternative in Autologous Breast Reconstruction. *British Journal of Plastic Surgery*, 1999 52, 185-193

[40] Alderman, AK; Wilkins, EG; Kim, HM; et al. Complications in Postmastectomy Breast Reconstruction: Two-Year Results of the Michigan Breast Reconstruction Outcome Study. *Plast Reconstr Surg,* 2002 June 109(7), 2265-2274.

[41] Gill, PS; John, P; Guerra, AB; et al. A 10-Year Retrospective Review of 758 DIEP Flaps for Breast Reconstruction. *Plast Reconstr Surg*, 2004 April 113(4), 1153-1160.

[42] DeBono, R; Thompson, A; Stenvenson, JH. Immediate Versus Delayed Free TRAM Breast Reconstruction: An Analysis of Perioperative Factors and Complications. *British Journal of Plastic Surgery*, 2002 55, 111-116.

[43] Pusic, AL, MHS; Cordeiro, PG. An Accelerated Approach to Tissue Expansion for Breast Reconstruction: Experience with Intraoperative and Rapid Postoperative Expansion in 370 Reconstructions. *Plast Reconstr Surg*, 2003 May 111, 1871-1875.

[44] Roth, RS; Lowery, JC; Davis, J et al. Quality of Life and Affective Distress in Women Seeking Immediate Versus Delayed Breast Reconstruction After Mastectomy for Breast Cancer. *Plast Reconstr Surg*, 2005 116, 993.

[45] Spear, SL; Majidian, A. Immediate Breast Reconstruction in Two Stages Using Textured, Integrated-Valve Tissue Expanders and Breast Implants: A Retrospective Review of 171 Consecutive Breast Reconstructions from 1989 to 1996. *Plast Reconstr Surg*, 1998 Jan 101, 53-63.

[46] Nahabedian, MY; Tsangaris, T; Momen, B; et al. Infectious Complications Following Breast Reconstruction with Expanders and Implants. *Plast Reconstr Surg*, 2003 Aug 112, 467-476.

[47] Pittet, B; Montandon, D; Pittet, D. Infection in Breast Implants. *Lancet Infectious Diseases*. 2005 Feb 5, 94-106.

[48] Spear, SL; Wolfe, AW. The Coincidence of TRAM Flaps and Prostheses in the Setting of Breast Reconstruction. *Plast Reconstr Surg*, 2002 Aug 110(2), 478-486.

[49] Goodwin, SJ; McCarthy, CM; Pusic, AL; et al. Complications in Smokers After Postmastectomy Tissue Expander/Implant Breast Reconstruction. *Ann Plast Surg*, 2005 July 55(1), 16-20.

[50] Andrade, WN; Baxter, N; Semple, J. Clinical Determinants of Patient Satisfaction with Breast Reconstruction. *Plast Reconst Surg*, 2001 Jan 107, 46-54.

[51] Shaikh-Naidu, N; Preminger, A; Rogers, K; et al. Determinants of Aesthetic Satisfaction Following TRAM and Implant Breast Reconstruction. *Ann Plast Surg*, 2004 May 52(5), 465-470.

[52] Losken, A; Carlson, GW; Schoemann, MB; et al. Factors That Influence the Completion of Breast Reconstruction. *Ann Plast Surg*, 2004 Mar 52(3), 258-262.

[53] Jabor, MA; Shayani, P; Collins DR Jr; et al. Nipple-Areola Reconstruction: Satisfaction and Clinical Determinants. *Plast Reconstr Surg*, 2002 Aug 110(2), 457-463.

[54] Benediktsson, K; Perbeck, L. Capsular Contracture Around Saline-Filled and Textured Subcutaneously-Placed Implants in Irradiated and Non-Irradiated Breast Cancer Patients: Five Years of Monitoring of a Prospective Trial. *J Plast Reconstr Aesthet Surg*, 2006 59(1), 27-34.

[55] Spear, SL; Ducic, I; Cuoco, F; et al. The Effect of Smoking on Flap and Donor-Site Complications in Pedicled TRAM Breast Reconstruction. *Plast Reconstr Surg*, 2005 Dec 116(7), 1873-80.

[56] Brandberg, Y; Malm, M; Blomqvist, L. A Prospective and Randomized Study, "SVEA," Comparing Effects of Three Methods of Delayed Breast Reconstruction on Quality of Life, Patient-Defined Problem Areas of Life, and Cosmetic Result. *Plast Reconstr Surg*, 2000 Jan 105(1), 66-74.

[57] Gabbay, JS; Eby, JB; Kulber, DA. The Midabdominal TRAM Flap for Breast Reconstruction in Morbidly Obese Patients. *Plast Reconstr Surg*, 2005 Mar 115(3), 764-70.

[58] Reaby, L. Reasons Why Women Who Have Mastectomy Decide to Have or Not to Have Breast Reconstruction. *Plast Reconstr Surg*, 1998 101, 1810.

[59] Rowland, JH; Holland, JC; Chaglassian, T; et al. Psychological Response to Breast Reconstruction. *Psychosomatics*, 1993 May-June 34(3).

[60] Dean, C; Chetty, U; Forrest, AP. Effects of Immediate Breast Reconstruction on Psychosocial Morbidity After Mastectomy. *Lancet*, 1983 1, 459.

[61] Harcourt, DM; Rumsey, NH; Ambler, NR; et al. The Psychological Effect of Breast Reconstruction: A Prospective Multicenter Study. *Plast Reconstr Surg*, 2003 111, 1060.

[62] Losken, A; Carlson, GW; Schoemann, MB; et al. Factors that Influence the Completion of Breast Reconstruction. *Ann Plast Surg*, 2004 52, 258-262.

[63] El-Mrakby, HH; Milner, RH; McLean, NR. Supercharged Pedicled TRAM Flap in Breast Reconstruction: Is It a Worthwhile Procedure. *Ann Plast Surg*, 2002 Sept 49(3), 252-7.

[64] Temple, CL; Strom, EA; Youssef, A; et al. Choice of Recipient Vessels in Delayed TRAM Flap Breast Reconstruction After Radiotherapy. *Plast Reconstr Surg*, 2005 Jan 115(1), 105-13.

[65] Rey, P; Martinelli, G; Petit, JY; et al. Immediate Breast Reconstruction and High-Dose Chemotherapy. *Ann Plast Surg*, 2004 Sept 55(3), 250-4.

[66] Mortenson, MM; Schneider, PD; Khatri, VP; et al. Immediate Breast Reconstruction After MAStectomy Increases Wound Complications: However, Initiation of Adjuvant Chemotherapy is Not Delayed. *Arch Surg*, 2004 Sept 139(9), 988-91.

[67] Woerdeman, LA; Van Schijndel, AW; Hage, JJ; et al. Verifying Surgical Results and Risk Factors of the Lateral Thoracodorsal Flap. *Plast Reconstr Surg*, 2004 Jan 113(1), 196-203.

[68] Wang, HT; Hartzell, T; Olbrich, KC; et al. Delay of Transverse Rectus Abdominis Myocutaneous Flap Reconstruction Improves Flap Reliability in the Obese Patient. *Plast Reconstr Surg*, 2005 Aug 116(2), 613-8.

[69] Moran, SL; Serletti, JM. Outcome Comparison Between Free and Pedicled TRAM Flap Breast Reconstruction in the Obese Patient. *Plast Reconstr Surg*, 2001 Dec 108(7), 1954-60.

[70] Ducic, I; Spear, SL; Cuoco, F; et al. Safety and Risk Factors for Breast Reconstruction with Pedicled Transverse Rectus Abdominis Musculocutaneous Flaps: 10-year Analysis. *Ann Plast Surg*, 2005 Dec 55(6), 559-64.

[71] Ascherman, JA; Hanasono, MM; Newman, MI; et al. Implant Reconstruction in Breast Cancer Patients Treated with Radiation Therapy. *Plast Reconstr Surg*, 2006 Feb 117(2), 359-65.

[72] Cligston, PA; Gingrass, MK; Azurin, D; et al. Ipsilateral Pedicled TRAM Flaps: The Safer Alternative? *Plast Reconstr Surg*, 2000 Jan 105(1), 77-82.

[73] Spear, SL; Ducic, I; Low, M; et al. The Effect of Radiation on Pedicled TRAM Flap Breast Reconstruction: Outcomes and Implications. *Plast Reconstr Surg*, 2005 Jan 115(1), 84-95.

[74] Chang, DW; Reece, GP; Wang, B; et al. Effect of Smoking on Complications in Patients Undergoing Free TRAM Flap Breast Reconstruction. *Plast Reconstr Surg*, 2000 June 105(7), 2374-2380.

[75] Cronin, T; Gerow, F. Augmentation Mammaplasty: A New "Natural Feel" Prosthesis In: Broadbent TR, ed. *Transactions of the Third International Congress of Plastic and Reconstructive Surgery*, 1963.

[76] Bohmert, H; Gabka, CJ. *Plastic and Reconstructive Surgery of the Breast: A Surgical Atlas*. 1997

SECTION 3: WOMEN AND COLORECTAL CANCER

In: Women and Cancer
Editor: Laurie Elit, pp. 109-127
ISBN: 978-1-60021-494-3

Chapter I

WOMEN AND COLORECTAL CANCER

Samantha Hendren*
Department of Surgery, University of Rochester, USA.

ABSTRACT

Colorectal cancer deaths are equally distributed among women and men. Prevention is possible using risk-stratified screening strategies and healthy lifestyle. Good outcomes are possible if the disease is discovered and treated at an early stage. Quality of life can be preserved but in rectal cancer patients, sexual function and changes in body image occur.

INTRODUCTION

It is a common misconception that colorectal cancer is a "male disease". On the contrary, colorectal cancer cases and deaths are approximately equally distributed between men and women in North America [1]. For women in Ontario, colorectal cancer (CRC) is the second most common cancer diagnosis, after breast cancer [2]. In terms of cancer deaths, it is third after breast and lung cancers. One in 16 Canadian women will develop CRC in her lifetime, compared to 1 in 14 men [3].

Table 1 displays American statistics for digestive system cancers [1]. These data illustrate that CRC is by far the most common digestive system cancer. It is also one of the most curable, as evidenced by the relatively low ratio of deaths to new cases diagnosed. Canadian statistics show that in 2006, an estimated 20,000 Canadians will be diagnosed with CRC and 8,500 will die of it [3].

* Correspondence concerning this article should be addressed to Dr. S. Hendren, 601 Elmwood Avenue, Box SURG, Rochester, New York 14642, USA. Phone: (585)275-0606; Email: *samantha_hendren@urmc.rochester.edu*.

Colorectal cancer diagnosis rates decreased in the USA between 1998 and 2002, by approximately 1.8% per year [4]. This may be due to improved cancer screening and the removal of pre-cancerous polyps. Death rates from CRC are also decreasing, probably due to improvements in early detection and treatment [4]. In Canada CRC rates have been decreasing since the mid-1980's, particularly in women, and in the distal colon and rectum [5]. In Ontario, an increase in incidence was seen more recently, from the mid-1990's to the present; the reason for this is not clear [2]. It is possible that improved detection from screening is a factor.

Table 1. Digestive Cancer Statistics for the USA, 2004*

	Estimated New Cases			Estimated Deaths		
	Both Genders	Male	Female	Both Genders	Male	Female
All Digestive System Cancers	255,640	135,410	120,230	134,840	73,240	61,600
Esophagus	14,250	10,860	3,390	13,300	10,250	3,050
Stomach	22,710	13,640	9,070	11,780	6,900	4,880
Small Intestine	5,260	2,750	2,510	1,130	610	520
Colon	**106,370**	**50,400**	**55,970**	**56730****	**28320****	**28410****
Rectum	**40,570**	**23,220**	**17,350**			
Anus	4,010	1,890	2,120	580	210	370
Liver and Extrahepatic Bile Duct	18,920	12,580	6,340	14,270	9,450	4,820
Gallbladder and Other Biliary	6,950	2,960	3,990	3,540	1,290	2,250
Pancreas	31,860	15,740	16,120	31,270	15,440	15,830
Other	4,740	1,370	3,370	2,240	770	1,470

*CA Cancer J Clin 2004; 54:8-29. **Estimated deaths combined for colon and rectum.

ANATOMY

As illustrated in Table 1, the vast majority of "bowel cancers" are colorectal cancers due to the low rates of small intestine and anal cancers. The majority of colorectal cancers are distal, in the sigmoid colon and rectum [2]. The rectum is the last 12-15 cm of the large bowel; it is defined by its pelvic anatomic location and its distinct muscular, lymphatic and vascular anatomy. Rectal cancers in the final 12 cm of the large bowel are treated somewhat differently from colon cancers, due to their location, the proximity of nerve and genitourinary structures, and more aggressive tumour behavior. However, rectosigmoid cancers are similar to sigmoid cancers, and the treatment is usually the same as for other colon cancers.

The term "colorectal cancer" refers to adenocarcinomas of the large bowel. These cancers arise from the glandular epithelial lining of the interior of the bowel. Other types of tumors of the bowel, such as lymphomas, carcinoid tumors, squamous cell cancers, melanomas and gastrointestinal stromal tumors are quite different, and are not discussed here.

Risk Factors and Prevention

Risk factors for colorectal cancer include: increasing age; a personal history of colorectal cancer or adenomatous polyps; a family history of CRC, particularly when the cancer is in a first-degree relative and/or the cancer was diagnosed at a young age; a family history of adenomatous polyps; inherited colorectal cancer syndromes; and having inflammatory bowel disease, including ulcerative colitis and Crohn's disease [4] (Table 2). However, in more than 75% of CRC, no specific risk factor is found [2].

There are several modifiable factors that may contribute to CRC and adenoma risk. The most important of these is cigarette smoking. Multiple cohort and case-control studies have also shown that former or current cigarette smoking increases the risk of colorectal cancer by a factor of 1.5 to 2 [6,7]. Several other dietary, lifestyle and pharmacologic interventions have been suggested to decrease colorectal cancer risk, and the data for these are reviewed below.

Table 2. Risk Factors for Colorectal Cancer

Age Over 50
Inflammatory Bowel Disease (Crohn's Disease, Ulcerative Colitis)
Personal History of CRC or Adenomatous Polyps
Family History of CRC or Adenomatous Polyps in a 1st Degree Relative
Genetic Syndromes (Familial Polyposis (FAP), Hereditary NonPolyposis Colon Cancer (HNPCC))

Diet, Vitamins and Exercise

Large cohort studies of women, such as the Nurses' Health Study have suggested that diet has a significant impact on the risk of CRC. Possible risk factors include low fruit intake [8], low legume intake [8], obesity, low physical activity, low folate intake, high red meat intake, high processed meat intake and high alcohol intake [9].

A case-control study of the diets of women found to have colorectal adenomas suggested that higher intake of calories, total fat, saturated fat, and red meat were risk factors for adenomas, while fish and chicken, vitamin A, and total fiber were protective [10]. It is interesting to note that these authors failed to find the same relationships between diet and adenomas in males. Meat, fat and fiber intake were prospectively studied in 88,000 women with a 6-year follow-up [11]. After adjusting for total calorie intake, several factors were associated with a higher risk of CRC: animal fat (not vegetable fat); red meat; processed meat and liver; and low intake of fruits. Fish and skinless chicken were protective. The same cohort study failed to show a protective effect of dietary fiber against CRC or adenomas [12]. A smaller cohort study with a 7-year follow-up showed an inverse relationship between protein intake and CRC risk in women [13]. Fish and dairy were protective in this study, but no relationship with total calories or fat was seen.

Prospective cohort studies have shown varying results with respect to dietary fiber and CRC risk. The large European EPIC study showed a significant protective effect of fiber

[14], while large American cohort studies have failed to show an effect [15]. Randomized trials of dietary fiber conducted to prevent recurrent adenomatous polyps in patients with prior polyps have had mixed results. A metaanalysis of randomized trials showed no effect of dietary fiber on polyp or cancer prevention [16], but studies had a relatively short follow-up of 2-4 years, and the possibility of a long-term benefit exists. Gender differences in the response to dietary fiber may exist, with a specific benefit for women [17].

Long-term (>15 years) multivitamin supplementation in women was associated with a decreased risk of colorectal cancer in the Nurses Health Study [18]. The pattern of benefit suggested that folate supplementation might be an important factor in the observed benefit. Antioxidant vitamins have also been studied in relatively short-term experimental studies, without a benefit observed [19,20]; however, these studies are limited by relatively short follow-up.

Calcium plus Vitamin D supplementation has been associated with lower risk of CRC in epidemiologic studies, and has been found to prevent adenomatous polyps [21,22]. In addition, dietary intake of milk and dairy foods has strong support from prospective cohort studies for a protective effect [23]. However a recent randomized trial of calcium plus Vitamin D supplementation in 36,000 post-menopausal women showed no effect on the risk of colorectal cancer in 7 years of follow-up [24]. It is possible that the long latency in the development of CRC and a very low-risk cohort may have led to this negative result, and longer follow-up is needed.

Physical exercise has been suggested to protect against the development of CRC [25]; however, the Physicians' Health Study failed to confirm this benefit after controlling for obesity and other risk factors [26]. Obesity may also predispose to CRC [9,25]. Finally, a pooled analysis of large, prospective cohort studies showed a moderate increase in CRC risk amongst people with high alcohol intake [27].

Table 3. Modifiable Factors in Colorectal Cancer Risk for Women

May Increase Risk of CRC	**May Decrease Risk of CRC**
Cigarette Smoking	Long-Term Multivitamin Supplementation
Obesity	High Fiber Intake
High Alcohol Intake	High Fruit Intake
High Intake of Animal, Saturated or Total Fat	Fish and Lean Chicken Intake
High Intake of Red or Processed Meat	Dairy Intake
	Calcium/Vitamin D Supplementation
	Folate Supplementation
	Physical Activity
Possible Chemoprevention for High-Risk Individuals	
Aspirin	
Calcium/Vitamin D	
Non-Steroidal Anti-Inflammatory Drugs	
Statins	
Hormone Replacement Therapy	
Ursodeoxycholic Acid	

In summary, there is some evidence suggesting that multivitamins, calcium/Vitamin D supplementation, dairy intake, fruit intake, fish and lean chicken intake, dietary fiber, a lean body weight, physical activity and avoidance of red and processed meats and excessive alcohol may reduce the risk of CRC. The evidence is mixed for most of these interventions; however, they are unlikely to have a deleterious effect on health if recommended (Table 3).

Chemoprophylaxis

Several medications have been shown to decrease the number of polyps in patients with familial adenomatous polyposis, the highest-risk individuals for polyp formation. The use of these agents in usual-risk persons has not been shown to be effective when rigorously tested. In high-risk individuals, chemoprevention may be considered, but risks of medications must be weighed against potential benefit. This issue was brought into focus with the recent finding of increased cardiovascular risk with COX-2 inhibitor medications.

Non-steroidal anti-inflammatory drugs and aspirin have been tested extensively for polyp- and cancer-prevention. A recent randomized trial of aspirin (100 mg) for the prevention of cancer in women contained 39,000 women, who were followed-up for 10 years. No reduction in colorectal cancer risk was demonstrated [28]. Therefore, low-dose aspirin does not appear to be useful for chemoprevention of CRC in healthy women, at least over a 10-year time frame. However, cohort studies have suggested a lower risk in healthy subjects who take aspirin, and both aspirin and NSAIDS are effective in decreasing the number of polyps in patients with FAP, although not sufficiently to avoid colectomy [29]. The most effective agents for use in the setting are sulindac and celecoxib [29].

Statins (HMG-CoA reductase inhibitors designed for cholesterol reduction) and ursodeoxycholic acid may reduce the risk of colorectal cancer [30]; however, studies have mixed results and further analysis is warranted. Hormone replacement therapy was associated with decreased risk of colorectal cancer in prospective cohort studies, but randomized trials have shown mixed results. HRT can not currently be recommended for chemoprophylaxis of CRC [29]. In summary, several medications may provide a protective effect against colorectal polyps and cancer. However their use in average-risk persons has not been shown to reduce risk in randomized trials, and use should only be considered in high risk people such as those with FAP or multiple prior polyps [4].

Summary Recommendations for CRC Prevention

For people at average risk, regular screening starting at age 50 combined with a healthy lifestyle will minimize the risk of developing colorectal cancer. Healthy lifestyle recommendations include: limiting fat and red meat; eating more fruits, vegetables and dairy; and increasing fiber and whole grains. A daily multivitamin containing folate, plus additional calcium and vitamin D should be considered. In addition, quitting smoking, physical exercise, avoiding excessive alcohol intake, and maintaining a healthy weight should be recommended.

Inherited Colorectal Cancer Syndromes

About 80% of patients with CRC have no family history for the disease, but about 20% have a genetic syndrome or a familial predisposition to the disease [31]. Identifying those few patients with familial syndromes is important, because prophylactic surgery will be required to prevent premature cancer in affected family members. The two autosomal-dominant colorectal cancer syndromes are the hereditary non-polyposis colon cancer syndrome (HNPCC or Lynch syndrome) and familial polyposis (FAP). These syndromes account for less than 4 percent of CRC [32]. Other patients with a positive family history may have the recessively-inherited MYH mutation, or hereditary colorectal adenomas.

Even if there is no definable genetic syndrome in a family, a person with a first degree relative with colorectal cancer has a 2.25 relative risk of developing CRC [32]. It is important to take a detailed family history for patients with colorectal cancer or adenomas, in order to identify those patients who should be referred for genetic counseling, and whose family members should be screened and counseled.

Patients with twenty or more adenomas should definitely be referred for genetic testing, and first-degree relatives should be screened with colonoscopy, because a hereditary syndrome is likely. A strongly positive family history meeting the Amsterdam or Bethesda criteria should also have genetic testing and relatives must be screened. Furthermore, any patient under the age of 50 with colorectal cancer, or under age 40 with adenomatous polyps, should be considered for genetic counseling and testing [31]. At the very least, first degree relatives of such a patient must be counseled to undergo colonoscopy, beginning at an age 10 years earlier than the earliest age of diagnosis in the family.

Screening for Colorectal Cancer

The rationale for colorectal cancer screening derives from the knowledge that colorectal cancers begin as pre-malignant adenomatous polyps. Early detection and removal of adenomatous polyps prevents cancers. There is strong evidence from randomized controlled trials to show that the cancer cases and mortality are decreased by screening, followed by the removal of pre-cancerous polyps or early treatment of cancers [33]. For fecal occult blood testing (FOBT), screening results in an absolute risk reduction for colorectal cancer death of between 0.8 and 4.6 per 1000. Seen another way, between 217 and 1250 persons will need to be regularly screened to prevent one death from colorectal cancer [33].

Women and men at average risk for the development of colorectal cancer are currently recommended to begin screening at age 50. The "best" method for population screening for colorectal cancer is a matter of considerable debate [34]. Options for screening average-risk patients include: annual or biennial FOBT (with a home testing kit such as Hemoccult II); flexible sigmoidoscopy every 5 years; colonoscopy every 10 years; a combination of FOBT and sigmoidoscopy; or double-contrast barium enema every 5 years [4]. In addition to these well-established tests, new tests such as "virtual colonoscopy" (also called CT colonography) and stool-based molecular screening are becoming available. There are pros and cons to each of these screening strategies; and the main issues are risk, sensitivity, cost, patient compliance and resource availability.

At present, Cancer Care Ontario, Health Canada and the Canadian Task Force on Preventive Health Care recommend annual or biennial FOBT for all people over age 50 [2]. Positive tests must be followed-up by a full colon examination with colonoscopy (preferably) or double-contrast barium enema. Rates of screening for colorectal cancer are much poorer than cancer screening for cervical cancer or breast cancer; approximately 20% of eligible persons are screened in Ontario [35]. A concerted effort to improve this statistic is underway in Ontario [2]. A recent study in Alberta showed that only 7.7% of people aged 50-59, and 12.5% of people 60-69 had an FOBT test in the last 2 years. Amongst women in the study, having a recent Pap test or mammogram, being employed or having a higher educational level were associated with a greater likelihood of having colorectal cancer screening [36].

In the USA, colorectal cancer screening rates have increased in recent years, and 43.1% of eligible women were screened in 2003 [37]. Much of the increase is attributable to increased colonoscopy rates. Women were slightly less likely than men to be screened, perhaps due to the perception of women that CRC is a "male" disease. Factors associated with being more likely to be screened included: having a higher educational level, having health insurance, older age (>65 years), having a "usual source" for health care, being a former smoker, having recently talked with a general doctor, having a greater number of recent doctors' visits, having a recent Pap test or mammogram, and having a non-Hispanic gender [37]. Women's preference for female practitioners may be another barrier to screening [38].

The above recommendations for CRC screening apply to asymptomatic people at average risk for colorectal cancer. Symptomatic patients or patients at increased risk of colorectal cancer (Table 2) should undergo colonoscopy at more frequent intervals.

Symptoms

Early colorectal cancers are usually asymptomatic, but may be detected by screening. Later signs and symptoms of colorectal cancer include rectal bleeding, a change in the bowel habits, abdominal pain and weight loss [4]. Microcytic anemia in an older person is colorectal cancer, until proven otherwise. Rectal cancers can cause rectal pain and bloody or mucus discharge. Symptoms may mimic hemorrhoids, but careful digital rectal examination will make the diagnosis clear in many cases.

Stage and Prognosis

When a person is diagnosed with colorectal cancer, the first priorities are addressing immediate risks to the patient such as bowel obstruction or bleeding, and determining the stage of the cancer. Chest X-ray, CT scan of the Abdomen and pelvis, and CEA level are routinely obtained to estimate stage. In addition, full colonoscopy or barium enema is required to determine if synchronous polyps or tumors elsewhere in the colon will require treatment, unless significant obstruction is present. PET scan is a valuable tool for staging a patient with questionable findings by CT scanning, but is not routinely used. For rectal cancer 12 cm or less from the anal verge, a transanal ultrasound or pelvis MRI is recommended to assess the status of mesorectal lymph nodes and the depth of wall-penetration of the primary tumor, because these factors will determine who should have preoperative chemoradiotherapy. A colorectal surgeon, surgical oncologist or general surgeon is the primary practitioner who coordinates the care of a patient with curable colorectal cancer.

Stages I and II colorectal cancer represent lymph node-negative disease, while Stage III is lymph-node positive ("regional"). Stage IV means that distant metastases are present. The most common location for distant metastasis is the liver. The distribution of stage at diagnosis and 5-year survival by stage are shown in Figure 1 (USA data) [1].

Figure 1. Stage at Diagnosis and Prognosis by Stage*.

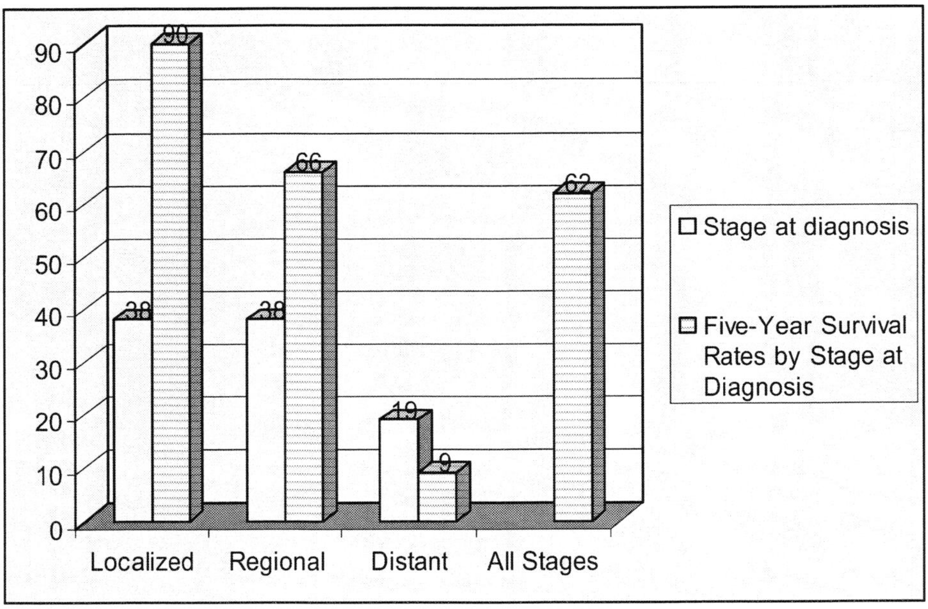

Table 4. Stage Definitions for Colorectal Cancer

AJCC Stage	TNM	Dukes Stage
I	T1/2, N0, M0	A
II	T3/4, N0, M0	B
III	Any T, N1/2, M0	C
IV	Any T, Any N, M1	

Treatment

The primary treatment for curable colorectal cancer is surgery. The exact combination of therapies used depends on the Tumor-Node-Metastasis (TNM) Stage of the cancer (Table 4), the overall health status of the patient and the patient's preferences [39]. Stage I colorectal cancer is curatively treated by surgery alone. Stage II disease is treated by surgery with or without adjuvant chemotherapy. The use of adjuvant chemotherapy for stage II colorectal cancer is established for low rectal cancers, in which case it is combined with pelvic radiotherapy. For Stage II colon cancer, adjuvant chemotherapy was not felt to be beneficial until recent evidence showed a small benefit in Stage II colon cancer patients, particularly with high-risk features such as poor differentiation, lymphovascular invasion or T4 tumors. Because the survival advantage is modest amongst Stage II patients, adjuvant chemotherapy is currently used selectively in this situation [39].

There is great research interest in identifying molecular markers that will help to stratify patients, particularly with Stage II colon cancer, into high and low risk groups. This would allow better selection of people likely to benefit from chemotherapy or biologic therapies. Microsatellite instability (MSI) and loss of heterozygosity at chromosome 18q are possible markers under study in clinical trials.

The benefit of adjuvant chemotherapy for Stage III CRC is well-established [40]. Recent trials have confirmed the superiority of FOLFOX (5-fluorouracil/leukovorin and oxaliplatin) over 5-FU/leukovorin in the adjuvant setting, showing an approximate 5% improvement in disease-free survival over 5-FU/leukovorin [41]. As a result, FOLFOX is becoming the standard adjuvant treatment in Stage III and selected Stage II patients.

For Stage IV colorectal cancer, treatment is highly individualized. Surgical resection of the primary tumor is recommended if it is symptomatic and/or the life expectancy is long. Limited metastatic disease may be treated for cure in good-risk patients with single-sided liver or lung metastases, in whom staged or synchronous surgical resection is performed. In highly-selected patients with surgical resection of liver metastases, five-year survival of approximately 30% has been achieved [42]. Even the use of a combination of liver resection and radiofrequency ablation for bi-lobar liver metastatic disease may be considered in selected, healthy patients.

Whether or not the disease is resectable, chemotherapy clearly improves survival in Stage IV CRC [43-45]. Standard chemotherapy for Stage IV CRC is FOLFOX or FOLFIRI (5-FU/leukovorin plus irinotecan), often with the addition of bevacizumab or cetuximab biologic therapy. Median overall survival of 20 months has been achieved using these treatments for Stage IV CRC [44]. The timing of surgical intervention, radiation and medical treatments must be individualized, and presentation of these patients in a multidisciplinary tumor board is essential when aggressive treatment is warranted.

Management of the "Malignant Polyp"

The finding of early invasive cancer (T1) within a completely-excised polyp is an area of controversy. If the polyp is completely excised as a single specimen, the margins are definitely negative, and the histologic features are uniformly favorable, selected patients can be observed, after marking the site with india ink on repeat endoscopy [46]. The rationale for this management strategy is that in such a situation the statistical likelihood of lymph node metastasis is very low. Specimens should be reviewed with the pathologist to confirm the histologic features.

Advances in Chemotherapy for Colorectal Cancer

Significant advances have been made in pharmacotherapy for colorectal cancer in recent years. Traditionally, 5-fluorouracil and leukovorin were used for adjuvant and palliative treatment of colorectal cancer. The most important new treatments are oxaliplatin and irinotecan as new chemotherapeutic agents, and the biologic agents bevacizumab (Avastin) and cetuximab. In addition, an oral form of fluorouracil, capecitabine (Xeloda), may have equivalent efficacy and allow for oral administration [44]. Increased sensory neurotoxicity with oxaliplatin had been dose-limiting in many patients, and neuroprotective treatments are under study.

Future directions in the treatment of colorectal cancer include: increased use of laparoscopic surgery; use of new biologic agents in the adjuvant setting; increased use of adjuvant therapy in Stage II disease; and increased surgical resection and/or ablation for stage IV disease.

Surgery for Colon Cancer

Surgery for colon cancer involves removal of a segment of the intestine, with re-connection of the two ends. The extent of resection depends primarily on the vascular supply of the involved part of the large intestine, because removal of accompanying lymph nodes requires division of the mesenteric blood vessels near their origins. Practically speaking, tumors of the ascending colon require right hemicolectomy, tumors of the descending colon require left hemicolectomy, sigmoid tumors may be treated by sigmoid colectomy, and the resection for transverse colon cancers varies depending on the relationship of the individual tumor to associated mesenteric blood vessels. Randomized trials have proven that laparoscopic surgery provides equivalent 5-year colon cancer outcomes to open surgery, at least when performed by surgeons experienced in the technique of laparoscopic colon surgery [47]. Tumors excluded from the multi-institutional, North American COST trial included tumors invading other organs or structures (T4 tumors), transverse colon tumors, and rectal tumors [47], and these tumors should be approached via conventional surgery for most patients at present. A "learning curve" of laparoscopic colon surgery for benign diseases should be completed by a surgeon prior to offering laparoscopic surgery for colon cancer.

Short-term quality of life is improved by laparoscopic surgery, compared to open surgery [48,49]. Advantages include decreased postoperative pain, a smaller scar, slightly reduced length of hospitalization, and slightly lower complication rates [48]. It should be noted that all of the information of laparoscopic surgery for colon cancer comes from specialized centers and surgeons, and the translation of these benefits to the surgical community as a whole has not been proven.

Surgery for colon cancer carries a very low risk of death within 30 days of surgery, ranging from about 1% for elective surgery in a specialized center [47,50] to about 4-5% when emergent procedures and patients with serious comorbidities are added into the population mix [51]. Complication rates for elective surgery are about 20%, most of which are minor [47]. After surgery for colon cancer, most patients will have normal bowel function, as the remainder of the intestine compensates for the segment removed. A temporary or permanent ostomy is rarely required for treatment of colon cancer. One exception is the case of an obstructing, left-sided cancer, in which case a temporary colostomy or ileostomy is selectively used [52].

SURGERY FOR RECTAL CANCER

Surgery for rectal cancer differs from surgery for colon cancer, due to the pelvic location of the tumor, which places nerves and reproductive organs at risk for temporary or permanent injury. In addition, removing part of the rectum may have a significant impact on the bowel function or, rarely, require a permanent colostomy. Another major difference is the use of radiation therapy before or after surgery to reduce the risk of local recurrence and improve survival.

There are three broad categories of surgery for rectal cancer: anterior resection (AR), abdominoperineal resection (APR), and trans-anal excision (TAE). AR is the operation of choice in healthy patients with rectal cancers, in whom the tumor is at least 1 cm above the anal sphincters. If the tumor is in the upper rectum, AR carries a lower risk of nerve damage and significant bowel function changes compared to a "low AR", in which the anastomosis is in the low rectum. Quality of life and bowel function are improved with a "pouch" reconstruction of the rectum [53]. Many patients having a low AR operation will require a temporary ileostomy for several months.

APR is required when technical or tumor factors require removal of the anus to achieve an adequate margin around the tumor. In this case, a permanent colostomy is required and the patient has an incision on the perineum as well as the abdomen. Newer surgical techniques and preoperative radiation therapy have greatly decreased the frequency with which this operation is required. Transanal excision of rectal cancers is limited to small, low, early-stage (T1) tumors with good histologic features. Even in these situations, transanal excision for rectal cancer has a higher recurrence rate than radical surgery, and radical surgery is the "gold standard" for treatment in good-risk patients [54]. This is a situation in which patients' preferences are important in the risk-benefit analysis.

Radiation therapy, usually combined with chemotherapy in North America, has become an important part of the treatment for low- and mid-rectal cancers with positive lymph nodes or full-thickness penetration through the rectal wall (T3/4). Preoperative (neoadjuvant) radiotherapy is preferred in cases where preoperative staging by transanal ultrasound, CT or MRI shows mesorectal lymphadenopathy or invasion of the tumor through the full-thickness of the muscular layer of the rectal wall [55-58]. In these situations, local recurrence rates and survival are both improved by neoadjuvant treatment [55-60]. Preoperative treatment may also improve the likelihood that an AR can be performed, rather than APR. If the stage is not clear, postoperative chemoradiotherapy can be given selectively based on the surgical pathology results [60].

Chemo-radiotherapy is clearly beneficial to selected patients with rectal cancer. However, the short-term and long-term toxicity of radiation treatment is significant, and patients should be well-informed.

Postoperative Recovery

After surgery for colorectal cancer, most patients spend between 3 and 7 days in the hospital. An epidural analgesia catheter, a patient-controlled narcotic pump (PCA), or intermittently-dosed pain medicine may be used for pain control. Thoracic epidural analgesia may be superior to PCA in terms of pain control and postoperative ileus, although these are not routinely done in all hospitals [61]. Early ambulation is encouraged after surgery, and clear liquids are often allowed within 48 hours of surgery. It is common for patients to feel fatigued for 4-6 weeks after surgery, and most will require extra help at home during recovery.

Bowel Function after Rectal Cancer Treatment

After colon cancer surgery, bowel changes are uncommon. However, rectal surgery frequently causes changes in the bowel function. The severity of these changes is determined by how low the anastomosis is, whether or not radiation treatment was given, the type of surgical reconstruction performed, and individual patient variation. With very low rectal anastomoses, median 24-hour bowel frequency is about 6.4 at 3 months and 3.5 at one year [62]. These numbers are improved to a median of 2 times per day at both time points if a pouch reconstruction is performed [62]. Other problems include nocturnal bowel movements, fecal urgency, incontinence or leakage of stool which requires wearing a pad, and a feeling of incomplete evacuation. Older patients and those with impaired continence preoperatively may have particular difficulty compensating for the bowel changes. Anti-diarrheal medication and fiber supplementation are frequently required, even one year postoperatively [62,63]. Patients can be reassured by evidence showing that most individuals see improvement in bowel function up to one year after surgery.

Ostomies

Permanent or temporary ostomies are infrequently required in the modern treatment of CRC. However, having an ostomy causes a change in the body image, and may negatively impact on the quality of life, although this is controversial [64]. Fortunately, modern ostomy appliances are excellent, and a completely normal lifestyle is possible for patients with ostomies. The services of a WOCN-certified enterostomal nurse is extremely valuable for preoperative and postoperative care of the patient with a temporary or permanent ostomy. Many support groups are also available.

Female Sexual and Urinary Function

Female sexual function has seldom been measured after treatment for rectal cancer, while male sexual problems due to nerve damage from surgery and radiation were recognized long ago. Recent research has finally begun to shed some light on this under-recognized problem. Our recent study of 81 women, curatively treated for rectal cancer, showed that almost 30% of women felt that their treatment had a negative impact on their sexual function [65]. Sexual problems varied, and included dyspareunia (in almost half of the women), loss of libido, problems with arousal, lubrication, and orgasm. The ostomy had a negative impact for about one-third of those with an ostomy. Older age, radiation therapy, and having an APR made sexual dysfunction more likely. Our hypothesis is that scarring of the pelvis, nerve damage, stress surrounding the cancer diagnosis and changes in body image each has a role in these problems. Of note, only 9% of the women remembered any preoperative discussion of potential sexual effects of surgery [65]. Greater awareness of this issue is needed.

For women with rectal cancer who receive pelvic radiation therapy, sexual dysfunction is probably worse. Possible therapeutic interventions for women with sexual dysfunction after radiation therapy (mixed cancer diagnoses) was performed by the Cochrane Collaboration, but the quality of the evidence was found to be poor. Nevertheless, the use of topical estrogens and benzydamine to the vagina is supported by randomized trials, for the treatment of acute radiation toxicity [66].

Quality of Life

After curative treatment for colorectal cancer, overall quality of life is excellent, particularly after 3 years, at which time full recovery from surgery and chemotherapy has been achieved. Most patients with long-term remission from colon cancer have a quality of life that is similar to age-matched controls [67]. Cancer recurrence is the most important factor impacting on the quality of life. For rectal cancer, numerous studies have confirmed that despite bowel and sexual changes, the overall quality of life is very high amongst survivors [65,68,89], including those with ostomies.

Surveillance

About 80% of curatively-treated patients who experience disease recurrence do so within the first 3 years [70]. Regular cancer surveillance (or "follow-up") is recommended for all patients with stage II/III disease, who are candidates for additional treatment, until 5 years. Stage I cancer patients have a very low risk of recurrence, and surveillance is not thought to improve outcome. Early-stage rectal cancer patients treated by transanal excision or whose tumors were pathologically down-staged by preoperative chemo-radiotherapy are exceptions, and should have intensive surveillance. The rationale for cancer surveillance is the early detection of recurrent CRC. While the majority of patients with disease recurrence will die of colorectal cancer, a minority can be treated for their recurrence with curative intent. It is these patients for whom surveillance is designed.

There is good evidence to show that "intensive" colorectal cancer surveillance improves overall survival for Stage II/III patients, and a 20-33% lower risk of death has been shown in metaanalyses [71,72]. However, the best surveillance regimen is not clear from existing evidence [72], and this is a controversial area. Surveillance should be performed by the surgeon or medical oncologist who is coordinating care. The American Society of Clinical Oncology currently recommends intensive surveillance for 3 years, and less intensive for 2 additional years [71]. For the first 3 years, CEA measurement is performed every 3 months, starting after completion of 5-FU-based chemotherapy, which can falsely elevate the CEA. History and physical examination are performed every 3-6 months for 3 years, then every 6 months for years 4-5. In addition, annual chest, abdomen and pelvis CT scan is performed for 3 years. Colonoscopy is recommended postoperatively if not complete preoperatively. If complete preoperatively it should be performed at 3 years, and then every 5 years if normal.

For rectal cancer patients, sigmoidoscopy should be performed about every 6 months, particularly if no radiation therapy was performed or if trans-anal excision was used as surgical therapy. Finally, all patients should be counseled to report symptoms or signs such as abdominal pain, bowel changes, anorexia, weight loss or a mass as soon as they occur. However, most patients who develop symptomatic recurrences are not curable.

Conclusion

Colorectal cancer is a significant public health concern for women. Prevention of CRC is possible with the use of a timely, risk-stratified screening strategy and a healthy lifestyle. High priority should be given to improving rates of CRC screening in North America. Women with CRC can expect a good outcome if the disease is discovered and treated at an early stage; and new advances in chemotherapy have improved the outlook even for women with advanced disease. Overall quality of life is preserved after curative treatment for colorectal cancer, but rectal cancer patients may experience sexual dysfunction and changes in body image. Recognition of these concerns and support for those affected is important.

References

[1] Jemal A, Tiwari RC, Murray T, et al. Cancer statistics, 2004. *CA Cancer J Clin* 2004;54:8-29.

[2] Website CCO. *Cancer Incidence and Mortality in Ontario* 1964-2002, 2006.

[3] Society CC. *Colorectal Cancer Stats*, 2006.

[4] Society AC. *Cancer Facts and Figures* 2006. Atlanta: American Cancer Society, 2006.

[5] Gibbons L, Waters C, Mao Y, Ellison L. Trends in colorectal cancer incidence and mortality. *Health Rep* 2001;12:41-55.

[6] Sturmer T, Glynn RJ, Lee IM, Christen WG, Hennekens CH. Lifetime cigarette smoking and colorectal cancer incidence in the Physicians' Health Study I. *Journal of the National Cancer Institute* 2000;92:1178-81.

[7] Larsen IK, Grotmol T, Almendingen K, Hoff G. Lifestyle as a predictor for colonic neoplasia in asymptomatic individuals. *BMC Gastroenterology* 2006;6:5.

[8] Michels KB, Giovannucci E, Chan AT, Singhania R, Fuchs CS, Willett WC. Fruit and vegetable consumption and colorectal adenomas in the Nurses' Health Study. *Cancer Res* 2006;66:3942-53.

[9] Wei EK, Giovannucci E, Wu K, et al. Comparison of risk factors for colon and rectal cancer. *Int J Cancer* 2004;108:433-42.

[10] Neugut AI, Garbowski GC, Lee WC, et al. Dietary risk factors for the incidence and recurrence of colorectal adenomatous polyps. A case-control study. [see comment]. *Annals of Internal Medicine* 1993;118:91-5.

[11] Willett WC, Stampfer MJ, Colditz GA, Rosner BA, Speizer FE. Relation of meat, fat, and fiber intake to the risk of colon cancer in a prospective study among women.[see comment]. *New England Journal of Medicine* 1990;323:1664-72.

[12] Fuchs CS, Giovannucci EL, Colditz GA, et al. Dietary fiber and the risk of colorectal cancer and adenoma in women. *N Engl J Med* 1999;340:169-76.

[13] Kato I, Akhmedkhanov A, Koenig K, Toniolo PG, Shore RE, Riboli E. Prospective study of diet and female colorectal cancer: the New York University Women's Health Study. *Nutrition & Cancer* 1997;28:276-81.

[14] Bingham SA, Day NE, Luben R, et al. Dietary fibre in food and protection against colorectal cancer in the European Prospective Investigation into Cancer and Nutrition (EPIC): an observational study. *Lancet* 2003;361:1496-501.

[15] Michels KB, Fuchs CS, Giovannucci E, et al. Fiber intake and incidence of colorectal cancer among 76,947 women and 47,279 men. *Cancer Epidemiol Biomarkers Prev* 2005;14:842-9.

[16] Asano TK, McLeod RS. Dietary fibre for the prevention of colorectal adenomas and carcinomas [Systematic Review]: *Cochrane Database of Systematic Reviews* 2006;(3).

[17] McKeown-Eyssen GE, Bright-See E, Bruce WR, et al. A randomized trial of a low fat high fibre diet in the recurrence of colorectal polyps. Toronto Polyp Prevention Group. [erratum appears in J Clin Epidemiol 1995 Feb;48(2):i]. *Journal of Clinical Epidemiology* 1994;47:525-36.

[18] Giovannucci E, Stampfer MJ, Colditz GA, et al. Multivitamin use, folate, and colon cancer in women in the Nurses' Health Study.[see comment]. *Annals of Internal Medicine* 1998;129:517-24.

[19] Greenberg ER, Baron JA, Tosteson TD, et al. A clinical trial of antioxidant vitamins to prevent colorectal adenoma. Polyp Prevention Study Group. [see comment]. *New England Journal of Medicine* 1994;331:141-7.

[20] Albanes D, Malila N, Taylor PR, et al. Effects of supplemental alpha-tocopherol and beta-carotene on colorectal cancer: results from a controlled trial (Finland) [see comment]. *Cancer Causes & Control* 2000;11:197-205.
[21] Weingarten MA, Zalmanovici A, Yaphe J. Dietary calcium supplementation for preventing colorectal cancer and adenomatous polyps. [update of Cochrane Database Syst Rev. 2004;(1):CD003548; PMID: 14974021]. *Cochrane Database of Systematic Reviews* 2005:CD003548.
[22] Shaukat A, Scouras N, Schunemann HJ. Role of supplemental calcium in the recurrence of colorectal adenomas: a metaanalysis of randomized controlled trials. [see comment]. *American Journal of Gastroenterology* 2005;100:390-4.
[23] Cho E, Smith-Warner SA, Spiegelman D, et al. Dairy foods, calcium, and colorectal cancer: a pooled analysis of 10 cohort studies. *J Natl Cancer Inst* 2004;96:1015-22.
[24] Wactawski-Wende J, Kotchen JM, Anderson GL, et al. Calcium plus vitamin D supplementation and the risk of colorectal cancer. [see comment]. *New England Journal of Medicine* 2006;354:684-96.
[25] Mao Y, Pan S, Wen SW, Johnson KC. Physical inactivity, energy intake, obesity and the risk of rectal cancer in Canada. *Int J Cancer* 2003;105:831-7.
[26] Lee IM, Manson JE, Ajani U, Paffenbarger RS, Jr., Hennekens CH, Buring JE. Physical activity and risk of colon cancer: the Physicians' Health Study (United States). *Cancer Causes & Control* 1997;8:568-74.
[27] Cho E, Smith-Warner SA, Ritz J, et al. Alcohol intake and colorectal cancer: a pooled analysis of 8 cohort studies. *Ann Intern Med* 2004;140:603-13.
[28] Cook NR, Lee IM, Gaziano JM, et al. Low-dose aspirin in the primary prevention of cancer: the Women's Health Study: a randomized controlled trial. *Jama* 2005;294:47-55.
[29] Raju R, Cruz-Correa M. Chemoprevention of colorectal cancer. *Dis Colon Rectum* 2006;49:113-24; discussion 124-5.
[30] Poynter JN, Gruber SB, Higgins PD, et al. Statins and the risk of colorectal cancer. *N Engl J Med* 2005;352:2184-92.
[31] American Gastroenterological Association medical position statement: hereditary colorectal cancer and genetic testing. *Gastroenterology* 2001;121:195-7.
[32] Church JM. A scoring system for the strength of a family history of colorectal cancer. *Dis Colon Rectum* 2005;48:889-96.
[33] Walsh JME, Terdiman JP. Colorectal cancer screening: scientific review. [see comment]. *JAMA* 2003;289:1288-96.
[34] McLeod RS, Canadian Task Force on Preventive Health C. Screening strategies for colorectal cancer: a systematic review of the evidence.[see comment]. *Canadian Journal of Gastroenterology* 2001;15:647-60.
[35] Rabeneck L, Paszat LF. A population-based estimate of the extent of colorectal cancer screening in Ontario. *American Journal of Gastroenterology* 2004;99:1141-4.
[36] McGregor SE, Bryant HE. Predictors of colorectal cancer screening: a comparison of men and women. *Can J Gastroenterol* 2005;19:343-9.

[37] Meissner HI, Breen N, Klabunde CN, Vernon SW. Patterns of colorectal cancer screening uptake among men and women in the United States. *Cancer Epidemiol Biomarkers Prev* 2006;15:389-94.

[38] Menees SB, Inadomi JM, Korsnes S, Elta GH. Women patients' preference for women physicians is a barrier to colon cancer screening. *Gastrointestinal Endoscopy* 2005;62:219-23.

[39] NCCN Practice Guidelines in Oncology v.2.2006: Colon Cancer. *NCCN Practice Guidelines in Oncology v.2.*2006, 2006.

[40] Gill S, Loprinzi CL, Sargent DJ, et al. Pooled analysis of fluorouracil-based adjuvant therapy for stage II and III colon cancer: who benefits and by how much? *J Clin Oncol* 2004;22:1797-806.

[41] Andre T, Boni C, Mounedji-Boudiaf L, et al. Oxaliplatin, fluorouracil, and leucovorin as adjuvant treatment for colon cancer. *N Engl J Med* 2004;350:2343-51.

[42] Simmonds PC, Primrose JN, Colquitt JL, Garden OJ, Poston GJ, Rees M. Surgical resection of hepatic metastases from colorectal cancer: a systematic review of published studies. *British Journal of Cancer* 2006;94:982-99.

[43] Jonker DJ, Maroun JA, Kocha W. Survival benefit of chemotherapy in metastatic colorectal cancer: a meta-analysis of randomized controlled trials. *British Journal of Cancer* 2000;82:1789-94.

[44] Meyerhardt JA, Mayer RJ. Systemic therapy for colorectal cancer. *N Engl J Med* 2005;352:476-87.

[45] Palliative chemotherapy for advanced or metastatic colorectal cancer. Colorectal Meta-analysis Collaboration. *Cochrane Database of Systematic Reviews* 2000:CD001545.

[46] Bond JH. Polyp guideline: diagnosis, treatment, and surveillance for patients with colorectal polyps. Practice Parameters Committee of the American College of Gastroenterology. *Am J Gastroenterol* 2000;95:3053-63.

[47] A comparison of laparoscopically assisted and open colectomy for colon cancer. *N Engl J Med* 2004;350:2050-9.

[48] Schwenk W, Haase O, Neudecker J, Muller JM. Short term benefits for laparoscopic colorectal resection. *Cochrane Database Syst Rev* 2005:CD003145.

[49] Abraham NS, Young JM, Solomon MJ. Meta-analysis of short-term outcomes after laparoscopic resection for colorectal cancer. [see comment]. *British Journal of Surgery* 2004;91:1111-24.

[50] Ko CY, Chang JT, Chaudhry S, Kominski G. Are high-volume surgeons and hospitals the most important predictors of in-hospital outcome for colon cancer resection? *Surgery* 2002;132:268-73.

[51] Schrag D, Panageas KS, Riedel E, et al. Surgeon volume compared to hospital volume as a predictor of outcome following primary colon cancer resection. *J Surg Oncol* 2003;83:68-78; discussion 78-9.

[52] De Salvo GL, Gava C, Pucciarelli S, Lise M. Curative surgery for obstruction from primary left colorectal carcinoma: primary or staged resection?[update of Cochrane Database Syst Rev. 2002;(1):CD002101; PMID: 11869622]. *Cochrane Database of Systematic Reviews* 2004:CD002101.

[53] Sailer M, Fuchs KH, Fein M, Thiede A. Randomized clinical trial comparing quality of life after straight and pouch coloanal reconstruction. [see comment]. *British Journal of Surgery* 2002;89:1108-17.

[54] Bentrem DJ, Okabe S, Wong WD, et al. T1 adenocarcinoma of the rectum: transanal excision or radical surgery? *Ann Surg* 2005;242:472-7; discussion 477-9.

[55] Mohiuddin M, Winter K, Mitchell E, et al. Randomized phase II study of neoadjuvant combined-modality chemoradiation for distal rectal cancer: Radiation Therapy Oncology Group Trial 0012. *Journal of Clinical Oncology* 2006;24:650-5.

[56] Allal AS, Bieri S, Pelloni A, et al. Sphincter-sparing surgery after preoperative radiotherapy for low rectal cancers: feasibility, oncologic results and quality of life outcomes. *British Journal of Cancer* 2000;82:1131-7.

[57] Improved survival with preoperative radiotherapy in resectable rectal cancer. Swedish Rectal Cancer Trial.[see comment][erratum appears in *N Engl J Med* 1997 May 22;336(21):1539]. *New England Journal of Medicine* 1997;336:980-7.

[58] Sauer R, Becker H, Hohenberger W, et al. Preoperative versus postoperative chemoradiotherapy for rectal cancer. *N Engl J Med* 2004;351:1731-40.

[59] Camma C, Giunta M, Fiorica F, Pagliaro L, Craxi A, Cottone M. Preoperative radiotherapy for resectable rectal cancer: A meta-analysis. *JAMA* 2000;284:1008-15.

[60] Glimelius B, Gronberg H, Jarhult J, Wallgren A, Cavallin-Stahl E. A systematic overview of radiation therapy effects in rectal cancer. *Acta Oncologica* 2003;42:476-92.

[61] Carli F, Trudel JL, Belliveau P. The effect of intraoperative thoracic epidural anesthesia and postoperative analgesia on bowel function after colorectal surgery: a prospective, randomized trial. *Diseases of the Colon & Rectum* 2001;44:1083-9.

[62] Hallbook O, Pahlman L, Krog M, Wexner SD, Sjodahl R. Randomized comparison of straight and colonic J pouch anastomosis after low anterior resection. *Ann Surg* 1996;224:58-65.

[63] Ho YH, Tan M, Seow-Choen F. Prospective randomized controlled study of clinical function and anorectal physiology after low anterior resection: comparison of straight and colonic J pouch anastomoses. *Br J Surg* 1996;83:978-80.

[64] Pachler J, Wille-Jorgensen P. Quality of life after rectal resection for cancer, with or without permanent colostomy. [update of Cochrane Database Syst Rev. 2004;(3):CD004323; PMID: 15266529]. *Cochrane Database of Systematic Reviews* 2005:CD004323.

[65] Hendren SK, O'Connor BI, Liu M, et al. Prevalence of male and female sexual dysfunction is high following surgery for rectal cancer. *Ann Surg* 2005;242:212-23.

[66] Denton AS, Maher EJ. Interventions for the physical aspects of sexual dysfunction in women following pelvic radiotherapy [Systematic Review]: *Cochrane Database of Systematic Reviews* 2006;(3).

[67] Ramsey SD, Andersen MR, Etzioni R, et al. Quality of life in survivors of colorectal carcinoma. *Cancer* 2000;88:1294-303.

[68] Camilleri-Brennan J, Steele RJ. Quality of life after treatment for rectal cancer. *Br J Surg* 1998;85:1036-43.

[69] Camilleri-Brennan J, Steele RJ. Prospective analysis of quality of life and survival following mesorectal excision for rectal cancer. *Br J Surg* 2001;88:1617-22.

[70] Sargent DJ, Wieand HS, Haller DG, et al. Disease-free survival versus overall survival as a primary end point for adjuvant colon cancer studies: individual patient data from 20,898 patients on 18 randomized trials. *J Clin Oncol* 2005;23:8664-70.

[71] Desch CE, Benson AB, 3rd, Somerfield MR, et al. Colorectal cancer surveillance: 2005 update of an American Society of Clinical Oncology practice guideline. *J Clin Oncol* 2005;23:8512-9.

[72] Jeffery GM, Hickey BE, Hider P. Follow-up strategies for patients treated for non-metastatic colorectal cancer [Systematic Review]: *Cochrane Database of Systematic Reviews* 2006;(3).

SECTION 4: GYNECOLOGIC CANCERS

Katharina E. Kieser*[1,*] *and Helen Steed*[2]

[1]Department of Obstetrics and Gynecology, Division of Gynecologic Oncology, Dalhousie University, Halifax, Nova Scotia, Canada;

[2]Department of Obstetrics and Gynecology, Division of Gynecologic Oncology, University of Alberta, Edmonton, Alberta, Canada.

ABSTRACT

With recent advancements in the diagnosis and treatment of cancer there has been a focus to individualize treatment. This has been the result of growing knowledge of cancer genetics, improvement in imaging technology and increasing evidence about adjuvant treatments.

In this chapter the diagnosis and treatment of gynecologic cancers will be discussed. The chapter will be divided into sections by anatomic tumor site; ovary and fallopian tube, uterus, cervix and vagina, and vulva. Each section will be subdivided into two major headings: diagnosis and treatment. The subsection on diagnosis will cover familial cancer syndromes, screening, signs and symptoms of disease, imaging techniques specific to that cancer site, biopsies and genetic testing. The new developments in familial cancer syndromes, genetic testing, and imaging will be emphasized. Diagnosis will be followed by a discussion of treatment options, focusing on the treatment of the most common tumor types of that site. A short discussion on the treatment of the rare pathologies will also be made. Each treatment strategy will be discussed in the context of the use of surgery, radiotherapy, chemotherapy and novel biologic therapies for the disease. For each strategy the expectations of response as well as side effects will be covered. In summary, in this chapter we will highlight the recent advances in the

* Correspondence concerning this article should be addressed to:
Katharina Kieser, Division of Gynecologic Oncology, Queen Elizabeth II Health Sciences Centre, VG Site 5th Floor, Room 5059, Dickson Building 5820 University Avenue, Halifax, Nova Scotia, Canada. B3H 1V7 Phone: 902 473-2366; Fax 902 473-7765; Email: katharina.kieser@cdha.nshealth.ca
Helen Steed, Division of Gynecologic Oncology, Cross Cancer institute 11560 University Ave NW Edmonton, Alberta, Canada. T6G 1Z2 Phone: 780 432-8560; Fax: 780 432-8888; Email: helenste@cancerboard.ab.ca.

diagnosis and treatment of gynecologic cancers orienting the contents to the scientific community who are involved in the education and treatment of these women.

INTRODUCTION

Gynecologic cancers include cancers that arise from the ovary, tubes, uterus, uterine cervix, vagina and vulva. These tumors are treated by a team of health care professionals interested in gynecologic oncology. Members of the team include oncology nurses, gynecologic pathologists, radiation oncologists, medical oncologists and gynecologic oncologists. Below we discuss the most common gynecologic malignancies; their epidemiology, diagnosis, treatment and follow-up along with specific recommendations for certain high risk groups such as germline mutation carriers in at risk families such as BRCA and, women with known premalignant conditions such as vulvar intraepithelial neoplasia.

In: Women and Cancer
Editor: Laurie Elit, pp. 131-146
ISBN: 978-1-60021-494-3

Chapter I

Ovarian Cancer

1. Incidence & Epidemiology

Epithelial ovarian cancer is the leading cause of death from gynecologic cancer in North America. In 2006, there will be an estimated 2500 new cases in Canada, and approximately 1500 women will die of this disease [1]. Ovarian cancer is the fourth most common cause of cancer death in woman and accounts for 4% of all cancer diagnoses. The lifetime risk of developing this disease is 1 in 70 and 1 in 100 women will die of ovarian cancer [2].

1.1. Risk Factors

The etiology of ovarian cancer is not known but risk factors include family history, Ashkenazi Jewish descent, infertility, low parity, and history of breast or colon cancer, Table 1. Use of oral contraceptives and history of tubal ligation are protective for ovarian cancer.

Table 1. Risk Factors for Ovarian Cancer

Risk Factor	Relative Risk
Nulligravidity	2-3
Infertility	2-5
North American/European	2-5
Family History	3-5
Ashkenazi Jewish descent	5
BRCA 1 carrier	50
Oral Contraceptive Use	0.3-0.6
Tubal Ligation	0.3

The incidence of ovarian cancer rises with increasing age and peaks in the fifth decade and then the rate plateaus [3]. There is a group of tumors called borderline or low malignant potential tumors that affect women of younger age, usually in their mid-forties. These tumors have a propensity to be confined to the ovary and have a good prognosis. They can recur many years later and thus, these women need appropriate follow up [4].

Ovarian cancer incidence varies among different ethnic backgrounds. It is highest among Caucasian women in Europe and North American and lower in women from South America and Asia [5].

Risk increases if there is a positive family history of ovarian cancer. Compared to the general population risk of 1.4%, a women with one relative affected has a 4-5% risk of ovarian cancer [6]. This risk increases to 7% if two related family members are affected. It is estimated that about 10% of ovarian cancers result from hereditary predisposition [7]. Women with hereditary cancer syndromes have an projected risk as high as 25-50% [8]. There are at least three genes that carry a genetic predisposition for ovarian cancer that have been identified. The most common of these is hereditary breast-ovarian cancer (HBOC). This syndrome accounts for 85-90% of all hereditary cases and the majority of cases are linked to the BRCA 1 locus located on chromosome 17 [9]. The second HBOC gene is BRCA 2 with a 27% risk of ovarian cancer [10]. Genetic studies have demonstrated that a higher carrier rate of BRCA1 and BRCA2 exists in women of Ashkenazi Jewish descent [11]. The appropriate management of women with increased risk is actively being studied. It has been suggested that they undergo screening ultrasound and follow up of CA125 levels, however, the value of this to alter prognosis has not be established. There is sufficient evidence to support prophylactic oophorectomy in known BRCA1 and 2 carriers [12,13]. Some clinicians advocate prophylactic hysterectomy in addition to oophorectomy due to the increased risk of tubal carcinoma and the proximal portion of the tube at the cornua can only truly be removed with a hysterectomy.

Ovarian cancer has been associated with nulliparity and infertility. Women who have been pregnant have a 30-60% reduction of ovarian cancer compared to women who have never carried a pregnancy [8]. This protective effect increases with increasing parity. The use of fertility enhancing drugs, such as clomiphene, and ovarian cancer risk is controversial. Results from most studies suggest that the higher risk in these women is related to infertility independent of drug use [14].

With regard to prevention, the use of the combined oral contraceptive pill has consistently demonstrated a 30-60% reduction in incidence for women who use the oral contraceptive for 5 or more years. It is the only currently proven preventative medication for ovarian cancer and may be recommended to women for this purpose [15]. Tubal ligation has also shown a decrease the incidence of ovarian cancer; however, for women at high risk of ovarian cancer considering a surgical option to decrease this risk an oophorectomy may be more appropriate.

2. Clinical Presentation

2.1. Signs and Symptoms

Unfortunately, the vast majority of women presenting with ovarian cancer have vague, nonspecific symptoms and lack early "warning signs" [16,17]. The earliest symptoms are often related to compression of surrounding organs. Patients may note pelvic pressure, urinary frequency or constipation. As the disease becomes more advanced affecting the upper abdomen, patients may experience symptoms such as abdominal distension, bloating, nausea, early satiety and altered bowel habits secondary to the accumulation of abdominal ascites, omental metastases or a growing abdominal mass [18]. Occasionally, a patient may have symptoms from a pleural effusion, such as shortness of breath, or may even present with a palpable inguinal or supraclavicular lymph node [19].

The most common sign is the finding of a pelvic mass on physical examination. The characteristics of the mass are important as malignancy must be differentiated from the many causes of benign ovarian masses. A solid, large, irregular and fixed pelvic mass is very suspicious for ovarian cancer, especially in the postmenopausal female. Other abdominal signs include a distended abdomen, presence of ascites or the palpation of an omental mass.

3. Screening Strategies

Many researchers are investigating methods that could be used to screen women at risk for ovarian cancer and to find ovarian cancer earlier. A significant way to improve overall survival for patients with ovarian cancer would be the ability to screen women and detect disease prior to its spread beyond the ovary.

Currently available methods that potentially could be used for screening include a pelvic examination, serum CA 125 measurements and pelvic/transvaginal ultrasonography. Unfortunately, the value of tumor markers and imaging to screen for ovarian cancer has not yet been determined.

Presently, there is no evidence that routine pelvic examination is effective in the early diagnosis of ovarian cancer [20].

CA 125 is a high-molecular weight glycoprotein that can be measured in patient sera. There are studies that support the suggestion that the use of CA 125 measurements may assist in the early diagnosis of ovarian cancer [21,22]. However, a literature review suggests that CA 125 is elevated in 50% of stage I and 60% of stage II ovarian cancers [23,24]. Therefore, alone it is unlikely to be an effective screening tool due to the low sensitivity for early disease and resultant false negatives. Another difficulty is its low specificity due to the many other gynecologic and non-gynecologic, benign and malignant causes of elevated CA 125 levels, Table 2.

Table 2. Conditions that may Elevate CA 125 Concentrations

Gynecologic	Non-gynecologic
Acute pelvic inflammatory disease	Acute hepatitis
Endometriosis	Acute pancreatitis
Uterine Leiomyomas	Cirrhosis
Functional ovarian cysts	Pneumonia
Menstruation	Pericarditis
Pregnancy	Congestive heart failure
Ovarian hyperstimulation	Diverticulitis
	Systemic lupus erythematosus
	Breast cancer
	Pancreatic cancer
	Lung cancer

CA 125 is a high-molecular weight glycoprotein that can be measured in patient sera. There are studies that support the suggestion that the use of CA 125 measurements may assist in the early diagnosis of ovarian cancer [21,22]. However, a literature review suggests that CA 125 is elevated in 50% of stage I and 60% of stage II ovarian cancers [23,24]. Therefore, alone it is unlikely to be an effective screening tool due to the low sensitivity for early disease and resultant false negatives. Another difficulty is its low specificity due to the many other gynecologic and non-gynecologic, benign and malignant causes of elevated CA 125 levels, Table 2.

Ultrasound is an effective method for visualizing the ovaries. Screening with transvaginal ultrasonography has been hopeful, yet there are still limitations with specificity. Sensitivity has been estimated at 95% for the detection of early ovarian cancer in the general population. However, due to low specificity ultrasonography alone may require up to 10-15 negative laparotomies for every ovarian cancer case found [25].

Thus, due to both the high false-positive and false-negative rates of both ultrasonography and serum CA 125 levels, it is not recommended that these tests be used routinely to screen the general population for ovarian cancer [26]. Current research is assessing new molecular markers and technologies, such as unique proteomic patterns that may better identify ovarian cancer as a screening test [27].

4. Diagnosis

4.1. Tumor Markers

As discussed above, the most commonly studied and currently available useful tumor marker for ovarian cancer is the CA 125 level. The preoperative determination of CA 125 may be helpful if there is a high suspicion of cancer. It is particularly useful in the postmenopausal women with an asymptomatic mass, where an elevated serum CA 125 (> 35U/ml) has a sensitivity of 97% and specificity of 78% [30].

However, its primary utility is in monitoring patient response to chemotherapy [28]. The serous histologic subtype of epithelial ovarian cancer has the highest incidence of elevated CA 125 levels (>85%), compared with mucinous tumors that rarely have elevated CA 125 levels [29]. If the CA 125 is markedly elevated prior to treatment then the decline can be useful in monitoring treatment. Recurrent elevation in CA125 can also be predictive of a recurrence.

4.2. Imaging

The actual diagnosis of ovarian cancer requires pathologic confirmation of cancer in ovarian tissue. However, ultrasonography is a very useful preoperative predictive tool in differentiating benign from malignant pelvic masses. There are features of the mass that combined with knowledge of the patient's age may suggest a higher likelihood of ovarian cancer. A high index of suspicion is warranted in women between the ages of 40 and 69 who have the following features on ultrasound, Table 3.

The use of other imaging tests is dictated by the initial history and physical exam findings to determine the extent of tumor or to help rule out other pelvic disorders. Helpful studies may be as follows. An CT pyelogram is used to assess the adjacent pelvic structures and the urinary system. A barium enema or colonoscopy is suggested in a postmenopausal woman with a pelvic mass and bowel complaints or elevated CEA marker indicative of possible colonic primary.

A CT scan or MRI should be individualized for each patient as it is not routinely valuable in the work up of a pelvic mass. If a women presents with only ascites and no mass, they can have a role in assessing other sites of primary cancer such as the liver and pancreas [31].

Other investigations that complete the preoperative work up include CBC, blood chemistries, chest film and any relevant consultations depending on personal history and physical examination.

Table 3. Ultrasonographic Findings concerning for Malignancy

Irregular borders
Multiple echogenic patterns within the mass
Dense multiple septae
Bilateral ovarian masses
Solid masses
Complex mass, size > 10 cm
Presence of ascites

4.3. Tissue biopsies

Due to the location of the ovaries deep within the pelvis, accessibility of preoperative biopsies is difficult. The definitive diagnosis usually comes from a staging laparotomy with multiple peritoneal biopsies performed at the time of surgery. Epithelial ovarian cancer is staged according to the International Federation of Gynecology and Obstetrics (FIGO) system. This is a surgical staging system based on the findings described at time of surgical exploration and the appropriate biopsies taken. The extent of disease spread can only be completely detected by exploratory laparotomy.

5. Prognostic Factors

5.1. Staging

Before planning any systemic treatment for a newly diagnosed ovarian cancer, accurate information about the surgical stage is required, Table 4. All patients who are medically fit for surgery should be considered for a full staging laparotomy performed by a gynecologic oncologist. The surgical procedure starts with an adequate midline incision to allow access to both the pelvis and upper abdomen. The ovarian tumor is removed intact without rupture if possible and free fluid is sent for cytology. In the absence of free fluid, peritoneal washings should be performed using normal saline. For most patients, a total abdominal hysterectomy and bilateral salpingoophorectomy is then performed. In patients who appear to have early disease with no visual disease beyond the ovary, all serosal surfaces should be inspected by palpation and biopsy samples taken from any suspicious areas. This includes assessment of the following: paracolic gutters, liver, gallbladder, both hemidiaphragms, both small and large intestine including its mesentery, appendix, and omentum. Several blind peritoneal biopsies are also performed as the most significant spread of ovarian cancer is exfoliation of cells into the peritoneal cavity. Also, a sampling from both the para aortic and pelvic lymph nodes should be completed [33]. The histology from these biopsies allows accurate staging according to the International Federation of Gynecology and Obstetrics (FIGO) system.

In a young woman who desires to maintain fertility, a unilateral salpingoophorectomy with staging may be performed if the tumor appears to be confined to the one ovary. A frozen section may be helpful to confirm malignancy. However, there can be false negatives; thus if high enough suspicion the surgeon should continue with detailed planned staging as outlined above [32].

Women with more advanced disease, as seen throughout the abdomen have at least FIGO stage IIIC and the extent of their surgery is outline in the section below under surgical treatment.

When surgical staging is performed adequately, a large number of patients thought to be early stage are often "upstaged". Young et al [34] reported that 30% of ovarian cancer patients considered stage I or II were upstaged to stage III or IV after a detailed staging laparotomy. There are also studies suggesting that this procedure should be performed by a gynecologic oncologist for proper surgical staging and improved patient outcomes [35].

When performed by a gynecologic oncologist, 97% of patients were properly staged versus less than 50% when surgery was performed by general gynecologists or general surgeons [36].

Table 4. FIGO Staging of Epithelial Ovarian Cancer

FIGO Stage		Features
I		Tumor confined to ovaries
	IA	Tumor limited to one ovary, capsule intact, no tumor on ovarian surface, no malignant ascites
	IB	Tumor limited to both ovaries, capsule intact, no tumor on ovarian surface, no malignant ascites
	IC	Tumor limited to one or both ovaries; with evidence of capsule ruptured, tumor on ovarian surface, malignant ascites
II		Tumor involves one or both ovaries with pelvic extension
	IIA	Extension on uterus and/or tubes, no malignant ascites
	IIB	Extension to other pelvic tissues, no malignant ascites
	IIC	Pelvic extension with malignant ascites
III		Tumor involves one or both ovaries with microscopically confirmed peritoneal metastasis outside the pelvis and/or regional lymph node involvement
	IIIA	Microscopic peritoneal metastasis beyond pelvis
	IIIB	Macroscopic peritoneal metastasis beyond pelvis, less than 2 cm in greatest dimension
	IIIC	Macroscopic peritoneal metastasis beyond pelvis, greater than 2 cm in greatest dimension, and/or regional lymph node involvement
IV		Distant metastasis (positive pleural effusions or intraparenchymal liver metastasis

Stage is the most important prognostic indicator in ovarian cancer. The 5-year survival of patients with epithelial ovarian cancer is directly correlated with the tumor stage. The majority of patients presents with advanced disease and have a poor prognosis. The 5-year survival of advanced stage III and IV disease is 15 to 20% and less than 5% respectively [37]. The early stage I tumors have a better prognosis. If it is confined to one ovary and early grade, 5 year survival can be greater than 90% for some subsets of patients with this disease.

5.2. Histology and Grade

Histologic grade has some prognostic significance especially in earlier stage disease. Stage I tumors with well-differentiated histology have a greater than 90% survival with surgery alone [37].

In general, the histologic subtype has little prognostic significance when compared with other factors such as stage and histologic grade. The vast majority of epithelial ovarian tumors are serous histology. The other types include mucinous, clear cell and endometrioid. Clear cell appears to have the worst prognosis when compared to the other types [38]. Endometrioid adenocarcinomas tend to have the best prognosis and are often associated with endometriosis [39]. This however is often related to the fact that endometrioid tumors present with lower grade and earlier clinical stage of disease.

5.3. Tumor Volume

Many studies have shown that the volume of residual disease after initial cytoreductive surgery correlates with overall survival [40,41]. Retrospective studies have suggested a 22 month improvement in median survival of patients who have been optimally cytoreduced [40,42]. The post-surgical macroscopic tumor-free status is an important prognostic factor for subsequent disease course.

6. Therapies

Treatment of ovarian cancer usually involves multi modality therapy. Surgical therapy is an important modality of treatment for all phases of ovarian cancer management. Nevertheless, it is unfortunately curative in only a small percentage of patients and usually adjunctive chemotherapy and sometimes radiotherapy are employed.

6.1. Surgery

For early stage I tumors confined to the ovary, surgical removal of the ovary with adequate surgical staging may be sufficient treatment of the disease. For properly staged low-risk epithelial ovarian cancer, survival is approximately 95% with no need for further therapy. Low risk patients have a stage IA, IB with a grade 1 or grade 2 tumor. Two recent randomized trials were recently reported on women with early-stage disease [44,45]. These studies included women with stage I and II, grade 2, 3 tumors. The final analysis of these 2 combined studies showed a survival benefit for the patients who received immediate postoperative chemotherapy amounting to a 7% absolute difference in overall survival at 5 years [44,45]. However a subgroup analysis suggested that there may be little benefit for patients who have been optimally staged.

Current treatment of advanced ovarian carcinoma consists of primary surgical tumor resection, "surgical debulking" followed by combination chemotherapy with carboplatin and paclitaxel. In patients who appear to have disease disseminated throughout the abdomen at laparotomy, all visible tumor deposits are removed where possible. The rationale for an aggressive surgical approach comes from several large retrospective studies, all of which have shown a survival advantage for patients who have had optimal debulking [40,42,43].

Despite advances in oncology surgery, optimal debulking is only possible ~ 50-70% of the time depending on surgical expertise [47,48]. There is a continuing debate as to whether the observed increased overall survival of individuals after optimal debulking is a result of surgical skill or inherent tumor biology [48,49].

An alternative to the standard approach of up front debulking surgery followed by chemotherapy is to treat initially with "neoadjuvant chemotherapy" followed by debulking surgery. Evidence suggests neoadjuvant chemotherapy decreases tumor volume and improves the chance of resectability of tumor deposits [50-53]. Chemotherapy can resolve pleural effusions and ascites, and improve performance status prior to surgery. Patients often have less intraoperative blood loss, shorter operative times, fewer admissions to intensive care post operatively and shorter lengths of stay in hospital. These issues are important in patients who often have medical co-morbidities that complicate surgical outcome. The EORTC (European Organization for Research and Treatment of Cancer) is currently conduction a randomized trial assessing the use of neoadjuvant chemotherapy. Until the conclusion of this trial, the standard of care should still be an attempt at initial cytoreductive surgery if the patient is medically fit for surgery.

6.2. Chemotherapy

The past 25 years have seen significant advances in the chemotherapy used to treat ovarian cancer that has spread beyond the ovary (Stage II-IV disease). A large number of clinical trials have led to the adoption of combination chemotherapy with carboplatin and paclitaxel as the international "standard of care". This choice is based on the results of sequential randomized controlled trials: from the synthesis of alkylating agents (chlorambucil and melphalan) in the 1950s; their use as single agents in the 1960s; the development of cisplatin and carboplatin in the 1970s and early 1980s, respectively; the controversies in the late 1980s about the addition of other drugs to cisplatin and the demonstration of the equal efficacy of cisplatin and carboplatin; through to the introduction of paclitaxel in the 1990s [54]. Randomized studies have demonstrated that cisplatin or carboplatin alone or in combination with other agents improve survival when used as first-line treatment of ovarian cancer compared with non-platinum-chemotherapy. In two randomized trials treatment with cisplatin plus paclitaxel resulted in improved survival compared with cisplatin plus cyclophosphamide [55,56].

At present, the standard of care in North America is to treat advanced ovarian cancer with carboplatin and paclitaxel after optimal debulking [57]. There is variation from center to center in terms of dose, duration of paclitaxel infusion, and the total number of cycles of treatment.

After more than 20 years of investigation, there are now three major North American phase III trials showing positive results for the use of intraperitoneal chemotherapy [58,60]. The most recent study observed an improvement in survival for those women treated with intravenous and intraperitoneal chemotherapy as adjuvant treatment following optimal cytoreductive surgery for ovarian cancer. These studies consistently show improved survival in a selected group of ovarian cancer patients. Intraperitoneal therapy can provide improved outcomes for patients with small-volume or no visible residual disease. The National Cancer Institute in the United States recently issued a clinical announcement in early 2006, supporting the use of intraperitoneal chemotherapy in this subset of ovarian cancer patients.

Intraperitoneal chemotherapy is appealing as the disease is most often confined to the intraperitoneal cavity and pharmacokinetic studies suggest an advantage to prolonged direct exposure of tumor to drug. However, there are treatment intricacies limiting acceptance primarily due to the presence of an intraperitoneal catheter, which may lead to short term potentially severe toxicities including infection, haemorrhage, bowel perforation, obstruction, and pain. Debate continues as to the optimal drug schedule of intravenous and intraperitoneal medications. In the most recent trial that showed a survival advantage for women who received intraperitoneal chemotherapy only 42% completed the 6 cycles.

Candidates for the intraperitoneal therapy include those in whom optimal surgical resection has been achieved. It is of crucial importance that the risks and complications of this therapy be discussed with the patient and this therapy offered by a team of medical professionals that have received appropriate training of this procedure.

6.3. Radiotherapy

Radiation therapy for ovarian cancer is not routinely used. However, whole abdominal radiotherapy is used in selected patients with metastatic ovarian cancer and no residual tumor in the upper abdomen [61]. There are no phase III trials comparing platinum-based chemotherapy with radiation therapy in low and intermediate risk patients. Most data comes from old retrospective studies.

There may also be a role for radiotherapy in women with a symptomatic isolated recurrence.

7. Follow-up & Recurrent Disease

Patients with early-stage ovarian cancer who had full staging and appropriate post operative care usually have a low recurrence rate. Suggested follow up consists of gynecologic examination every 3-4 months for the first two years and every 6 months for the next 3 years [62]. There is controversy about the use of CA 125 levels and ultrasounds in conjunction with the physical examination in follow up. The use of additional testing may increase patient anxiety due to false positive results and not improve the long term outcome by initiating treatment at the earliest opportunity [63]. These should be used at the discretion of the treating physician based on their center's philosophy and guidelines.

The survival of patients with advanced epithelial ovarian cancer has improved since the introduction of paclitaxel and carboplatin/cisplatin into first-line chemotherapy [55,56]. Unfortunately, between 50-80% of patients with advanced ovarian cancer relapse after achieving a complete clinical response to regimens such as paclitaxel plus carboplatin, and most of these patients are incurable. CA 125 levels are used to follow patient response during chemotherapy treatments. The value of continuing CA 125 levels during follow up is controversial given that the goal of treatment in the incurable patient should be to prolong the symptom free survival time, close follow of the CA 125 levels may be non-contributory.

When ovarian cancer recurs, the treatment goal shifts from cure to palliation and symptom-management. Since second-line treatments have limited curative potential, patients are offered therapy that may slow disease progression and supportive care emphasizing control of symptoms [64]. There are several cytotoxic agents shown to have significant activity in the setting of relapsed disease that help slow the progression of disease. There is no best second-line treatment agreed on for patients with recurrent disease [65].

When the interval from standard, initial treatment to recurrence is longer than 6 months, the disease is referred to as "platinum-sensitive" and many clinicians will re-treat patients with either carboplatin or cisplatin [66]. The response rate in this scenario is directly related to the length of the disease-free interval. The longer the disease free interval, the better the response.

Patients who relapse less than six months after the initial treatment with carboplatin or cisplatin are considered "platinum-resistant". There are numerous options available for subsequent chemotherapy. Topotecan [67], gemicitabine [68], oral etoposide [69], encapsulated doxorubicin [70] and docetaxel [71] have all been show to have activity in platinum-resistant disease and platinum-sensitive. Recently, Gordon et al [72] showed a survival advantage of pegylated liposomal doxirubicin in comparison to topotecan. The advantage for pegylated liposomal doxirubicin was more significant in platinum-sensitive disease in terms of progression free survival (PFS) and overall survival (OS). Patients also tolerated pegylated liposomal doxirubicin better than topotecan with fewer adverse events.

Numerous factors must be evaluated prior to the selection of the appropriate second-line drug, including extent of disease, patient performance status, and toxicity of treatment. Treatment is usually administered over 3 cycles and response assessed prior to continuing therapy.

Palliation and symptom control are managed by a multidisciplinary team including gynecologic oncology, palliative care, and family physicians. Symptoms such as pain, nausea, emesis, and constipation are common. Conservative therapy is the goal. Commonly prescribed therapies include opoids for pain, antinauseants such as ondansetron, metoclopramide, and bowel routines for constipation. Eventually many recurrent ovarian cancer patients have bowel obstructions which need decompression with either nasogastric tubes, surgery or permanent percutaneous enterogastric tubes.

8. Germ Cell Ovarian Cancer

Non epithelial ovarian cancers are rare and account for less than 10% of all ovarian cancers [73]. The most common non epithelial ovarian cancer is germ cell malignancies, specifically dysgerminomas. These tumors tend to affect young girls in their teens and twenties. The presentation can be acute with pain related to rupture and hemorrhage of the tumor. Tumor markers are especially helpful with these tumors and should include βHCG, AFP, and LDH.

The treatment is primarily surgical with removal of the ovarian tumor. Fertility sparing surgery is performed even if there is spread of disease, as these tumors are very sensitive to chemotherapy. The most frequently used chemotherapy for metastatic germ cell tumors is bleomycin, etoposide and cisplatin [74]. The prognosis is very positive with patients being diagnosed in early stage IA having greater than 95% survival. Even patients with advanced disease are achieving 90% survival after treatment with both surgery and chemotherapy.

References

[1] McGuire, V; Jesser, CA; Whittemore, AS. Survival among US women with invasive epithelial ovarian cancer. *Gynecol Oncol*, 2002 84, 399-403.

[2] Jemal, A ; Murray, T ; Samuels, A ; et al. Cancer Statistics 2003. *CA Cancer J Clin*, 2003 53, 2-26.

[3] Zanetta, G; Rota, S; Chiari, S; et al. Behavior of borderline tumors with particular interest to persistence, recurrence and progression to invasive carcinoma. A prospective study. *J Clin Oncol*, 2001 19, 2658-2664.

[4] Ferlay, J; Bray, F; Pisani, P; Parkin, D. GLOBOCAN 2000: *Cancer incidence, mortality and prevalence worldwide*. Version 1.0 IARC Cancer Base No. 5 Lyon, IARC Press, 2001.

[5] Whittemore, AS. Characteristics relating to ovarian cancer risk: implications for prevention and detection. *Gynecol Oncol*, 1994 55, S15-S19.

[6] Whittemore, AS; Gong, G; Itnyre J. Prevalence and contribution of BRCA1 mutations in breast and ovarian cancer: results from three US population-based case-control studies of ovarian cancer. *Am J Hum Genet*, 1997 60, 496-504.

[7] Daly, M, Obrams GI. Epidemiology and risk assessment for ovarian cancer. *Semin Oncol*, 1998 25, 255-264.

[8] Easton, DF; Ford, D; Bishop, DT. Breast Cancer Linkage Consortium: breast and ovarian cancer incidence in BRCA1-mutation carriers. *Am J Hum Genet*, 1995 56, 265-271.

[9] Frank, TS. Testing for hereditary risk of ovarian cancer. *Cancer Control* 1999 6, 327-334.

[10] Struewing, JP; Hartge, P; Wacholder, S; Baker, SM; Berlin, M McAdams, M; et al. The risk of cancer associated with specific mutations of BRCA1 and BRCA2 among Ashkenazi Jews. *N Engl J Med*, 1997 336, 1401-1408.

[11] Kauff, ND; Satagopan, JM; Robson, ME; Scheuer, L; Hensley, M; Hudis, C; et al. Risk-reducing salpingo-oophorectomy in women with BRCA1 or BRCA2 mutation. *N Engl J Med*, 2002 346, 1609-1615.

[12] Rebbeck, TR; Lynch, HT; Neuhausen, SL; Narod, SA; Vant Veer, L; Garber, JE; et al. Prophylactic oophorectomy in carriers of BRCA1 or BRCA2 mutations. *N Engl J Med*, 2002 346, 1616-1622.

[13] Ness, RB; Cramer, DW; Goodman, MT; Kjaer, SK; Mallin, K; Mosgaard, BJ; et al. Infertility, fertility drugs, and ovarian cancer : a pooled analysis of case-control studies. *Am J Epidemiol*, 2002 155, 217-224.

[14] Hankinson, SE ; Colditz, GA ; Hunter, DJ ; et al. A prospective study of reproductive factors and risk or epithelial ovarian cancer. *Cancer*, 1995 76, 284-290.

[15] Goff, BA; Masnedel, L; Muntz, HG; Melancon, CH. Ovarian carcinoma diagnosis. *Cancer*, 2000 9, 2068-2075.

[16] Olson, SH; Mignone, L; Nakraseive, C; Caputo, TA. Symptoms of ovarian cancer. *Obstet Gynecol*, 2001 98, 212-217.

[17] Vine, MF; Calingaert, B; Berchuck, A; Schildkraut, JM. Characterization of prediagnostic symptoms among primary epithelial ovarian cancer case and controls. *Gynecol Oncol*, 2003 90, 75-82.

[18] Berek, JC; Bast, RC. Ovarian cancer. In: Kufe, DW; Pollock, RE; Weichsebaum, RR; Bast, RC; Gansler, TS; Holland, JF; Frei, E. *Cancer medicine 6th Ed*. Hamilton ON: BC Decker; 2004; 1831-1861.

[19] De Preist, PD ; van Nagell, JR Jr ; Gallion, HH ; Shenson, D ; Hunter JE ; Andrews, SJ ; et al. Ovarian cancer screening in asymptomatic postmenopausal women. *Gynecol Oncol*, 1993 51, 205-209.

[20] Jacobs, IJ; Skates, S; Davies, AP; Woolas, RP; Jeyerajah, A; Weidemann, P; et al. Risk of diagnosis of ovarian cancer after raised serum CA 125 concentration: a prospective cohort study. *BMJ*, 1996 313,1355-1358.

[21] Skates, SJ; Wu, FJ; Yu, YH; Sjovall, K; Einhorn, N; Chang, Y; et al. Towards an optimal algorithm for ovarian cancer screening with longitudinal tumor markers. *Cancer*, 1995 76, 2004-2010.

[22] Einhorn, N; Sjovall, K; Knapp, RC; Hall, P; Scully, RE; Bast, RC Jr; Zurawski, VR Jr. A Prospective evaluation of serum CA 125 levels for early detection of ovarian cancer. *Obstet Gynecol*, 1992 80, 14-18.

[23] Zurawski, VR Jr; Orjaseter, H; Andersen, A; Jellum, E. Elevated serum CA 125 levelss prior to diagnosis of ovarian neoplasia: relevance for early detection of ovarian cncer. Int J *Cancer*, 1988 42, 677-680.

[24] Jacobs, I; Oram, D; Fairbanks, J; Turner, J; Frost, C; Grudzinskas, JF. A risk of malignancy index incorporating CA 125, ultrasound and menopausal status for the accurate preoperative diagnosis of ovarian cancer. *BJOG*, 1990 97, 922-929.

[25] National Institute of Health Consensus Development Conference Statement. Ovarian cancer: screening, treatment and follow-up. *Gynecolo Oncol*, 1994 55, S4.

[26] Petricoin, EF; Ardekani, AM; Hitt, BA; Levine, PJ; Fusaro, VA; Steinberg, SM; et al. Use of proteomic patterns in serum to identify ovarian cancer. *Lance*t, 2002 359, 572-577.

[27] Olt, GJ; Berchuck, A; Bast, RC. Gynecologic tumor markers. Semin Surg Oncol, 1990 6, 305-313.

[28] Niloff, JM; Bast, RC Jr; Schaetzl, EM; et al. Predictive value of CA 125 antigen levels in second-look procedures for ovarian cancer. *Am J Obstet Gynecol*, 1985 151, 981-986.

[29] Malkasian, GE Jr; Knapp, RC; Lavin, PT; et al. Preoperative evaluation of serum CA 125 levels in premenopausal and postmenopausal patients with pelvic masses: discrimination between benign and malignant disease. *Am J Obstet Gynecol*, 1988 159, 341-346.

[30] Togashi, K. Ovarian cancer; the clinical role of US, CT, and MRI. *Eur Radiol*, 2003 13 [Suppl 4], L87-104.
[31] Rose, PG; Rubin, RB; Nelson, BE; Hunter, RE; Reale, FR. Accuracy of frozen section (intraoperative consultation) diagnosis of ovarian tumors. *Am J Obstet Gynecol*, 1994 171(3), 823-826.
[32] Wu, PC; Lang, JH; Huang, RL; et al. Lymph node metastatsis and retroperitoneal lymphadenectomy in ovarian cancer. *Bailleres Clin Obstet Gynecol*, 1989 3, 143-155.
[33] Young, RC; Decker, DG; Wharton, JR; et al. Staging laparotomy in early ovarian cancer. *JAMA*, 1983 250, 3072-3076.
[34] Giede, C; Kieser, K; Dodge, J; Rosen, B. Who should operate on patients with ovarian cancer? An evidence-based review. *Gynecol Oncol*, 2005 99, 447-461.
[35] McGowan, L; Lesher, LP; Norris, HJ; et al. Misstaging of ovarianc cancer. *Obstet Gynecol*, 1985 65, 568-572.
[36] Heintz, APM; Odicino, F; Maisonneuve, P; Beller, U; Benedet, JL; Creasman, W; et al. Carcinoma of the ovary. 25th annual report on the results of treatment of gynecological cancer. *Int J Gynecol Obstet*, 2003 83, 135-166.
[37] Tammela, J; Geisler, JP; Eskew, PNJ; et al. Clear cel carcinoma of the ovary: poor prognosis compared to serous carcinoma. *Eur J Gynecol Oncol*, 1998 19, 438-440.
[38] Steed, H; Chapman, WB; Laframboise, S. Endometriosis associated ovarian cancer: A clinicopathologic review. *JOGC*, 2004 26(8), 709-15.
[39] Hacker, NF; Berek, JS; Lagasse, LD; et al. Primary cytoreductive surgery for epithelial ovarian cancer. *Obstet Gynecol*, 1983 61, 413-420.
[40] Delgado, G; Oram, DH; Petrilli, ES. Stage III epithelial ovarian cancer: the role of maximal surgical cytoreduction. *Gynecol Oncol*, 1984 18, 293-298.
[41] Hoskins, WJ; Bundy, BN; Thigpen, JT; et al. The influence of cytoreductive surgery on recurrence-free interval and survival in small-volume stage III epithelial ovarian cancer: a Gynecologic Oncology Group study. *Gynecol Oncol*, 1992 47, 159-66.
[42] Hoskins, WJ; McGuire, WJ; Brady, MF; et al. The effect of diameter of largest residual disease on survival after primary surgery in patients with sub optimal residual epithelial ovarian carcinoma. *Am J Obstet Gynecol*, 1994 170, 974-80.
[43] ICON 1: a randomized trial of adjuvant chemotherapy in women with early-stage ovarian cancer. *J Natl Cancer Inst*, 2003 95(2), 125-132.
[44] Impact of adjuvant chemotherapy and surgical staging in early-stage ovarian carcinoma: European Organization for Research and Treatment of Cancer –Adjuvant Chemotherapy in Ovarian Neoplasm Trial (ACTION). *J Natl Cancer Inst*, 2003 95(2), 113-125.
[45] ICON 1 and ACTION: two parallel randomized phase III trials of adjuvant chemotherapy in patients with early-stage ovarian carcinoma. *J Natl Cancer Inst*, 2003 95(2), 105-112.
[46] Hunter, RW; Alexander, ND; Soutter, WP. Meta-analysis of surgery in advanced ovarian carcinoma: is maximum cytoreductive surgery and independent determinant of prognosis? *Am J Obstet Gynecol*, 1992 166, 504-11.

[47] Huober, J; Meyer, A; Wagner, U; Wallwiener, D. The role of neoadjuvant chemotherapy and interval laparotomy in advanced ovarian cancer. *J Cancer, Res Clin Oncol*, 2002 128, 153-60.
[48] Covens, AL. A critique of surgical cytoreduction in advanced ovarian cancer. *Gynecol Oncol*, 2000 78, 269-84.
[49] Vergote, I; De Wever, I; Tjalma, W; et al. Neoadjuvant chemotherapy or primary debulking surgery in advanced ovarian carcinoma: a retrospective analysis of 285 patients. *Gynecol Oncol*, 1998 71, 431-6.
[50] Jacob, JH; Gershenson, DM; Morris, M; et al. Neoadjuvant chemotherapy and interval debulking for advanced epithelial ovarian cancer. *Gynecol Oncol*, 1991 42, 146-50.
[51] Schwartz, PE; Rutherford, TJ; Chambers, JT; et al. Neoadjuvant chemotherapy for advanced ovarian cancer: long-term survival. *Gynecol Oncol*, 1999 72, 93-9.
[52] Mazzeo, F; Berliere, M; Kerger, J; et al. Neoadjuvant chemotherapy followed by surgery and adjuvant chemotherapy in patients with primarily unresectable, advanced-stage ovarian cancer. *Gynecol Oncol*, 2003 90, 163-9.
[53] Harries, M; Gore, M. Part I: chemotherapy for epithelial ovarian cancer-treatment at first diagnosis. *Lancet Oncol*, 2002 3, 529-36.
[54] McGuire, WP; Hoskins, WJ; Brady, MF; et al. Cyclophosphamide and cisplatin compared with paclitaxel and cisplatin in patients with stage III and stage IV ovarian cancer. *N Engl J Med*, 1996 334, 1-6.
[55] Piccart, MJ; Bertelsen, K; James, K; et al: Randomized intergroup trial of cisplatin-paclitaxel versus cisplatin-cyclophosphamide in women with advanced epithelial ovarian cancer: three-year results. *J Natl Cancer Inst*, 2000 92, 699-708.
[56] Ozols, RF. Update on the management of ovarian cancer. *Cancer J*, 2002 8 Suppl 1, S22-30.
[57] Alberts, DS; Liu, PY; Hannigan, EV; O Toole, R; et al. Intraperitoneal cisplatin plus intravenous cyclophosphamide versus intravenous cisplatin plus intravenous cyclophosphamide for stage III ovarian cancer. *N Engl J Med*, 1996 335, 1950-1955.
[58] Markman, M; Bundy, BN; Alberts, DS; Fowler, JM; et al. Phase III trial of standard-dose intravenous cisplatin plus paclitaxel versus moderately high-dose carboplatin followed by intravenous paclitaxel and intraperitoneal cisplatin in small-volume stage III ovarian carcinoma: an intergroup study a of the gynaecologic oncology group, south western oncology group, and eastern cooperative oncology group. *J Clin Oncol*, 2001 19, 1001-1007.
[59] Armstrong, DK; Bundy, B; Wenzel, L; Huang, HO; Baergen, B; et al. Intraperitoneal cisplatin and paclitaxel in ovarian cancer. *N Engl J Med*, 2006 354(1), 34-43.
[60] Thomas, GM. Radiotherapy in early ovarian cancer. *Gynecol Oncol*, 1994 55, S73-S79.
[61] Kew, F.M; Cruikshank, DJ. Routine follow up after treatment for a gynecologic cancer: a survey of practice. *Int J Gynecol Cancer*; 2006 16, 380-384.
[62] Parker, PA; Kudelka, A; Basen-Enquist, K; Kavanagh, J; de Moor, J; Cohen L. The associations between knowledge, CA 125 preoccupation, and distress in women with epithelial ovarian cancer. *Gyn Onc*, 2006 100, 495-500.
[63] Donovan, KA; Greene, PG; Shuster, JL; Partridge, EE; Tucker, DC. Treatment preferences in recurrent ovarian cancer. *Gynecol Oncol*, 2002 86, 200-211.

[64] Cannistra, SA. Is there a "best" choice of second-line agent in the treatment of recurrent, potentially platinum-sensitive ovarian cancer? *J Clin Oncol*, 2002 20(5), 1158-60.

[65] Parma,r MK; Ledermann, JA; Colombo, N; et al. Paclitaxel plus platinum-based chemotherapy versus conventional platinum-based chemotherapy in women with relapsed ovarian cancer: the ICON4/AGO-OVAR-2.2 trial. *Lancet*, 2003 361(9375), 2099-106.

[66] Bookman, MA; Malmstrom, H; Bolis, G; et al. Topotecan for the treatment of advanced epithelial ovarian cncer: An open-label phase II study in patients treated after prior chemotherapy that contained cisplatin or carboplatin and paclitaxel. *J Clin Oncol*, 1998 16, 3345-3352.

[67] Lund, B; Paaske Hansen, O; Theilade, K; et al. Phase II study of gemcitabine in previously treated ovarian cancer patients. *J Natl Cancer Inst*, 1994 86, 1530-1533.

[68] Rose, PG; Blessing, JA; Mayer, AR; Homesley, HD. Prolonged oral etoposide as second-line therapy for platinum-resistant and platinum-sensitive ovarian cancer: a GOG study. *J Clin Oncol*, 1998 16, 405-410.

[69] Muggia, FM; Hainsworth, JD; Jeffer, S; et al. Phase II study of liposomal doxorubicin in refractor ovarian cancer: Antitumor activity and toxicity modification by liopsomal encapsulation. *J Clin Oncol*, 1997 15, 987-983.

[70] Piccart, JM; Gore, M; ten Bokkel, Huinink; et al. Docetaxel: An active new drug for treatment of advanced epithelial ovarian cancer. *J Natl Cancer Inst*, 1995 87, 676-681.

[71] Gordon, AN; Tonda, M; Sun, S; Rackoff, W. Long-term survival advantage for women treated with pegylated liposomal doxorubicin compared with topotecan in a phase 3 randomized study of recurrent and refractory epithelial ovarian cancer. *Gynecol Oncol*, 2004 95(1), 1-8.

[72] Berek, JS; Hacker, NF. Nonepithelial ovarian and fallopian tube cancers. In: Berek, JS; Hacker, NF eds. *Practical Gynecologic Oncology*. Philadelphia: Lippincott, Williams and Wilkins; 2005; 341-343.

[73] Williams, SD; Blessing, JA; Hatch, K; Homesley, HD. Chemotherapy of advanced ovarian dysgerminoma: trials of the Gynecologic Oncology Group. *J Clin Oncol*, 1991 9, 1950-1955.

In: Women and Cancer
Editor: Laurie Elit, pp. 147-158
ISBN: 978-1-60021-494-3

Chapter II

UTERINE CANCER

1. INCIDENCE & EPIDEMIOLOGY

Uterine cancer is the most common gynecologic tumor of Canadian women and the fourth most common tumor overall. In 2005, 3,900 Canadian women or 19/100,000 women were diagnosed with uterine cancer and 3/100,000 women died of uterine cancer [1]. It primarily affects women in the postmenopausal years and incidence peaks in the 7th decade [2].

The majority of uterine cancers are endometrial in origin arising from the lining of the uterus. These endometrial cancers are typically of endometrioid histology. As a group, endometrial, endometrioid cancer comprises 87% of uterine cancers [3]. These tumors will be discussed here. Small proportions of uterine cancers arise from the endometrium but have a different histology and others originate from the myometrium or muscle of the uterus. These tumors are quite rare and some will be reviewed individually at the end of this section.

1.1. Risk Factors

There are multiple risk factors for endometrial cancer but the most common risk factor is exposure to unopposed estrogen, see Table 1. Unopposed estrogen can be the result of many causes but commonly is due to increased body mass index, and/or abnormal menstrual cycles. Patients with a family history of colon cancer or endometrial cancer are also at increased risk. This is discussed further in section 8.

2. SCREENING STRATEGIES

In women taking tamoxifen as prevention or treatment for breast cancer, there is no evidence that routine endometrial sampling will detect endometrial cancer at an earlier stage and alter subsequent treatment. Of 159 patients that were followed prospectively with 635 endometrial biopsies, one diagnosis of complex hyperplasia was made. However 9 women required a D&C for further investigation of persistent bleeding or abnormal office biopsy [5].

Table 1. Risk Factors for Endometrial Cancer [4]

Risk factor	Relative Risk
Obesity >30lbs >50lbs	 3 10
Unopposed estrogen	9
Nulliparity	4
Atypical hyperplasia	29
Late menopause	4
Tamoxifen	2-3
Family history of colon cancer	9
Family history of endometrial cancer	6

3. Clinical Presentation

In 90% percent of women, endometrial cancer presents with abnormal vaginal bleeding [6]. In the premenopausal patients this manifests as irregular menses or spotting, while in postmenopausal patients any vaginal bleeding should be considered abnormal and appropriately investigated.

Occasionally, women present with glandular cells on routine Pap smear. Women over 40 year of age with glandular tissue on a Pap smear should be seen for further investigation of the cervix and endometrum [7]. Of these women 13% will have hyperplasia or carcinoma [7].

4. Diagnosis

4.1. Tissue Biopsies

The mainstay of diagnosing endometrial cancer is by tissue sampling. Tissue is most effectively and promptly obtained by endometrial sampling with an endometrial pipelle during an office visit. Both pipelle and dilatation & curettage (D&C) have been shown to have greater than 85% sensitivity for diagnosing endometrial cancer and atypical endometrial hyperplasia in women with abnormal vaginal bleeding [8,9]. As compared to D&C or hysterectomy the Pipelle has 91% and 99.6% sensitivity in pre- and post-menopausal women respectively [9]. If the pipelle is feasible in the office then it avoids the risks of general anesthetic and the delay of waiting for surgical time required to achieve adequate cervical dilatation for a D&C.

Hysteroscopy can be used to visualize the endometrial cavity. This is useful in combination with endometrial sampling to detect endometrial polyps or other gross anatomic abnormalities which may be the cause of the abnormal bleeding [10]. Given that there is a significant false-negative endometrial biopsy rate, any woman with persistent abnormal bleeding should have repeat tissue sampling in combination with hysteroscopy and ultrasound screening [11].

4.2. Imaging

In postmenopausal women with abnormal bleeding or spotting a trans-vaginal ultrasound may be helpful during triage. Trans-vaginal ultrasound has been used to detect a thickened endometrial lining or endometrial polyp in postmenopausal woman. It has been well shown that in the postmenopausal woman a cut off of 5mm will detect 90% of the endometrial cancers [8]. It must be remembered however that in women with an endometrial thickness greater than 5mm the majority will not have a malignancy. This is not the case for premenopausal women with abnormal bleeding. In the menstruating woman the specificity of this test is lost due to the normal physiologic endometrial thickness, which will often be greater than 5mm [12]. In two studies of women at high risk for endometrial cancer with hereditary non-polyposis colorectal cancer (HNPCC), see section 8, no cancer was detected through ultrasound screening but of 225 screening ultrasounds done 3 carcinomas were missed [13,14].

In premenopausal women with endometrial cancer there is a high incidence of synchronous ovarian cancer, 20-25% [15,16]. For these women ultrasound screening may assist in detecting ovarian abnormalities, thereby assisting in surgical planning.

Although not required in the routine planning of treatment for endometrial cancer, CT scanning can be helpful in select cases. Women who are difficult to examine by ultrasound or if history and physical examination are abnormal, CT imaging may further delineate the extent of disease. It is particularly helpful in imaging the large bowel, upper abdomen and retroperitoneal areas.

5. Prognostic Factors

5.1. Staging

Stage of cancer is assigned according to the 1988 International Federation of Gynecology and Obstetrics (FIGO) criteria with early stage being understood as confined to the uterine body and cervix, Table 2 [17]. Advanced stage disease is considered as FIGO stages III and IV or recurrent disease. In FIGO stage III or IV the disease has spread beyond the uterus to adnexa, retroperitoneal lymph nodes or more distant sites. Tumor stage at diagnosis is the most important prognostic factor. Eighty-five percent of women present with early stage disease and of these, 80% are cured of their disease [18,19]. Women who present with stage III or IV endometrial cancer have a poor prognosis with 30% 5-year survival, except those women with stage III diseases whose metastases are limited to the ovary, these women have a >70% 5-year survival [20,21].

Table 2. FIGO Staging of Endometrial Cancer [17]

FIGO Stage		Features
I		Tumor confined to uterus
	IA	Tumor limited to endometrium
	IB	Invasion to less than one-half of myometrium
	IC	Invasion to more than one-half of myometrium
II		
	IIA	Endocervical gland involvement
	IIB	Endocervical stromal involvement
III		
	IIIA	Tumor invades serosa or adnexa or positive cytology
	IIIB	Vaginal metastases
	IIIC	Pelvic or paraaortic lymphnode metastasese
IV		
	IVA	Tumor invading bowel or bladder mucosa
	IVB	Distant metastases

5.2. Histology

After stage of disease, histology is the next most important prognostic factor. Most endometrial cancers are of endometrioid histology. This is pathologically graded from 1 to 3 based on the percentage of solid growth and nuclear atypia (FIGO) and grade 1 endometrioid adenocarcinoma has the most favorable prognosis. With increasing grade, the 5-year overall survival decreases from 83% in FIGO stage Ic, Grade 1 to 58% 5-year overall survival in FIGO stage Ic, Grade 3 endometrioid adenocarcinoma [22]. Other histologies like papillary serous carcinoma, clear cell carcinomas carry a poorer prognosis.

Endometrial biopsies should be read by pathologists with gynecologic pathology experience to establish the correct preoperative diagnosis. Patients with uterine papillary serous pathology had the correct preoperative diagnosis only 77% of the time [23]. Having accurate preoperative histology is important as it may change the planned surgical management.

Another pathologic feature that is associated with a poorer prognosis is lymphvascular space invasion [24,25].[3]

6. THERAPIES

6.1. Surgery

Surgical therapy is the mainstay of treatment for endometrial cancer. In most centers women have a hysterectomy and bilateral salpingo-ophorectomy. Whether the role of lymphadenectomy is for accurate surgical staging or both staging and therapy is controversial. Good retrospective evidence shows that patients with high grade tumors who had more than 11 pelvic lymph nodes removed had improved overall survival compared to those who had less than 11 pelvic lymph nodes removed [26].

In advanced disease a hysterectomy should be done, if possible, to improve pelvic control. There may also be a role for removing the uterus and debulking intra-abdominal tumor to improve survival [27].

6.2. Radiotherapy

The role of whole pelvis radiotherapy in FIGO stage I has been well studied in large randomized controlled trials. In women with intermediate risk disease there is a reduction in the number of pelvic recurrences. There has been no improvement however in long term survival or distant relapse [28,29]. Given that no increase in survival has been shown with the addition of whole pelvic radiotherapy, some centers advocate for vaginal vault brachytherapy in this group to decrease the morbidity from whole pelvis radiotherapy. Evidence suggests that both the vaginal vault recurrence and distant recurrence rates are similar in patients who receive whole pelvis radiotherapy as compared to vaginal vault brachytherapy [30,31].

Women who have not received adjuvant radiotherapy and have only a locoregional recurrence are usually treated with curative intent. Treatment is usually with whole pelvis radiotherapy, and 89% of patients have a complete response to therapy [32].

6.3. Systemic Therapy

Conventionally, systemic treatment includes hormone therapy or chemotherapy, which is used in the treatment of recurrent or metastatic disease.

6.31. Hormonal Therapy

Endometrioid endometrial cancer has long been associated with states of estrogen excess, as a result a variety of anti-estrogens have been used for systemic treatment [33].

Based on the theory of estrogen excess as a carcinogenic promoter, progestogens have been used in the treatment of advanced endometrial cancer for their anti-estrogenic effects on the endometrium. Thigpen's trial reinforced the biologic plausibility of progestin use, lower grade tumors had a better response to progesterone than higher grade tumors, and tumors with higher progesterone receptor levels also had a better response rate. In this population of women with poor prognosis tumors progestogens are often used for palliative treatment to extend the symptom free time given their excellent tolerability as compared to chemotherapy. Traditionally progestins alone have had favorable short-term response rates but have not greatly impacted long term results. One of the reasons for this is that the progestin receptors become down regulated with exposure to progestin and the effect is lost. The estrogen agonist/antagonist, tamoxifen alone has been studied in early trials with a minimal response rate of 10% [34]. For these reasons combinations of progestins with tamoxifen have been studied, theorizing that tamoxifen will prevent the down regulation of the progestin receptors. In 2004, two studies with maestro acetate and tamoxifen were reported [35,36]. The response rates in these trials were 33% and 27% respectively.

6.32. Chemotherapy

Traditional chemotherapeutics have been used primarily for the treatment of distant, metastatic disease.

Women who have FIGO stage I or II endometrial cancer with poor prognostic features have up to 30% recurrence rates for distant metastases with poor response to further treatment [22]. Traditionally whole pelvic radiotherapy has been used to provided local pelvic control but with no improvement on long-term survival [28,29]. It is becoming increasingly clear that patients with high-risk features are at equal or greater risk of having a distant relapse as a local relapse [22,37]. However, at this stage, there is no prospective randomized trial to guide decisions for adjuvant systemic therapy in early stage disease.

A well-designed retrospective trial looked at surgically staged patients with stage I and II endometrioid, endometrial carcinoma. All patients had a total abdominal hysterectomy, bilateral salpingo-ophorectomy and retroperitoneal lymph node dissection performed. Patients were divided into high and low risk groups. The high-risk group had grade 3 histology, greater than 50% myometrial invasion, lymph vascular space invasion or cervical involvement. Those high-risk patients who had adjuvant cisplatin, doxorubicin and cyclophosphamide had 88.5% vs. 50% 5-yr progression free survival compared with those who received no adjuvant therapy. In this trial no patients had adjuvant radiotherapy [38].

Recent chemotherapy trials in advanced endometrial cancer have focused on a variety of combinations of agents that have shown activity as single agents in endometrial cancer. A major difficulty in these trials is how to balance the increasing toxicity with increasing numbers of chemotherapeutic agents. Currently the primary outcomes in many of these clinical trials are response rates. One comparison of doxorubicin and cisplatin with or without paclitaxel used survival as the primary outcome and showed a modest survival difference of 3 months [39]. However, this regimen has not been universally adopted due to the toxicity and requirement for routine growth factor support. Therefore there are presently trials looking at other more tolerated chemotherapies such as a carboplatin and paclitaxel combination.

In a randomized comparison of whole abdominal radiotherapy and systemic chemotherapy women who had presented with Stage III or IV disease and had undergone optimal debulking with less than 2 cm maximum size of residual disease both progression free and overall survival were significantly improved with chemotherapy over radiation, with a 30% reduction in the risk of progression and a 34% reduction in the risk of death. Those who did receive chemotherapy had more toxicity. The short-term toxicity was primarily hematologic and cardiac and long-term toxicity was neurologic.[38]. Seventeen percent of patients discontinued chemotherapy because of toxicity as opposed to 3% discontinuing radiation.

6.4. Novel Therapies

Targeted agents are those agents that act on specific population of cells or on a specific molecule of the cell cycle. Many of these novel agents are being discovered and trialed in the phase I/II settings. There is a paucity of phase II studies exploring novel therapies in gynecologic malignancies and endometrial cancer in particular. We are now entering an era of rationally designed therapies based on tumor biology. Impressive activity has been demonstrated in many malignancies such as breast, lung and colorectal cancers. Targeting the EGFR pathway or mTOR (mammalian target of rapamycin) would be appropriate based on the biologic characteristics of endometrial cancer or possibly VEGF based on anti-angiogenic effects seen in other malignancies including ovarian cancer. It is likely that these will need to be combined with systemic therapy to assess synergy and improve outcome.

7. Follow-up & Recurrent Disease

Women treated for endometrial cancer are routinely seen in follow up. Routine visits are usually scheduled every 3months in the first year, every 4 months in the second year, every 6 months in the third year and then annually [41]. Visits should include history and physical exam. Any unusual findings should be followed with the appropriate imaging and biopsies.

In women with isolated recurrent vaginal disease who have not had previous radiotherapy, there will be an 89% complete remission and 65% 5-year survival [32]. In women with stage one disease who received adjuvant pelvic radiotherapy 27% will have their 1st relapse distantly. For these women systemic treatment as discussed above will be more appropriate.

8. HNPCC

Hereditary non-polyposis colorectal cancer (HNPCC) is a familial cancer syndrome with an autosomal dominant inheritance pattern caused by germline mutations of one of the DNA mismatch repair genes. Five percent of endometrial cancers are associated with HNPCC. The most commonly mutated mismatch repair genes are MLH1, MSH2 and MSH6. Members of HNPCC families who inherit a germline mutation are at increased risk of cancers of the colon, endometrium, ovary, stomach, small bowel, ureter and renal pelvis [42]. The most common cancers in these families originate in the colorectum and endometrium. The lifetime risk of either cancer is dependent on the type of germline mutation but can be between 40 and 80% [42,43]. Both cancers present 15 years earlier than their sporadic counterparts.

It is unknown whether the presentation, pathology and survival of endometrial cancer in women with HNPCC are different from those with sporadic cancer. Most studies would indicate that there is no difference in stage at presentation, however these have not had a non-HNPCC control group [44,45]. In an at risk population like the HNPCC population there are controversial screening recommendations. Ultrasound screening will result in many false positive results given that the majority of women are menstruating and therefore their endometrium will be physiologically thickened with their cycles. In the current literature, no carcinomas were detected in 225 ultrasounds but 3 carcinomas were missed [13,14].

Women who are known carriers of a germline mutation may benefit from prophylactic hysterectomy and bilateral salpingoophorectomy to decrease the risk of both endometrial and ovarian cancer. A retrospective review of women who had prophylactic surgery suggests a significant decrease in the number of endometrial cancers and perhaps a significant decrease in the number of ovarian cancers in this at risk population [46].

9. Uterine Papillary Serous Carcinoma

Uterine papillary serous carcinoma is an aggressive epithelial tumor that arises in the endometrium. Its pattern of spread is similar to ovarian cancer, with its dissemination to the peritoneal surfaces. Ultrasound is less helpful in the diagnosis of this tumor as 17% of patients have an endometrial thickness of < 4mm [47]. It is controversial which patients with early stage papillary serous carcinoma of the uterus should be treated with adjuvant therapy, and which type of adjuvant therapy, radiotherapy or chemotherapy, is most useful.

Patients who have had extensive surgical staging in the form of hysterectomy, bilateral salpingo-ophorectomy, omental biopsy and lymph node sampling with peritoneal biopsies and have stage I disease were found to have an 82% overall 5 year survival and may not benefit from additional treatment [23,48]. Those whose surgery was not as extensive or who have more advanced disease have a much poorer prognosis [23,49]. For these patients there is increasing evidence for treating with chemotherapy in addition to their surgery [50].

10. Sarcoma

Uterine sarcomas are a group of tumors which arise from the mesenchymal cells or body of the uterus. Uterine sarcomas are a heterogeneous group of endometrial stromal sarcomas and leiomyosarcomas, both can be classified as high grade or low grade. Previously malignant mixed Muellerian tumors were classified as a sarcoma but they are now felt to arise from the same precursors as endometrioid carcinoma and can be treated in a similar fashion as an aggressive endometrioid histology [51].

Uterine sarcomas are rare. They usually affect women in their 50's who present with abnormal uterine bleeding or an increasing pelvic mass. The primary treatment is surgery. In endometrial stromal sarcomas the treatment is often hormonal. The efficacy of both chemotherapy and radiotherapy is controversial. Survival for high-grade uterine sarcomas is poor with 50% of stage I surviving at 5 years.

REFERENCES

[1] Canadian Cancer Statistics 2005, pg27, 29.

[2] Public Health, Purdie, 2001.

[3] Wilson, TO; Podratz, KC; Gaffey, TA; Malkasian, GD Jr; O'Brien, PC; Naessens, JM. Evaluation of unfavorable histologic subtypes in endometrial adenocarcinoma. *Am J Obstet Gynecol*, 1990 162(2), 418-23, discussion 423-6.

[4] Farquhar, CM; Lethaby, A; Sowter, M; Verry, J; Baranyai, J. An evaluation of risk factors for endometrial hyperplasia in premenopausal women with abnormal menstrual bleeding. *Am J Obstet Gynecol*, 1999 181(3), 525-529.

[5] Barakat, RR; Gilewski, TA; Almadrones, L; et al. Effect of adjuvant tamoxifen on the endometrium in women with breast cancer: A prospective study using office endometrial biopsy. *J Clin Oncol*, 2000 18(20), 3459-3463.

[6] Berek, JS; Hacker, NF. *Practical Gynecologic Oncology*. 3rd ed. Philadelphia: Lippincott Williams & Wilkins; 2000.

[7] Fadare, O, Ghofrani, M; Chacho, MS; Parkash V. The significance of benign endometrial cells in cervicovaginal smears. *Adv Anat Pathol*, 2005 12(5), 274-287.

[8] Deckardt, R; Lueken, RP; Gallinat, A; et al. Comparison of transvaginal ultrasound, hysteroscopy, and dilatation and curettage in the diagnosis of abnormal vaginal bleeding and intrauterine pathology in perimenopausal and postmenopausal women. *J Am Assoc Gynecol Laparosc*, 2002 9(3), 277-282.

[9] Dijkhuizen, FP; Mol, BW; Brolmann, HA; Heintz, AP. The accuracy of endometrial sampling in the diagnosis of patients with endometrial carcinoma and hyperplasia: A meta-analysis. *Cancer*, 2000 89(8), 1765-1772.

[10] Ben-Yehuda, OM; Kim, YB; Leuchter, RS. Does hysteroscopy improve upon the sensitivity of dilatation and curettage in the diagnosis of endometrial hyperplasia or carcinoma? *Gynecol Oncol*, 1998 68(1),4-7.

[11] Loffer, ED. Hysteroscopy with selective endometrial sampling compared with D&C for abnormal uterine bleeding: The value of a negative hysteroscopic view. *Obs Gyn*, 1989 73, 16-20.

[12] Goldstein SR. The endometrial echo revisited: Have we created a monster? *Am J Obstet Gynecol*, 2004 191(4), 1092-1096.

[13] Dove-Edwin, I; Boks, D; Goff, S; et al. The outcome of endometrial carcinoma surveillance by ultrasound scan in women at risk of hereditary nonpolyposis colorectal carcinoma and familial colorectal carcinoma. *Cancer*, 2002 94(6), 1708-1712.

[14] Rijcken, FE; Mourits, MJ; Kleibeuker, JH; Hollema, H; van der Zee, AG. Gynecologic screening in hereditary nonpolyposis colorectal cancer. *Gynecol Oncol*, 2003 91(1), 74-80.

[15] Walsh, C; Holschneider, C; Hoang, Y; Tieu, K; Karlan, B; Cass, I. Coexisting ovarian malignancy in young women with endometrial cancer. *Obstet Gynecol*, 2005 106(4), 693-699.

[16] Soliman, PT; Oh, JC; Schmeler, KM; et al. Risk factors for young premenopausal women with endometrial cancer. *Obstet Gynecol*, 2005 105(3), 575-580.

[17] Benedet, JL; Bender, H; Jones, H3rd; Ngan, HY; Pecorelli, S. FIGO staging classifications and clinical practice guidelines in the management of gynecologic cancers. FIGO committee on gynecologic oncology. *Int J Gynaecol Obstet*; 2000 70(2), 209-262.

[18] Kosary, CL. FIGO stage, histology, histologic grade, age and race as prognostic factors in determining survival for cancers of the female gynecological system: An analysis of 1973-87 SEER cases of cancers of the endometrium, cervix, ovary, vulva, and vagina. *Semin Surg Oncol* 1994, 10(1), 31-46.

[19] Purdie, DM; Green, AC. Epidemiology of endometrial cancer. *Best Pract Res Clin Obstet Gynaecol*, 2001 15(3), 341-354.

[20] Greven, KM; Lanciano, RM; Corn, B; Case, D; Randall, ME. Pathologic stage III endometrial carcinoma. prognostic factors and patterns of recurrence. *Cancer*, 1993 71(11), 3697-3702.

[21] Connell, PP; Rotmensch, J; Waggoner, S; Mundt, AJ. The significance of adnexal involvement in endometrial carcinoma. *Gynecol Oncol*, 1999 74(1), 74-79.

[22] Creutzberg, CL; van Putten, WL; Warlam-Rodenhuis, CC; et al. Outcome of high-risk stage IC, grade 3, compared with stage I endometrial carcinoma patients: The postoperative radiation therapy in endometrial carcinoma trial. *J Clin Oncol*, 2004 22(7), 1234-1241.

[23] Bristow, RE; Asrari, F; Trimble, EL; Montz, FJ. Extended surgical staging for uterine papillary serous carcinoma: Survival outcome of locoregional (stage I-III) disease. *Gynecol Oncol*, 2001 81(2), 279-286.

[24] Pitson, G; Colgan, T; Levin, W; et al. Stage II endometrial carcinoma: Prognostic factors and risk classification in 170 patients. *Int J Radiat Oncol Biol Phys*, 2002 53(4), 862-867.

[25] Briet, JM; Hollema, H; Reesink, N; et al. Lymphvascular space involvement: An independent prognostic factor in endometrial cancer. *Gynecol Oncol*, 2005 96(3), 799-804.

[26] Cragun, JM; Havrilesky, LJ; Calingaert, B; et al. Retrospective analysis of selective lymphadenectomy in apparent early-stage endometrial cancer. *J Clin Oncol*, 2005 23(16), 3668-3675.

[27] Lambrou, NC; Gomez-Marin, O; Mirhashemi, R; et al. Optimal surgical cytoreduction in patients with stage III and stage IV endometrial carcinoma: A study of morbidity and survival. *Gynecol Oncol*, 2004 93(3), 653-658.

[28] Creutzberg, CL; van Putten, WL; Koper, PC; et al. Surgery and postoperative radiotherapy versus surgery alone for patients with stage-1 endometrial carcinoma: Multicentre randomised trial. PORTEC study group. post operative radiation therapy in endometrial carcinoma. *Lancet*, 2000 355(9213), 1404-1411.

[29] Keys, HM; Roberts, JA; Brunetto, VL; et al. A phase III trial of surgery with or without adjunctive external pelvic radiation therapy in intermediate risk endometrial adenocarcinoma: A gynecologic oncology group study. *Gynecol Oncol*, 2004 92(3), 744-751.

[30] Horowitz, NS; Peters, WA3rd; Smith, MR; Drescher, CW; Atwood, M; Mate, TP. Adjuvant high dose rate vaginal brachytherapy as treatment of stage I and II endometrial carcinoma. *Obstet Gynecol*, 2002 99(2), 235-240.

[31] Pearcey, RG; Petereit, DG. Post-operative high dose rate brachytherapy in patients with low to intermediate risk endometrial cancer. *Radiother Oncol*; 2000 56(1), 17-22.

[32] Creutzberg, CL; van Putten, WL; Koper, PC; et al. Survival after relapse in patients with endometrial cancer: Results from a randomized trial. *Gynecol Oncol*, 2003 89(2), 201-209.

[33] Persson, I. Estrogens in the causation of breast, endometrial and ovarian cancers - evidence and hypotheses from epidemiological findings. *J Steroid Biochem Mol Biol*, 2000 74(5), 357-364.

[34] Thigpen, T; Brady, MF; Homesley, HD; Soper, JT; Bell, J. Tamoxifen in the treatment of advanced or recurrent endometrial carcinoma: A gynecologic oncology group study. *J Clin Oncol*, 2001 19(2), 364-367.

[35] Whitney, CW; Brunetto, VL; Zaino, RJ; et al. Phase II study of medroxyprogesterone acetate plus tamoxifen in advanced endometrial carcinoma: A gynecologic oncology group study. *Gynecol Oncol*, 2004 92(1), 4-9.

[36] Fiorica, JV; Brunetto, VL; Hanjani, P; et al. Phase II trial of alternating courses of megestrol acetate and tamoxifen in advanced endometrial carcinoma: A gynecologic oncology group study. *Gynecol Oncol*, 2004 92(1), 10-14.

[37] Mariani, A; Dowdy, SC; Keeney, GL; Long, HJ; Lesnick, TG; Podratz, KC. High-risk endometrial cancer subgroups: Candidates for target-based adjuvant therapy. *Gynecol Oncol*, 2004 95(1), 120-126.

[38] Aoki, Y; Watanabe, M; Amikura, T; et al. Adjuvant chemotherapy as treatment of high-risk stage I and II endometrial cancer. *Gynecol Onco*l, 2004, 94(2), 333-339.

[39] Fleming, GF; Filiaci, VL; Bentley, RC; et al. Phase III randomized trial of doxorubicin + cisplatin versus doxorubicin + 24-h paclitaxel + filgrastim in endometrial carcinoma: A gynecologic oncology group study. *Ann Oncol*, 2004, 15(8), 1173-1178.

[40] Randall, ME; Filiaci, VL; Muss, H; et al. Randomized phase III trial of whole-abdominal irradiation versus doxorubicin and cisplatin chemotherapy in advanced endometrial carcinoma: A gynecologic oncology group study. *J Clin Onco*l, 2006 24(1), 36-44.

[41] Kew, FM; Cruickshank, DJ. Routine follow-up after treatment for a gynecological cancer: A survey of practice. *Int J Gynecol Cancer*, 2006, 16(1), 380-384.

[42] Sharma, A; James, M; Donaldson, A; Fox, R. Hereditary non-polyposis colorectal cancer syndrome: Combined risk of gastrointestinal and gynaecological cancer. *BJOG*. 2001, 108(7), 671-677.

[43] Lynch, HT; Lynch, JF. Lynch syndrome: History and current status. *Dis Markers*. 2004, 20(4-5), 181-198.

[44] Boks, DE; Trujillo, AP; Voogd, AC; Morreau, H; Kenter, GG; Vasen, HF. Survival analysis of endometrial carcinoma associated with hereditary nonpolyposis colorectal cancer. *Int J Cancer*, 2002 102(2), 198-200.

[45] Parc, YR; Halling, KC; Burgart, LJ; et al. Microsatellite instability and hMLH1/hMSH2 expression in young endometrial carcinoma patients: Associations with family history and histopathology. *Int J Cancer*, 2000 86(1), 60-66.

[46] Schmeler, KM; Lynch, HT; Chen, LM et al. Prophylactic surgery to reduce the risk of gynecologic cancers in the lynch syndrome. *N Engl J Med*, 2006 354(3), 261-269.

[47] Wang, J; Wieslander, C; Hansen, G; Cass, I; Vasilev, S; Holschneider, CH. Thin endometrial echo complex on ultrasound does not reliably exclude type 2 endometrial cancers. *Gynecol Oncol*, 2006 101(1), 120-125.

[48] Elit, L; Kwon, J; Bentley, J; Trim, K; Ackerman, I; Carey, M. Optimal management for surgically stage 1 serous cancer of the uterus. *Gynecol Oncol*, 2004 92(1), 240-246.

[49] Slomovitz, BM; Burke, TW; Eifel, PJ; et al. Uterine papillary serous carcinoma (UPSC): A single institution review of 129 cases. *Gynecol Oncol*, 2003 91(3), 463-469.

[50] Kelly, MG; O'malley, DM; Hui, P; et al. Improved survival in surgical stage I patients with uterine papillary serous carcinoma (UPSC) treated with adjuvant platinum-based chemotherapy. *Gynecol Oncol*, 2005 98(3), 353-359.

[51] McCluggage, WG. Uterine carcinosarcomas (malignant mixed mullerian tumors) are metaplastic carcinomas. *Int J Gynecol Cancer*, 2002 12(6), 687-690.

In: Women and Cancer
Editor: Laurie Elit, p. 159
ISBN: 978-1-60021-494-3

Chapter III

GESTATIONAL TROPHOBLASTIC DISEASE

Gestational trophoblastic diseases include molar pregnancies, gestational choriocarcinoma and placental site trophoblastic tumors. The quoted incidence varies widely from 23/100,000 pregnancies in Paraguay to 1299/100,000 pregnancies in Indonesia [1]. Most molar pregnancies are diagnosed by elevated βHCG levels and/or ultrasound. Patients who are suspected to have GTD require a serum quantitative βHCG, pelvic ultrasound, chest x-ray, complete blood count, renal and liver function tests.

Eighty percent of patients are fully treated after their suction dilatation and curettage. It is important however for all of these patients to have serial screening of their quantitative bHCG every week until the levels are negative and monthly thereafter for 6-12 months. During this time contraception is important so that the βHCG levels can be accurately followed, as they are the most sensitive indicator of persistent disease. If the levels of βHCG rise the patients must be referred for a metastatic work up and consideration of chemotherapy. GTD is very sensitive to chemotherapy with excellent long-term results.

There is a 10-fold increased risk of GTD in a subsequent pregnancy. Thus, these patients should have an early ultrasound and quantative βHCG in ensuing pregnancies. After delivery the placenta should also be sent to pathology for histologic examination and a 6-week post-partum βHCG level should be drawn to assure that the βHCG levels are negative.

REFERENCES

[1] Altieri, A; Franceschi, S; Ferlay, J; Smith, J; La Vecchia, C. Epidemiology and aetiology of gestational trophoblastic diseases. *Lancet Oncol*, 2003 4(11), 670-678.

In: Women and Cancer
Editor: Laurie Elit, pp. 161-172
ISBN: 978-1-60021-494-3

Chapter IV

CERVIX CANCER

1. INCIDENCE & EPIDEMIOLOGY

Invasive cervical cancer accounts for approximately 5-6% of all cancers in women in North America. In 2006, there will be an estimated 1350 new cases and 450 women will die of this disease. Worldwide, cervical cancer is second only to breast cancer as the most common malignancy in both incidence and mortality. More than 471 000 new cases are diagnosed each year, predominantly in economically challenged and developing nations [1]. It is a very important cancer for female patients as screening can help prevent this cancer. During the past 50 years, the utilization of screening programs in North America has led to a steep decline in both the incidence and death rate from cervical cancer.

A number of risk factors predispose women to cervical cancer. Cervical cancer is associated with chronic infection by oncogenic types of human papilloma virus (HPV). Therefore, risk factors for cervical cancer are similar to those for sexually transmitted diseases, including early age at onset of sexual activity, multiple sexual partners, and having a documented infection of HPV. Smoking has also been a significant risk factor for cervical cancer [2]. Women with immunosuppression are also at increased risk. This includes women with human immunodeficiency virus (HIV) infection [3], whole-organ transplant patients on immunosuppressant therapies and women with Hodgkin's lymphoma.

2. CLINICAL PRESENTATION

2.1. Signs and Symptoms

The most common finding discovered on physical examination is a grossly visible lesion on the cervix seen during the speculum examination. The primary tumor may arise high in the endocervical canal, and thus the cervix appears normal but feels abnormal on palpation during bimanual examination. The vagina should also be visualized and palpated for direct extension of tumor. A rectovaginal examination allows a better appreciation of size of cervix and for the detection of any extension of disease into the surrounding parametrial tissues.

A common complaint is abnormal vaginal bleeding. This includes post coital bleeding in sexually active women, postmenopausal bleeding in older women and any menstrual irregularities. Women may complain of an increased vaginal discharge that is foul–smelling, especially in advanced cases.

In patients with advanced disease, pelvic pain secondary to extension into lumbosaccral nerve roots or hydronephrosis may be reported. Pelvic pressure, hematuria and hematochezia may suggest advanced disease with spread into bladder and rectum.

3. Screening Strategies

Cytologic evaluation of cells obtained from the cervix using the Papanicolaou (Pap) smear is the standard screening test for lower female genital tract neoplasia. The Pap smear was first propsed by Papanicolaou and Traut in the 1940's [4]. Since that time, cervical cytology has proved to be a very efficacious and cost-effective method of cancer screening. The current recommendation is that all women who are or have been sexually active should have an annual Pap test and pelvic examination. Some regions are fortunate to have Pap smear registries and strict follow up. Thus, they can screen less frequently such as every 3 years.

The Pap smear using a competent laboratory and personnel results in false-negative rates of 15% for high grade lesions [5]. Most laboratories operate with a very low false-positive rate of 2-5% [6]. Specimen collection is key to the accuracy of cytologic diagnosis as there is much sample-to-sample variation depending on collection techniques. Best results are obtained by use of both spatula and cytobrush and ensuring that both the ectocervix and endocervix are sampled. The samples are smeared immediately onto slides and fixed promptly to avoid air-drying. There are new liquid-based cytology techniques emerging that have proven to be very efficacious and cost-effective also [7].

The results of the Pap smear cannot be used to make a diagnosis or formulate a treatment plan as it functions solely as a "screening tool". The Pap smear screens for abnormalities and depending on the report often leads to further investigation using colposcopy. Colposcopy is the visual examination of the cervix and lower genital tract using a magnified illumination system. It detects abnormal appearances suggestive of a preinvasive lesion or neoplasia. It is most frequently performed in response to an abnormal pap smear. Colposcopic-directed biopsies are required to confirm the findings.

4. Diagnosis

4.1. Tumor Markers

There is currently no biomarker used in the evaluation and work-up of cervical cancer. There are multiple biomarkers that are currently being researched. Many of these biomarkers have prognostic potential, however, results at present are often conflicting and inconsistent [8]. Many researchers are investigating epidermal growth factor, vascular endothelial growth factor and cyclooxygenase- (COX-2) in relation to hypoxia and apoptosis [9]. Translational research continues in this area with the goal of finding useful diagnostic biomarkers that could eventually be used in the clinical work up.

4.2. Imaging

Imaging studies are useful tools to evaluate the extent of disease and assist with treatment planning.

The lymphagiogram was used in the 1960's and 1970's to predict possible lymphatic spread. However, a review of the literature revealed a high false positive rate of 32%, false negative rate of 10% and only 84% accuracy [10]. Most centers no longer use this modality.

The three most commonly used imaging studies include computed tomography (CT), magnetic resonance imaging (MRI), and positron emission tomography (PET).

CT scanning allows evaluation of other organs such as the liver, kidneys and urinary tract and bony structures. It is important in assessing changes in the size of the lymph nodes and the possibility of lymph node invasion. The radiographic and surgical-pathologic findings have been correlated showing that 75% of the enlarged pelvic lymph nodes detected on CT scan contained metastases [11].

MRI has recently been used to assess the extension of disease into parametria, vagina and uterine ligaments. There have also been reports suggesting MRI is valuable in estimating tumor volume, diameter and size assisting with treatment decisions in bulky cervical carcinomas [12].

Finally, depending on availability at certain centers, PET has been increasingly used in cervical cancer to assess lymphatic involvement and distant metastatic spread of disease. It uses metabolic changes rather than anatomic alterations for detection of disease. It appears to have a sensitivity of 86%, specificity of 94% and accuracy of 92% at experienced centers [13].

4.3. Tissue Biopsies

Diagnostic biopsy is essential in the diagnosis of cervical cancer. Any suspicious lesion of the cervix should be biopsied to confirm diagnosis and determine depth of invasion in early disease and histologic cell type. This can be performed in the office under direct visualization if a gross lesion is seen, or at the time of colposcopy if colposcopic findings suggestive of invasive disease.

5. Prognostic Factors

Important prognostic factors for patients with cervical cancer include stage of disease, status of lymph nodes, size/tumor volume, depth of stromal invasion, histologic cell type, lymphovascular space invasion and parametrial extension.

5.1. Staging

Clinical

Staging of cervical cancer is based on clinical evaluation, thus, a careful clinical examination, including speculum, bimanual and rectovaginal examination, should be performed [14]. This is often performed by both the surgical gynecologic oncologist and the radiation oncologist, as a team to help guide treatment decisions. Some centers still perform an examination under anesthesia to allow assessment of parametrial and pelvic sidewall involvement with the patient fully relaxed. This can also include cystoscopy, proctoscopy, and hysteroscopy if indicated but is rarely indicated in early stage cervical cancer.

Table 1. FIGO Staging of Cervical Cancer

FIGO Stage		Features
I		Tumor confined to cervix
	IA	Invasive cancer identified microscopically
	IA1	Stromal invasion is limited to a maximum depth no greater than 3 mm and no wider than 7mm
	IA2	Stromal invasion is greater than 3 mm but less than 5 mm, and no wider than 7mm
	IB	Clinical lesions confined to the cervix
	IB1	Clinical lesions less than 4 cm in size
	IB2	Clinical lesions greater than 4 cm in size
II		Tumor extends beyond cervix but has not extended onto the pelvic sidewall or lower vagina
	IIA	Extension upper third of vagina, negative parametria
	IIB	Extension with obvious parametria involvement

Table 1. (Continued)

FIGO Stage		Features
III		Tumor extends onto pelvic sidewall, no cancer-free space between tumor and pelvic side wall; tumor involves lower third vagina, any case with hydronephrosis of unknown cause
	IIIA	Extension lower third vagina, no extension on to the pelvic sidewall
	IIIB	Extension on to pelvic sidewall or hydronephrosis
IV		Extension beyond the pelvis or biopsy proven involvement of bladder or rectal mucosa
	IVA	Spread of carcinoma to adjacent organs, bladder and bowel
	IVB	Distant spread

The International Federation of Gynecology and Obstetrics (FIGO) staging system is listed below. It should be noted that this is a clinical staging system and does not take into account lymph node status. Stage of disease is an important prognostic indicator.

Surgical

Due to the fact that the available diagnostic tests cannot detect small lymph node metastases, many clinicians argue that cervical cancer should be surgically staged prior to treatment to identify patients with positive pelvic and para-aortic lymph nodes. This can be performed via transperitoneal approach, extraperitnoeal or laparoscopically. The transperitoneal approach is least favorable due to the associated risk of postoperative bowel complications and an increased risk of postradiation morbidity [15,16].

5.2. Lymph Node Status

Positive lymph nodes appear to be the most important prognostic factor in most studies [17]. Patients with negative lymph nodes have higher 5-year survival (90% or higher) compared to patients with positive pelvic lymph nodes (60%) or para-aortic nodes (20-40%) [18,19].

5.3. Tumor Size, Depth of Invasion and lymph-vascular Involvement

A large prospective study was performed by the Gynecology Oncology Group in 1990 that demonstrated tumor size, depth of invasion and lymph-vascular involvment are three independent prognostic factors significantly affect survival in cervical cancer patients [20]. Another study was later performed assessing the use of postoperative adjuvant whole pelvis radiotherapy in this group of patients who are node-negative but high risk with a combination of at least two of the following risk factors: large tumor size, greater than one third stromal invasion, and lymphvascular invasion. The addition of radiation significantly reduced recurrence with a recurrence-free survival of 88% versus 79% for observation alone [21].

5.4. Histologic Cell Type

The most common histologic cell type is squamous cell carcinoma. Adenocarcinoma is second and the prognostic significance of Adenocarcinoma is controversial. Some studies suggest it has a poorer prognosis [22], however, other authors argue that there is no difference compared with survival rates for squamous cervical carcinoma [23].

Small cell carcinoma is quite rare. It is known to be a much more aggressive carcinoma with poor prognosis [24].

5.5. Parametrial Involvement

Cervical cancer is known to spread laterally into parametrial tissues either by direct extension or by lymphatic embolization. The incidence of pathological parametrial involvement has been reported between 6-31% [25-27]. A study found that 5-year survival was significantly lower for patients with positive parametria, 62.4% versus those with no parametrial involvement 85.8% [28]. It should be noted however, that reporting of parametria depends on pathologic processing techniques and the giant section technique has been argued to be most effective [26].

6. Therapies

Gynecologic oncologists and radiation oncologists should collaborate in planning therapy for patients with cervical cancer. For patients with early stage disease, surgery and radiotherapy provide comparable survival rates [15]. The selection of treatment modality depends on patient age, medical and surgical risk factors, and both patient and physician preference.

6.1. Surgery

Patients with a stage IA1 tumor (less than 3 mm depth of invasion) have a microinvasive tumor and can be adequately treated with a simple hysterectomy, or if continued fertility is desired conization only, provided surgical margins are free of cancer. The chance of lymph node involvement is less than 0.5% and death rate less than 0.1% [29]. There is some debate amongst gynecologic oncologists as to how best to treat patients with stage IA1 tumors that have positive lymphvascular involvement. Most agree that it can be disregarded unless it is extensive which there may then be an argument for including a lymph node dissection.

For the smaller tumors confined to the cervix (stages IA2 and IB1) the treatment usually consists of surgery if the patient is medically fit with 5-year survival rates of 85-95% [15]. The advantages of a primary surgical approach include preservation of ovarian function in young women, avoidance of long-term radiation effects on normal tissues, such as vaginal atrophy and dyspareunia [30,31], and to define surgically the extent of disease. Also, the patient's history or physical status influences the decision as patients with a history of ulcerative colitis, regional ileitis, or pelvic inflammatory disease may experience serious postradiation complications [32,33]. Therefore, most healthy, young patients are treated by radical surgery consisting of a radical hysterectomy and bilateral pelvic lymphadenectomy reserving radiation for the surgically unfit patient. Radical hysterectomy is a procedure that should be performed by a skilled surgeon with subspecialty training in gynecologic oncology and sufficient experience to ensure adequate removal of surrounding parametrial tissues with an acceptable morbidity rate. The procedure involves removal of the uterus, upper vagina, a portion of the uterosacral and uterovesical ligaments and parametria. A pelvic lymph node dissection is also performed removing all nodal tissue along the iliac vessels and within the obtuator fossa. The ovaries may be preserved if they are disease free. Due to the radicality of the procedure, there are increased risk of postoperative complications including urinary tract injury, lymphocyst formation, obturator nerve injury, postoperative infection, bladder dysfunction and sexual dysfunction [34,35].

This procedure traditionally has been performed via laparotomy. However, with recent advances in technology, the applications for laparoscopy have expanded and the techniques to perform radical hysterectomy with pelvic lymph node dissection laparoscopically have been described [36,37]. The cited advantages of laparoscopic pelvic lymphadenectomy combined with an assisted-radical vaginal hysterectomy over radical abdominal hysterectomy are decreased blood loss, superior cosmetic results, quicker patient recovery and shorter length of hospital stay with decreased costs to the healthcare system [38].

6.2. Radiotherapy

As discussed above, radiotherapy has similar survival rates to radical surgery [15]; however, surgery is the preferred modality in the younger healthy patient population. Conversely, there will always be a subgroup of patients at risk for recurrence because of adverse prognostic factors, such as lymph node metastasis, positive margins, and a combination of large tumor size, lymphvascular space involvment, and depth of invasion [20, 39-41]. It has been suggested that postoperative adjuvant radiation therapy improves survival for these high-risk patients. Morrow et al. showed an improved 5-year survival in patients with positive nodes treated with adjuvant radiotherapy [42]. A randomized study of adjuvant pelvic radiotherapy versus no further treatment after radical hysterectomy for patients with high-risk features but negative lymph nodes, also showed a reduced risk of recurrence with recurrence-free survival of 88% versus 79% respectively [21].

For patients with advanced stage IIB to IVA, radical external beam pelvic radiotherapy combined with intracavitary brachytherapy is the gold standard for advanced disease. More recently, the use of chemoradiation has become the treatment of choice after three larger randomized controlled trials all confirmed the survival advantage of concurrent chemotherapy with radiation therapy in advanced cervical cancer [44-46]. The optimal dose of chemotherapy and frequency may vary from center to center, but the majority use cisplatin weekly during the five weeks of external beam therapy.

6.3. Chemotherapy

As described above, the use of concurrent chemotherapy has become the gold standard treatment for advanced cervical carcinoma.

Chemotherapy is also used for recurrent or metastatic disease with the goal being palliative. Cisplatin is the single most active and preferred agent for metastatic cervical cancer. Unfortunately, the response rates are poor with only 20-25% and duration of response is often less than 6 months [47]. Combination cisplatin-based chemotherapy is more toxic without an associated survival benefit. The search for more effective systemic chemotherapy continues [48].

7. Follow-up & Recurrent Disease

After therapy, either radiation or surgery, patients should be followed every 3 months for 2 years, every 6 months for 3 years and then annually after that. However, the role of routine follow up has been challenged because most recurrences are discovered when patients self-refer due to symptoms such as new onset vaginal bleeding, discharge or pain [49]. Patients should be questioned about symptoms and a physical exam performed including a rectovaginal examination. Due to the risk of distant metastases, supraclavicular and inguinal nodes should be palpated also.

Recurrent cervical carcinoma is devastating as these patients have a poor prognosis with a one year survival of approximately 15% and 5 year survival of less than 5% [50]. Treatment decisions are made after patients are evaluated for local and distant metastases. Patients can be considered in one of two categories: those who may be treated with hope of cure or those for which only palliative therapy is available. The type of therapy offered depends on the mode of primary therapy and the location of the recurrence.

First, potentially curable lesions include isolated central pelvic recurrences, or solitary lung metastasis. An isolated pelvic recurrence after primary radiotherapy is treated with radical pelvic surgery involving an exenterative procedure removing usually both the bladder and rectum in addition to the uterus, cervix, vagina and supporting ligaments. It is imperative that there is biopsy-proven recurrence and distant metastatic disease has been excluded. The complication rate is as high as 50% including both gastrointestinal and genitourinary complications [51]. Five-year survival and quality of life have both improved since this procedure was originally performed. Five year survival has been reported as high as 60% [52].

If the primary treatment was surgery, radiation therapy is the treatment of choice. Most centers use concurrent chemotherapy, such as cisplatin or 5-fluoruracil, with the radiation. If patients have central recurrences, curative intent radiotherapy has survival rate of 30-70% [53].

For patients with distant metastatic disease, palliative chemotherapy and radiotherapy have been employed. Symptom management should also be addressed including pain management and control of bleeding.

REFERENCES

[1] National Institutes of Health Consensus Development Conference Statement on Cervical Cancer. *Gynecol Oncol*, 1997 66, 351-361.

[2] Winkelstein W. Smoking and cervical cancer: current status-a review. *Am J Epidemiol*, 1990 131, 945-957.

[3] Jay, N; Moscicki, AB. Human papillomavirus infections in women with HIV disease: prevalence, risk and management. *AIDS Read*, 2000 10, 659-668.

[4] Papanicolaou, GN; Traut, HF. The diagnostic value of vaginal smears in carcinoma of the uterus. *Am J Obstet Gynecol*, 1941 42, 193-7.

[5] Gay, JD; Donaldson, LD; Goellner, JR. False-negative results in cervical cytologic studies. *Acta Cytol*, 1985 29, 1043-1046.

[6] Corkill, M; Knapp, D; Hutchinson, ML. Improved accuracy for cervical cytology with the ThinPrep method and the endocervical brush-spatula collection procedure. *Journal of Lower Genital Tract Disease*, 1998 2, 12-16.

[7] Saslow, D; Runowicz, C; Solomon, D; Moscicki, AB; Smith, RA; Eyre, HF; et al. American Cancer Society cervical cancer screening guidelines 2002. *CA Cancer J Clin*, 2002 52, 375-376.

[8] Lee, IJ; Park, KR; Lee, KK; et al. Prognostic value of vascular endothelial growth factor in stage IB carcinoma of the uterine cervix. *Int J Radiat Oncol Biol Phys*, 2002 54, 768-779.

[9] Gaffney, DK; Haslam, D; Tsokidov, A; et al. Epidermal growth factor receptor (EDFR) and vascular endothelial growth factor (VEGF) negatively affect overall survival in carcinoma of the cervix treated with radiotherapy. *Int J Radiat Oncol Biol Phys*, 2003 56, 922-928.

[10] Hacker, NF; Berek, JS. Surgical staging of cervical cancer. In: Surwit, EA; Alberts, DS; eds. *Cervix cancer*. Boston: Martinus Nijhoff; 1987; 43-47.

[11] Camilien, L ; Fordon, D ; Frucher, RG ; et al. Predictive value of computerized tomography in the presurgical evaluation of primary carcinoma of the cervix. *Gynecol Oncol*, 1988 30, 209-214.

[12] Wagenaar, HC; Trimbos, JB; Postema, S; Anastasopoulou, A; van der Geest, RJ; Reiber, JHC; et al. Tumor diameter and volume assessed by magnetic resonance imaging in the prediction of outcome for invasive cervical cancer. *Gynecol Oncol*, 2001 82, 474-482.

[13] Lin, WC; Hung, YC; Yeh, LS; et al. Usefulness of 18F-fluorodeoxyglucose positron emission tomography to detect para-aortic lymph nodal metastasis in advanced cervical cancer with negative computed tomography findings. *Gynecol Oncol*, 2003 89, 73-76.

[14] Hacker, NF. Cervical Cancer. In: Berek, JS; Hacker, NF; eds. *Practical Gynecologic Oncology*. Philadelphia: Lippincott, Williams and Wilkins; 2005; 341-343.
[15] Landoni, F; Maneo, A; Colombo, A; et al. Randomized study of radical surgery versus radiotherapy for stage IB-IIA cervical cancer. *Lancet*, 1997 350, 535-540.
[16] Nelson, JF Jr ; Boyce, J ; Macasanet, M ; Lu, T ; et al. Incidence, significance and follow-up of para-aortic lymph node metastases in late invasive carcinoma of the cervix. *Am J Obstet Gynecol*, 1977 128, 336-340.
[17] Randall, ME; Michael, H; Ver Morken, J; Stehman, F. Uterine cervix. In: Hoskins, WJ; Perez, CA eds. *Principles and practice of gynecologic oncology*. Philadelphia: Lippincott, Williams and Wilkins; 2005; 743-761.
[18] Tinga, DR ; Timmer, PR ; Bouma, J; et al. Prognostic significance of single versus multiple lymph node metastases in cervical carcinoma stage IB. *Gynecol Oncol*, 1990 39, 175-180.
[19] Hacker, NF; Wain, GV; Nicklin, JL. Resection of bulky positive lymph nodes in patients with cervical cancer. *Int J Gynecol Cancer*, 1995 5, 250-256.
[20] Delgado, G; Bundy, B; Zaino, R; et al. Prospective surgical-pathological study of disease-free interval in patients with stage IB squamous cell carcinoma of the cervix: a Gynecologic Oncology Group study. *Gynecol Oncol*, 1990 38, 352-357.
[21] Sedlis, A; Bundy, BN; Rotman, M; Lentz, S; Muderspach, LI; Saino, R. A randomized trial of pelvic radiation therapy versus no further therapy in selected patients with stage IB carcinoma of the cervix after radical hysterectomy and pelvic lymphadenectomy: a Gynecologic Oncology group study. *Gynecol Oncol*, 1999 73, 177-183.
[22] Eifel, PJ; Burke, TW; Morris, M; Smith, TL. Adenocarcinoma as an independent risk factor for disease recurrence in patients with stage IB cervical cancer. *Gynecol Oncol*, 1995 59, 38-44.
[23] Shingleton, HM; Bell, MC; Fremgen, A; et al. Is there really a difference in survival of women with squamous cell carcinoma, adenocarcinoma and adenosquamous cell carcinoma of the cervix? *Cancer*, 1995 76, 1948-1955.
[24] Van Nagel, JR; Powell, DE; Gallion, HH; et al. Small cell carcinoma of the uterine cervix. *Cancer*. 1988 62, 1586-1593.
[25] Covens, A; Rosen, B; Murphy, J; Laframboise, S; DePetrillo, D; Lickrish, G; et al. How important is removal of the parametrium at surgery for carcinoma of the cervix? *Gynecol Oncol*, 2002 84(1), 145-9.
[26] Benedetti-Panici, P; Maneschi, F; D'Andrea, F; Cutillo, G; Rabittti, C; Congiu, M; et al. Early cervical carcinoma: the natural history of lymph node involvement redefined on the basis of thorough parametrectomy and giant section study. *Cancer*, 2000 88(10), 2267-74.
[27] Delgado, G; Bundy, BN; Fowler, WC; Stehman, FB; Sevin, B; Creasman, WT; et al. A prospective surgical pathological study of stage I squamous carcinoma of the cervix: a Gynecologic Oncology Group Study. *Gynecol Oncol*, 1989 35(3), 314-20.
[28] Burghardt, E; Baltzer, J; Tulusan, AH; Haas, J. Results of surgical treatment of 1028 cervical cancers studied with volumetry. *Cancer*, 1992 70, 648-655.

[29] Ostor, AG. Pandora's box or Ariadne's thread? Definition and prognostic significant of microinvasion in the uterine cervix: squamous lesions. In: *Pathology annual, part II. Melbourne: Dept. of Pathology*; 1995; 103-136.

[30] Fiorica, MD; Roberts, WS; Greenberg, H; Hoffman, MS; LaPolla, JP; Cavanagh, D. Morbidity and survival patterns in patients after radical hysterectomy and postoperative adjuvant pelvic radiotherapy. *Gynecol Oncol*, 1990 36, 343-347.

[31] Flay, LD; Matthew, JH. The effects of radiotherapy and surgery on the sexual function of women treated for cervical cacner. *Int J Radiat Oncol Biol Phys*, 1995 31, 399-404.

[32] Van Nagell, JR ; Maruyama, Y ; Parker, JC ; et al. Small bowel injury following radiation therapy for cervical cancer. *Am J Obstet Gynecol*, 1974 118, 163-167.

[33] Van Nagell, JR; Parker, JC; Maruyama, Y; et al. The effect of pelvic inflammatory disease on enteric complications following radiation therapy for cervical cancer. *Am J Obstet Gynecol*, 1977 128, 767-771.

[34] Samlal, RAK; van der Velden, J; Ketting, BW; Gonzalez, DG; Ten Late, FJW; et al. Disease-free interval and recurrence pattern after the Okabayashi varian to Wertheim's radical hysterectomy for stage IB and IIAcervical carcinoma. *Int J Gynecol Cancer*, 1996 6, 120-127.

[35] Sivanesaratnam, V; Sen, DK; Jayalakshmi, P; Ong G. Radical hysterectomy and pelvic lymphadenectomy for early invasive cancer of the cervix: 14 years experience. *Int J Gynecol Cancer*, 1993 3, 231-238.

[36] Spirtos, NM; Eisenkop, SM; Schlarth, JB; Ballon, SC. Laparoscopic radical hysterectomy (type III) with aortic and pelvic lymphadenectomy in patients with stage I cervical cancer: Surgical morbidity and intermediate follow-up. *Am J Obstet Gynecol*, 2002 187, 340-8.

[37] Steed, H; Rosen, B; Murphy, J; Laframboise, S; De Petrillo, D; Covens, A. A comparison of laparoscopic-assisted radical vaginal hysterectomy and radical abdominal hysterectomy in the treatment of cervical cancer. *Gynecol Oncol*, 2004 93, 588-593.

[38] Hertel, H; Kohler, C; Michels, W; Possover, M; Tozzi, R; Schneider, A. La paroscopic-assisted radical vaginal hysterectomy (LARVH): prospective evaluation of 200 patients with cervical cancer. *Gynecol Oncol*, 2003 90, 505-11.

[39] Burghardt, E; Pickel, H; Haas, J; et al. Prognostic factors and operative treatment of stages IB to IIB cervical cacner. *Am J Obstet Gyncol*, 1987 156, 988-996.

[40] Lai, CH ; Change, HC ; Change, TC ; et al. Prognostic factors and impacts of adjuvant therapy in early-stage cervical carcinoma with pelvic node metastases. *Gynecol Oncol*, 1993 51, 390-6.

[41] Fuller, AF Jr, Elliott, N; Kosloff, C; Hoskins, WJ; Lewis, JL. Determinants of increased risk for recurrence in patients undergoing radical hysterectomy for stage IB and IIA carcinoma of the cervix. *Gynecol Oncol*, 1989 33, 34-39.

[42] Morrow, CP; Shingleton, HM; Austin, JM; et al. Panel report: Is pelvic radiation beneficial in the postoperative management of stage IB Squamous cell carcinoma of the cervix with pelvic node metastasis treated by radical hysterectomy and pelvic lymphadenectomy. A report from the Presidential Panel at the 1979 annual meeting of the SGO. *Gynecol Oncol*, 1980 10, 105-110.

[43] Hacker, NF. Cervical cancer. In: Hacker, NF; Berek, JS eds. *Practical Gynecologic Oncology*. Philadelphia: Lippincott, Williams, & Wilkins; 2005; 337-389.

[44] Rose, PG; Bundy, B; Watkins, Eb; Thigpen, T; Deppe, G; et al. Concurrent cisplatin-based radiotherapy and chemotherapy for locally advanced cervical cancer. *N Engl J Med*, 1999 340, 1144-1153.

[45] Morris, M; Eifel, PJ; Lu, J; Grigsby, PW; Levenback, C; Stevens, RE; et al. Pelvic radiation with concurrent chemotherapy compared with pelvic and paraaortic radiation for high-risk cervical cancer. *N Engl J Med*, 1999 340, 1137-1143.

[46] Whitney, CW; Sause, W; Bundy, BN; Malfetano, JH; et al. Randomized comparison of fluorouracil plus cisplatin vs hydroxyurea as an adjunct to radiation therapy in stage IIB-IVA carcinoma of the cervix with negative paraortic nodes: a gynecologic oncology group study. *J Clin Oncol*, 1999 17, 1339-1348.

[47] Vermoken, JB. The role of chemotherapy in squamous cell carcinoma of the uterine cervix: a review. *Int J Gynecol Cancer*, 1993 3, 129-142.

[48] Rose, PG; Blessing, JA; Gershensen, DM; McGehee, R. Paclitaxel and cisplatin as first-line therapy in recurrent or advanced squamous cell carcinoma of the cervix: a Gynecologic Oncology Group study. *J Clin Oncol*, 1999 17, 2676-2680.

[49] Duyn, A, van Eijkeran, M; Kenter, G; Zwinderman <; Anskink, A. Recurrent cervical cancer: detection and prognosis. *Acta Obstet Gynecol Scand*, 2002 81, 759-763.

[50] Thomas, G; Dembo, AJ; Black, B; et al. Concurrent radiation and chemotherapy for carcinoma of the cervix recurrent after radical surgery. *Gynecol Oncol*, 1987 27, 254-264.

[51] Miller, B; Morris, M; Gershenson, CM Levenback, CL; Burke, TW. Intestinal fistulae formation following pelvic exenteration: a review of the University of Texas MD Anderson Cancer Center experience, 1956-1990. *Gynecol Oncol*, 1995 56, 207-210.

[52] Morley, GW; Hopkins, MP; Lindenauer, SM; Roberta, JA. Pelvic exenteration, University of Michigan: 100 patients at 5 years. *Obstet Gynecol*, 1989 74, 934-943.

[53] Lanciano R. Radiotherapy for the treatment of locally recurrent cervical cancer. *J Natl Cancer Inst Monogr*, 1996 21, 113-11.

In: Women and Cancer
Editor: Laurie Elit, pp. 173-178
ISBN: 978-1-60021-494-3

Chapter V

VULVAR CANCER

1. INCIDENCE & EPIDEMIOLOGY

Vulvar cancer accounts for less than 5% of gynecologic malignancies. The most common histologic cell type is squamous cell carcinoma followed by melanoma and basal cell carcinoma. Squamous cell carcinoma usually affects the labia major in postmenopausal women. Many women with vulvar cancer have, unfortunately, delayed seeking medical attention for their lesions. Also, they are often treated medically with topical creams for presumed benign conditions. Vulvar cancer can be difficult to distinguish visually from other benign skin lesions of the area and therefore women with persistent symptoms should be examined and any abnormalities should be biopsied. Partially as a result of various delays, of patients who undergo surgical staging only 25% have stage I disease. As with other gynecologic malignancies, prognosis declines with advancing stage [1].

Peak incidence of vulvar cancer is in the postmenopausal population. There are two peaks in incidence, the 6th and the 8th decade. Women who present at a younger age often have concomitant vulvar intraepithelial neoplasia (VIN) [2,3]. VIN is related to human papilloma virus (HPV) and smoking. HPV DNA is found in 80% of vulvar cancers associated with VINIII [2]. These tumors can be multi-focal. An increase in secondary cancers has been reported in women with vulvar cancer and these cancers are also often smoking related [4]. In the 8th decade it is usually not linked with HPV.

1.1. Risk Factors

Because cancer of the vulva is rare there are few known modifiable risk factors. However, a known medical risk factor is infection with HPV and history of VIN. Vulvar epithelial neoplasia is graded from I-III depending on severity. In women with untreated VIN III 87% progressed to vulvar cancer compared to only 3% of those women who received treatment [5,6]. Therefore women with biopsy proven VIN should be treated with laser therapy or surgery and followed for recurrence.

Smoking has been associated with an increased risk both VIN III and vulvar cancer in people with a known HPV16 infection [7].

Another potentially modifiable risk factor is lichen sclerosis. Lichen sclerosis is an epithelial disorder which affects the vulva in women of all ages but primarily postmenopausal women. It results in atrophy and scarring. It is controversial whether this is a true risk factor for vulvar cancer and whether it's treatment modifies the risk of subsequent cancer [8,9]. In women with lichen slerosis followed prospectively the incidence of vulvar cancer was 2-9% [9,10]. This condition is often treated with high dose topical steroids.

2. Clinical Presentation

Most women with vulvar cancer have a history of vulvar itching. The most common symptoms in both VIN and carcinoma are itching and irritation. Many will have a palpable lesion, which is occasionally associated with bleeding. Most vulvar cancers arise on the labia majora. When examining the genitalia, the size, location and mobility of a visible lesion should be recorded.

3. Diagnosis

3.1. Tissue Biopsies

The mainstay of diagnosis is a tissue biopsy of the lesion. Vulvar lesions suspicious for vulvar cancer should be either biopsied or removed with adequate tissue margins. Office biopsies using the Keys punch biopsy technique removes adequate tissue for assessment of depth of invasion while leaving the visible tumor for radical resection. This information is useful when planning surgical management. Depth of invasion is the most important information for surgical planning, as tumors with greater than 1mm of tumor invasion from the most superficial dermal papillae of the epithelial-stromal junction should have ipsilateral groin node dissection. The risk of groin metastasis when the depth is >1mm is 9% and increases with increasing depth of invasion [11,12].

3.2. Imaging

Routine imaging is not ordered for all patients with vulvar lesions. If there are palpable groin nodes on examination, CT imaging of the chest, abdomen, and pelvis may identify distant disease. The knowledge of distant disease may help in tailoring the therapy to the appropriate radiation fields or chemotherapy may be considered as a part of treatment.

4. Prognostic Factors

Staging is of the most important prognostic factor in vulvar cancer. Individual prognostic factors are tumor size, depth of invasion, nodal metastases and lymphovascular space invasion [1,12,13]. All of these are reflected in the FIGO stage except lymphovascular space invasion.

Melanoma is the second most common type of vulvar cancer and has a poorer prognosis than squamous cell carcinoma of the vulva over all. Melanoma of the vulva is staged based on a description by Chung, which uses depth of invasion [14].

Table 1. FIGO Staging of Vulvar Cancer

FIGO Stage		Features
I		
	IA	Tumor ≤2cm with ≤ 1mm invasion
	IB	Tumor ≤2cm with > 1mm invasion
II		Tumor confined to the vulva/perineum and > 2cm
III		Any tumor with: Adjacent spread to lower urethra, vagina or anus Unilateral groin node metastases
IV	IVA	Tumor invades upper urethra, bladder mucosa, rectal mucosa, pelvic bone or bilateral regional node metastases
	IVB	Any distant metastases

5. Therapies

5.1. Surgery

Primary surgery is the treatment of choice for lesions that do not involve the urethra or anus. Surgery should include complete excision of the tumor with at least 1cm margins. Pathologic margins of <8mm have been shown to have a local recurrence risk of 50% [15].

Surgical resection includes a radical resection of the vulvar tumor with or without groin node resection. The risk of having positive groin nodes increases primarily with the depth of invasion. Tumors of ≤ 1mm of tumor invasion have a 3% risk of having positive groin nodes. At increasing depth, the risk increases substantially; therefore tumors with depth of invasion beyond 1mm of require a groin node resection [11]. Tumors within one centimeter of the midline require bilateral node dissection.

Groin node dissection has a high postoperative complication rate. Wound breakdown and lymph edema occur in approximately 25% and 35% of patients respectively [16]. Recently there has been an interest in sentinel node dissection for vulvar cancer. This may provide the information on lymph node status and guide adjuvant therapy while decreasing the complication rate from a full groin node dissection. Currently this method is being actively investigated. Most studies still perform a full groin node dissection for comparison. Recent data reassuringly indicates a low false negative rate with good sensitivity [17,18]. There is no long-term data on the outcome of sentinel node dissection alone and whether the morbidity is less than a groin node dissection.

5.2. Radiotherapy

Radiotherapy is used both as a primary modality and adjuvant treatment in vulvar cancer. Women who have one micrometastasis in a single inguinal lymph node do not require further treatment. All others with greater than one positive groin node or extranodal metastases should have whole pelvis radiotherapy to complete therapy. Radiotherapy alone is not felt to be adequate for treatment of the inguinal area [19].

For women whose tumor approaches the urethra or anus and a complete resection is not possible radiotherapy can be used as a primary treatment to preserve these structures. Given the lack of evidence for radiotherapy alone in the groins surgery for the inguinal nodes may be discussed [19].

5.3. Chemotherapy

Chemotherapy has also been used in both for adjunctively with radiotherapy and as treatment for recurrent disease [20].

6. Follow-up & Recurrent Disease

Women with vulvar cancer are commonly followed with routine office visits every 3 months in the first year, every 4 months in the second year, every 6 months in the third and fourth years, and eventually annual visits. If a recurrence is suspected at the time of the office visit, biopsies should be performed. Imaging is also helpful to detect distant disease.

Women with negative lymph nodes have a greater than 90% five-year survival compared to 50% of all women with positive lymph nodes [13,21,22]. Patients who have not undergone a inguinal node dissection and have a nodal recurrence have a 90% death rate [23].

Depending on the location and extent of disease, recurrent tumor on the vulva is usually treated with surgical resection. More distant recurrences may be more difficult to treat, radiotherapy can be used if there has been no radiotherapy previously.

7. Paget's Disease of the Vulva

Also known as extramammary Paget's disease is characterized by adenocarcinoma in-situ on the vulva. Women with Paget's disease of the vulva disorder are in their 7th decade and usually present with vulvar itching and discomfort. At the time of examination the area is reddened and can be velvety in appearance. The treatment is surgical excision of the visibly affected area with 15-20mm lateral margins and 5mm deep to include the apocrine structures. This wide exision is required because the histologic extent of the lesion may not be easy to appreciate. Attempts should be made to spare the clitoris, urethra and anus and for this reason local recurrences are frequent regardless of the size of the surgical margins and repeat re-excision is the treatment of choice. In 4% of patients there is an underlying adenocarcionma, in these patients a radical vulvectomy and lymphadenectomy is required [24].

References

[1] Kosary; CL. FIGO stage, histology, histologic grade, age and race as prognostic factors in determining survival for cancers of the female gynecological system: An analysis of 1973-87 SEER cases of cancers of the endometrium, cervix, ovary, vulva, and vagina. *Semin Surg Oncol*; 1994 10(1), 31-46.

[2] Hording, U; Junge, J; Daugaard, S; Lundvall, F; Poulsen, H; Bock, JE. Vulvar squamous cell carcinoma and papillomaviruses: Indications for two different etiologies. *Gynecol Oncol*, 1994 52(2), 241-246.

[3] Toki, T; Kurman, RJ; Park, JS; Kessis, T; Daniel, RW; Shah, KV. Probable nonpapillomavirus etiology of squamous cell carcinoma of the vulva in older women: A clinicopathologic study using in situ hybridization and polymerase chain reaction. *Int J Gynecol Pathol*, 1991 10(2), 107-125.

[4] Sturgeon, SR; Curtis, RE; Johnson, K; Ries, L; Brinton, LA. Second primary cancers after vulvar and vaginal cancers. *Am J Obstet Gynecol*, 1996 174(3), 929-933.

[5] Jones, RW; Rowan, DM. Vulvar intraepithelial neoplasia III: A clinical study of the outcome in 113 cases with relation to the later development of invasive vulvar carcinoma. *Obstet Gynecol*, 1994 84(5), 741-745.

[6] McNally, OM; Mulvany, NJ; Pagano, R; Quinn, MA; Rome, RM. VIN 3: A clinicopathologic review. *Int J Gynecol Cancer*, 2002 12(5), 490-495.

[7] Madeleine, MM; Daling, JR; Carter, JJ; et al. Cofactors with human papillomavirus in a population-based study of vulvar cancer. *J Natl Cancer Inst*, 1997 89(20), 1516-1523.

[8] Hart, WR; Norris, HJ; Helwig, EB. Relation of lichen sclerosus et atrophicus of the vulva to development of carcinoma. *Obs Gyn*, 1975 45(4), 369-377.

[9] Cooper, SM; Gao, XH; Powell, JJ; Wojnarowska, F. Does treatment of vulvar lichen sclerosus influence its prognosis? *Arch Dermatol*, 2004 140(6), 702-706.

[10] Renaud-Vilmer, C; Cavelier-Balloy, B; Porcher, R; Dubertret, L. Vulvar lichen sclerosus: Effect of long-term topical application of a potent steroid on the course of the disease. *Arch Dermatol*, 2004 140(6), 709-712.

[11] Sedlis, A; Homesley, H, Bundy, BN; et al. Positive groin lymph nodes in superficial squamous cell vulvar cancer. *Am J Obstet Gynecol*, 1987 156(5), 1159-1164.

[12] Homesley, HD; Bundy, BN; Sedlis, A; et al. Prognostic factors for groin node metastasis in squamous cell carcinoma of the vulva (a gynecologic oncology group study). *Gynecol Oncol*, 1993 49(3), 279-283.

[13] Origoni, M; Sideri, M; Garsia, S; Carinelli, SG; Ferrari, AG. Prognostic value of pathological patterns of lymph node positivity in squamous cell carcinoma of the vulva stage III and IVA FIGO. *Gynecol Oncol*, 1992 45(3), 313-316.
[14] Chung, AF; Woodruff, JM; Lewis, JLJ. Malignant melanoma of the vulva; A report of 44 cases. *Obstet Gynecol*, 1975 45, 638.
[15] Heaps, JM; Fu, YS; Montz, FJ; Hacker, NF; Berek, JS. Surgical-pathologic variables predictive of local recurrence in squamous cell carcinoma of the vulva. *Gynecol Oncol*, 1990 38(3), 309-314.
[16] Rouzier, R; Haddad, B; Dubernard, G; Dubois, P; Paniel, BJ. Inguinofemoral dissection for carcinoma of the vulva: Effect of modifications of extent and technique on morbidity and survival. *J Am Coll Surg*, 2003 196(3), 442-450.
[17] Dhar, KK; Woolas, RP. Lymphatic mapping and sentinel node biopsy in early vulvar cancer. *BJOG*. 2005 112(6), 696-702.
[18] Merisio, C; Berretta, R; Gualdi, M; et al. Radioguided sentinel lymph node detection in vulvar cancer. *Int J Gynecol Cancer*, 2005 15(3), 493-497.
[19] Stehman, FB; Bundy, BN; Thomas, G; et al. Groin dissection versus groin radiation in carcinoma of the vulva: A gynecologic oncology group study. *Int J Radiat Oncol Biol Phys*, 1992 24(2), 389-396.
[20] Montana, GS; Thomas, GM; Moore, DH; et al. Preoperative chemo-radiation for carcinoma of the vulva with N2/N3 nodes: A gynecologic oncology group study. *Int J Radiat Oncol Biol Phys*, 2000 48(4), 1007-1013.
[21] Kirby, TO; Rocconi, RP; Numnum, TM; et al. Outcomes of stage I/II vulvar cancer patients after negative superficial inguinal lymphadenectomy. *Gynecol Oncol*, 2005 98(2), 309-312.
[22] Mariani, L; Lombardi, A; Atlante, M; Atlante, G. Radiotherapy for vulvar carcinoma with positive inguinal nodes. adjunctive treatment. *J Reprod Med*, 1993 38(6), 429-436.
[23] Homesley, HD. Vulva. *Am J Obstet Gyn*, 1991 84, 741-745.
[24] Fanning, J; Lambert, HC; Hale, TM; Morris, PC; Schuerch, C. Paget's disease of the vulva: Prevalence of associated vulvar adenocarcinoma, invasive paget's disease, and recurrence after surgical excision. *Am J Obstet Gynecol*, 1999 180(1 Pt 1), 24-27.

Section 5: Psychosocial Issues of Cancer for Women

In: Women and Cancer
Editor: Laurie Elit, pp. 181-202

ISBN: 978-1-60021-494-3

Chapter I

DISTRESS, BODY IMAGE, SEXUALITY AND SELF-IDENTITY AND IMPLICATIONS FOR TREATMENT

Mary Jane Esplen[*]
Department of Psychiatry, Faculty of Medicine, University of Toronto, Canada.

ABSTRACT

Objective: To provide an overview of the the major stressors related to having a cancer diagnosis and the emotional impact and quality of life issues associated with survivorship.

Results: The prevalence of distress following a cancer diagnosis and specific predictors of adjustment difficulties will be explored. In addition, a number of quality of life impacts and the specific impacts of cancer on body image , sexuality and identity are reviewed. The implications for assessment and treatment include psychosocial assessment, support resources and counseling approaches.

Conclusion: The diagnosis of cancer has psychosocial impacts on women and their families from the time of diagnosis, during treatment and recovery and through survivorship. Psychosocial screening, education and empirically-based treatment can address specific issues. Future work is needed to test innovative treatments.

[*] Correspondence concerning this article should be addressed to Mary Jane Esplen, PhD, RN Program of Psychosocial and Psychotherapy Research in Cancer Genetics, University Health Network, 200 Elizabeth Street, Eaton N 9-242 A, Toronto, Ontario, M5G 2C4. Tel: (416) 340-3024; Fax: (416) 340- 4739; Email: mesplen@uhnres.utoronto.ca.

INTRODUCTION

Cancer is one of the most frequently diagnosed illnesses among women and a leading cause of female death [1]. Cancer is well known to be a challenging disease affecting cancer patients and their families. This chapter describes the major stressors related to having a cancer diagnosis and the emotional impact and quality of life issues associated with survivorship. A specific focus on body image and sexual functioning impacts will be included. Finally, implications for screening and treatment will be discussed.

Distress and the Nature of the Specific Stressors Following a Diagnosis of Cancer

Over the past 20 years with an increase in the number of survivors due to advances in treatment and early detection, scientific attention has turned to considerations of the patient's quality of life during and after treatment, rather than solely issues of disease-free and overall survival. The process of a cancer diagnosis, treatment, recovery, and survivorship has inevitable psychosocial consequences in terms of physical, psychological and social functioning [2]. In fact, evidence exists for significant psychosocial distress at all stages of cancer.

The majority of cancer survivors do well after the initial adjustment within the first 2 years post-treatment [3,4]. However, depending on when they were assessed, a broad range of cancer survivors either score at levels suggestive of a psychiatric diagnosis or are diagnosed with a psychological problem [5,6,7]. And, an important subset of survivors experience adjustment problems long after treatment completion.

Emotional distress levels (typically measured in terms of anxiety and depression symptoms) vary across the disease trajectory and between cancer disease sites [7]. The incidence of emotional distress in North America ranges from 24% to 50% [5-12]. Up to 58% of patients in palliative care experience significant levels of emotional distress [13]. In addition to symptoms of depression or anxiety, distress has been documented in terms of stress response symptoms. For example, in the literature conceptualizing cancer as "trauma", among women with breast cancer, 44% reported being "super alert, watchful or on guard" as a consequence of being diagnosed and treated for cancer with 4% to 24% reporting other Post-traumatic stress disorder (PTSD)-like symptoms [14]. Even by a mean of 20 years after their diagnosis, the prevalence of PTSD can be considerable among cancer survivors, with 15% reporting two or more PTSD symptoms that are "moderately" to "extremely" bothersome [6].

The presence of heightened distress is associated with a number of negative outcomes including greater non-adherence to treatment recommendations [15], poorer satisfaction with care [16] and reduced quality of life across multiple domains [17-19].

Psychological distress among women with cancer stems from multiple sources: the fear of recurrence and an early death; treatments and their effects; disfigurement; emotional disturbance triggered by stimuli that remind them of their cancer experience; cancer-related sexual problems; long-term medical sequelae; and employment problems [15,20,21]. Other concerns include feelings of uncertainty about the future [21-25] fears of being unable to do things [22-24]; concerns of being a burden to the family [26,27]; and doubts about treatment and its side effects [22,23,28]. Although further study is needed and it remains uncertain whether or not certain chemotherapies affect cognitive function, some women report experiencing diminished cognitive functions (e.g. verbal and visual memory, attention, language and motor skill alteration) during and after adjuvant cancer chemotherapy referred to in the literature as "chemo-fog" or chemo-brain" [29,30].

Feelings of being marginalized or of being "different"[24], discomfort with unwanted sympathies [31], embarrassment, and shame have also been documented among cancer patients and can impact on sexuality and relationships with others [24,25,28,31].

A diagnosis of cancer in many ways continues to be a culturally taboo topic for discussion, which can result in isolation or silence, further creating emotional distress in patients [32,33]. For many individuals (e.g. the woman herself or her family) a cancer diagnosis is equated with an experience of "being given a death sentence," and is experienced as a "jarring" of one's awareness to the full realization that existence is finite [34]. Individuals can fear burdening others through the "opening up" of emotional expressions or be uncertain in how to have conversations around the illness. In addition, sometimes women or family members feel that maintaining a positive attitude is important or even fear that by expressing negative emotions the disease can further progress or return. Such beliefs and fears can result in women and their friends and family members feeling isolated, and lead to missed opportunities for support and result in increased distress.

In addition to the factors noted above, women in particular have unique challenges as they face a potentially life-threatening illness. Most women fulfil the primary parenting role for children and more than 50% of women work outside the home [35]. Gender proscribed roles or social demands place additional challenges in getting through cancer treatments with the competing needs to maintain balance and ongoing responsibilities. Women may also have fewer financial resources or face challenges in seeking access to care [35].

Factors Associated With Distress

Some research has been done to examine what factors place women with a cancer diagnosis at increased risk for distress. Factors examined often focus primarily on demographic and medial factors. Having more physical symptoms and worse physical functioning are associated with greater psychological distress. Women with more advanced or recurrent disease and those more recently diagnosed tend to have higher levels of distress [7,21,24,36]. For example, in a study of 121 individuals treated for colorectal cancer [37], the time since treatment, perception of illness severity, and activity level accounted for 45% of variance in a self-reported instrument to measure the demands of illness. Demands of illness were perceived greater and more distressing in the younger age group (26-45 years old), when more recently completing treatment, and if the illness was reported to cause greater impairment of activity. The 10 most intense illness-related demands were reported to be mainly psychosocial and existential concerns [37].

Particular subgroups, for example, younger women or minority groups may also be at increased risk for distress [7,38-40]. Younger women or specific cultural groups can feel isolated as they often are unable to relate to older women or other cultures in cancer settings, due to their uniquely experienced challenges. For example, it has been suggested that younger women with cancer have fewer expectations of disease or disability being normative than women at a later life stage, which may cause a greater sense of emotional distress in response to their cancer [41]. They have added concerns around self-image, fertility and subsequent pregnancy, or fears around their survival in their felt need to be there for young children. Other issues include impacts on dating or future relationships and concerns around work opportunities. As in other health areas pre-existing emotional difficulties or a past history of mental health illnesses may exacerbate adjustment difficulties following a cancer diagnosis and are related to long-term distress [42,43].

Social support is another important factor. Generally, higher levels of social support and greater satisfaction are associated with positive adjustment [44-46]. Social support is believed to buffer the impact of stress and provides assistance in coping with a challenging illness. Individuals with cancer most often request emotional support from spouses, family, friends, healthcare professionals, and peers who have experiential knowledge about how to survive [47]; or for some, allow them to compare their positions to others (not as well off) to feel more secure and less vulnerable [48]. Social and cultural values and structures, as well as individual variables, such as age, previous experience and coping styles are associated with behaviors of avoidance towards people with cancer [49]. Women can often be surprised by reactions of others who have not visited or offered support. Individuals may avoid contact due to unease in discussing the illness, being unsure "how to help" or may experience personal feelings of fear of death and dying as evoked through a friend or family member's life threatening diagnosis [47]. As a consequence, many individuals during and following treatments report feeling separate from others and alone, with resulting psychosocial impacts [50].

Positive adjustment is predicted by an active, rather than avoidant coping style [51,52]. During the early stages following a cancer diagnosis, individuals use several coping strategies [53] and the number of strategies used reflects total coping efforts [54]. Coping effort tends to decrease markedly across the first year post diagnosis [55,56]. Sustained high coping effort is associated with poor long-term adjustment to cancer [54]. Coping styles involving helplessness are associated with greater distress and have been shown to relate to cancer outcomes. Women having a repertoire of coping mechanisms and who have flexibility in their use tend to experience more positive adjustment [45].

Important "anniversary" markers have been identified. For example, it is common for women to view the "5 year survival" mark as an important event. While this is generally experienced as positive in their survivorship, it is a time when past memories associated with the cancer diagnosis and its illness are aroused and communication barriers may occur as family members see it as a time to clearly put the traumatic event behind them [57]. There are also other marked time points to note that can be associated with increased feelings of vulnerability or distress. One well-known marker is the end of treatment where on the one hand women feel relief that the treatments are completed and they can move on to recovery, while on the other, experience feelings of abandonment, increased anxiety or concern that there is decreased structure and attention on the "fight" against cancer, and experience feelings of loss around the earlier sense of protection gained through the treatments.

QUALITY OF LIFE IMPACTS

Quality of life is multidimensional and covers a number of life domains [19]. Traditionally, quality of life has been focused primarily on aspects of physical functioning to compare different treatments, rather than to extend the meaning of quality of life to include psychosocial or existential concerns. However, there is growing evidence that quality of life is a complex concept that involves not only physical well-being, but psychological, social, and spiritual well-being [57,58]. For each domain, quality of life may be perceived and weighted differently by various women. Changes in one domain can influence perceptions in others. For example, any changes in the physical domain are likely to affect a woman's psychological or social functioning [57].

Within the *physical domain*, women may vary in the kinds of treatments they receive, depending on the severity of illness, age and other medical factors. Treatment or disease impacts include fatigue, scarring, pain, loss of or altered function (e.g. arm movement in lymphedema), and other physiological effects such as induced menopause and its associated side effects (e.g. vaginal dryness, decreased libido, hot flashes). These short, and in some cases longer effects, can affect emotional and social well-being of cancer survivors which impact on quality of life. For example, physical and social problems that may not be relieved include menopause, menstrual changes, infertility, sleep problems, lymphedema, pain, problems with physical and recreational activities and weight changes (gains or losses) [57,59]. Ganz found arm problems among breast cancer survivors 2 and 3 years post treatment related to the initial surgical procedures (e.g. numbness, tightness and pulling in the arm and intermittent mild pan). Furthermore, 70% reported reduced energy and 60% reported difficulties in doing physical activities [60].

In the *psychological domain*, studies suggest that for most women improvements in mood and overall quality of life occur during the first year. However, further improvement may not necessarily occur when 2 to 3 year follow ups are conducted [57,60]. Psychological issues continue to be a source of great distress at least for a significant subset of cancer survivors. Depending on the age and disease site, up to 1/3 of long-term survivors may report significant distress (e.g. depression) [61]. Other studies suggest lower rates of anxiety and depression over the long term [62]. Inconsistent findings may reflect the use of varying measurement tools and time points among studies. While concerns about the future are a dominant problem, other concerns about the cancer diagnosis and treatment, medical follow-up and issues of self image appear to be common [57]. For example, individuals may continue to experience difficulties coping with feelings of fatigue, alterations in weight (gain or losses) or experience cognitive changes that are troubling. These treatment or illness impacts can lead to loss of confidence and self-esteem and impair quality of life.

Within the *social domain* relationships and work-related issues are important. Work-related issues include "subtle discrimination" in promotional opportunities and being laid off because supervisors do not believe they can do the work [57,63]. Racial differences have been found in functioning which may be explained by differences in upper body disability, physical demands on the job and the fact that minority groups of women are more likely to be employed in service occupations or as labourers or fabricators [35,57].

Cancer survivors may also experience problems in accessing medical care and in communication with physicians [35,57]. Some women report feeling abandoned by medicine, or experience challenges in discussing their health with others, feel social stigma associated with having a cancer diagnosis, or are unable to receive or ask for assistance [57].

Other areas to consider within the social domain include family impacts. For example, concern for offspring and their risk for cancer, challenges in discussing illness with family members and concern about how the family will cope, difficulties in delegating or carrying out social roles (e.g. management of parenting issues), challenges with partners in communicating about the illness or in dealing with a partner's attitude or woman's altered body image and priorities have been documented [57,62,64-66].

Spiritual Domain-There is increased interest among researchers in the spiritual well-being of cancer survivors and its measurement [67]. Concerns for women with cancer often include a re-examining of life priorities and of spiritual and philosophical perspectives of life, given the threat of mortality that comes along with the diagnosis. A common thread throughout the illness trajectory, irrespective of cancer type, race/ethnicity, or length of time since diagnosis are existential themes that include spirituality and religiosity to maintain a sense of hope, to find meaning and purpose, and which involve issues of personal growth [68].

Existential health or spirituality refers to seeking meaning through being harmoniously engaged and connected to family, friends, nature, or a higher being (e.g. God) beyond oneself [69]. Existential distress is spiritual or philosophical suffering that may or may not include issues of intrinsic religiosity [69]. Existential and psychological health are confounded, however, existential distress in cancer patients has been found in an exploratory survey [70] to be strongly correlated with end-of-life despair even after controlling for the effect of depressive symptoms, physical symptoms, and social support. Though existential concerns are pervasive in the cancer population, existential issues do not necessarily lead to significant distress and may enhance a deepened meaning of life [20,28]. Spirituality can enable a sense of hope through transcendence, and empower individuals to be whole and live life fully once more. Although spirituality can be expressed through religion, the practice of religion does not necessarily lead to feelings of transcendence. Non-religious activities such as meditation, creative activities, or contact with nature may assist with spiritual well-being [71]. Studies have found higher levels of hope and lower total negative mood states in individuals with high spiritual and intrinsic religiosity compared to individuals with low spiritual and intrinsic religiosity [69].

There are also positive aspects of quality of life following a cancer diagnosis among survivors. Several studies have documented the positive coping strategies and processes used by cancer survivors and the ways that quality of life may be enhanced rather than diminished by the experience of having faced a life-threatening illness, undergone toxic and painful treatments and survival [45,62]. Women frequently feel empowered and have a sense of renewed life priorities. These positive changes are life enhancing as women feel permitted and "free" and less restrained by social or cultural expectations in choosing to use their time for activities that they value, having a renewed sense of which relationships are most important, thereby leading to increased quality of life. Other experiences include a sense of resilence and "survivorship" in getting through a difficult illness experience and its associated personal growth and learning.

LONG TERM QUALITY OF LIFE IMPACTS

The largest numbers of studies focusing on long-term impacts are conducted with breast cancer survivors or include a high proportion of breast cancer survivors in heterogeneous samples [62]. Most studies document considerable physical, psychological and social problems among these women. Although individuals move beyond treatment effects and the initial coping with life-threatening illness additional challenges may emerge over time, and these problems can be some of the most persistent and resistant to treatment [5]. The aspects of quality of life that pose the most difficulty for survivors are likely to vary by cancer site, but the literature indicates specific challenges, such as alterations in body image, decreased self esteem and lower satisfaction and difficulties with sexual functioning, intimacy and social situations, regardless of diagnosis or treatment [62,66,72,73,74].

PERSISTENT SURVIVORSHIP ISSUES: BODY IMAGE, SEXUAL FUNCTIONING AND SELF-IDENTITY

The diagnosis of cancer and its subsequent treatment can have a profound impact on body image and sexual functioning. For a list of factors contributing to body and self image and sexual functioning see Table I. As individuals attempt to improve their quality of life after treatment, recovery of sexual health and body image become more important. It is significant that approximately 20% to 40% of survivors experience sexual and body image problems following cancer and treatment, and these difficulties can persist for several years after treatment completion [5,61,74].

In the earlier phases of the cancer experience when survival is a major goal, issues of sexual functioning, body image and intimacy are not usually given the same attention as treatment protocols and procedures [75]. Furthermore, body image and sexual functioning problems are often sidestepped and not raised by health professionals due to their highly private nature. In addition, women may feel "less permitted" to raise these personal issues, given the highly valued and more frequent focus on the treatment of the illness and its threat of mortality. Women may fear being judged or perceived as being vain if they focus on such personal issues, given that they "should" (and of course do) feel gratitude to have survived the treatment or illness. Failure to provide opportunity for women to discuss more personal issues such as challenges around their sexual functioning and to express the emotional impact of changes they are experiencing can create less opportunity for developing supportive relationships with a health care professional [76] and lead to increased isolation and distress.

Table 1. Cancer Treatment –Related Factors Contributing to Body Image and Psychosexual Difficulties

- Fatigue, nausea, hair loss
- Loss of libido
- Loss of fertility, induced menopause
- Reduced/lack of vaginal lubrication
- Reduced/lack of orgasmic response
- Loss of/altered to body parts, sexual organs
- Incontinence
- Lymphoedema
- Weight gain or loss
- Scarring
- Pain
- Fatigue
- Reduced Sensation
- Cognitive Changes (e.g. memory)

Adapted from Sundquist and Yee (2003). Sexuality and body image after cancer. *Australian Family* Physician, 32(1-2), 1922.

Body Image

Surgical treatments for cancer alter one's sense of body image. For example, breast cancer surgery can negatively impact breast sensitivity [72]. Chemotherapy treatments can lead to premature menopause and hormonal treatments can worsen menopausal symptoms, such as vaginal dryness and dysparaunia. Sexual dysfunction and body image can be persistent problems; for example, 20% to 30% of survivors develop sexual problems following a breast cancer diagnosis and treatment, and these difficulties tend to persist for several years after treatment completion [5,61,74]. Additional survivorship issues cited as being problematic include intimate situations (36%) and social contacts (28%) [73]. For younger women concerns around infertility and premature menopause are common [40].

In breast cancer, studies comparing types of surgery have shown that in comparison to mastectomy, breast-conserving surgery surprisingly results in minor to no advantage in terms of survivors' psychological distress, fear of recurrence, body image concerns, sexual functioning, social and marital-sexual adjustment, and overall quality of life [3,77-79]. In one study, 25% of women who had undergone only breast-conserving surgery had serious body image problems [80]. Distress over scars, feeling less sexually attractive, being uncomfortable in more revealing clothes, such as bathing suits [74,77] and avoidance of leisure activities were common expressions of body image problems. In terms of mastectomy, a number of studies report that women may continue to have significant problems with body image many years following their surgery, ranging from a mean of 3.4 to 8 years [5,80,81]. Not surprisingly, a poorer body image among both subgroups is significantly related to worse adjustment [74,80].

While it had been anticipated that breast reconstruction would provide survivors with a significant advantage in terms of their body image, psychosexual adaptation and overall adjustment, at least two studies report no significant psychosocial or sexual advantage of breast reconstruction compared to that of the other breast cancer surgeries [74,82]. While it is unclear why those choosing breast construction may not benefit psychosexually, it has been speculated that survivors choosing breast reconstruction may be the most concerned about body image and therefore the most disappointed if the breast reconstruction did not return the patient to full psychosexual functioning [73].

In the gynaecological cancers the resulting loss of reproductive functioning forces a woman to adjust her sense of self worth and feminine identity. Surgery that results in premature menopause can result in women feeling older, in addition to other physical effects associated with menopause.

Cancer causes a strain on relationships often as a result of a woman's altered body image or sense of self. Sometimes partners fear harming a woman. While intuitively it would seem that a partner's acceptance of bodily changes is important, a partner's acceptance of body changes may not reduce the woman's anxiety or perception of sexual concerns [66,83]. Furthermore, there can be differences within the relationship in terms of focus of concern. For example, partners may focus on intimacy and relationships, whereas women may be more attentive to their concerns of their future and the natural course of the illness [76]. These issues are best resolved through open communication between women and their partners. For some women a couple approach to treatment and/or individual and group counselling are recommended to facilitate this process.

Sexual Functioning

Sexual health is considered multidimensional and changes that occur in one dimension may produce changes in another [76]. Three dimensions of sexual health that have been identified include: sexual function, sexual self-concept and sexual relationships [76,84]. Intimacy, self esteem, attitudes, knowledge, satisfaction, participation and interest have also been identified as dimensions within a biopsychosocial framework to assess sexual health [85]. Gender roles, traditional, cultural and religious beliefs may also influence one's sexual health [86]. Therefore, sexual functioning is not viewed simply as an isolated component but is highly dependent on how a woman perceives changes imposed on her life as a result of having cancer and its treatment [66,76].

Rates of general sexual disruption, decreased frequency of sexual intercourse and difficulties with orgasm range from 21% to 39% [6]. Dorval [61] found that breast cancer survivors at 8 years post diagnosis were significantly less satisfied with their sexual life compared to controls. Ganz [87] found similar rates of sexual activity to age-matched samples of women without a history of breast cancer, however, significantly fewer patients were moderately to extremely satisfied with their sexual relationship at the time of the survey than they recalled having been prior to breast cancer diagnosis. A subsequent study found that vaginal dryness and treatment with chemotherapy were associated with sexual dysfunction, and sexual satisfaction was related to the strength of the partner relationship and the absence of sexual problems in the partner [88]. Studies on the effect of type of surgery on sexual adjustment have been more mixed, with some studies finding that women who have breast conserving surgery reporting better sexual adjustment [81,89] and other studies not finding a relationship between type of surgery and sexual adjustment [61,91]. The wide variety of measures of sexual adjustment may account for these inconsistent findings.

Research that has addressed quality of life issues after gynaecological cancer identifies sexuality as the major components of one's life that is affected by the cancer and related treatments [66,76,90]. Although the literature more often focuses on cervical cancer, there is some indication that experiences with endometrial cancer have similar effects on women's feelings of intimacy and sexual functioning [76]. In the gynaecological cancers treatments induce invisible assaults to femininity and can permanently affect one's sexual identify and functioning [76]. In ovarian cancer vasomotor symptoms and vaginal dryness associated with menopause may lead to physical discomfort and sexual dysfunction that can also contribute to the onset of mood symptoms [90].

Women with pre-existing relationship problems, those who receive chemotherapy and who undergo hormonal changes during treatment may be at particular risk for developing these problems [87,88,91].

Self-Identity/ Alterations in the Self

Self-identity (including body image) and its relationship to illness is a complex subject [92], however, we know that extreme experiences, such as a cancer illness can produce discontinuities in the sense of self. Contemporary theory stresses the persistence of embodiment in explaining personal identity [93,94]. A diagnosis of cancer threatens the element of continuity because it brings bodily changes as well as cognitive changes that challenge central values [92,95]. Experiences of loss (related to body parts or functioning) and the need to restore or preserve continuity is a major task for women with cancer. Little [92] described the term "resumption" referring to survivors of extreme experience being able to re-construct their identities in ways that accommodate the experience and its sequelae-that is, they *resume* a version of their former lives within the context of their changed embodiment and new insights.

Individuals bring a pre cancer self concept to the situation that is unique in terms of the exact configuration of content and structure (e.g. personality, cognitive self beliefs and schemas, self perceptions of physical appearance). Models suggest that individuals crossover into the "cancer self", and that the "self" continues to shift over time [95,96]. For example, the self concept at diagnosis may be quite different from the self concept during treatment or during survivorship. Individuals tend to manage discontinuity by reference to stable "anchor points" in their self beliefs and values (e.g. I value inner wisdom; I value outward attractiveness). Individuals who cannot achieve a sense of continuity may feel alienated from themselves, their friends and family and have negative self views [92]. These feelings of alienation can result in increased psychosocial distress and impact relationships with partners, other family or friends.

The shift in personal identity is important in understanding the self and body image experiences that occur as a result of physical changes resulting from surgery and the emotional "jarring" impact of being diagnosed with a life-threatening illness. When a woman experiences physical losses and changes that result in her feeling less attractive and feminine, or when she feels emotional shifts in her inner values and priorities due to the increased realization that life is finite and precious (that comes as a result of being diagnosed with a life-threatening illness) her sense of identity shifts. This shift often has an impact on her relational patterns, self-esteem and her comfort level in intimate situations, and may impact on her day to day social functioning (e.g. social withdrawal). Therefore, while the physical alterations obviously lead to body image changes, shifts in life priorities as a result of having faced a life-threatening illness are also relevant, regardless of the disease site and treatments. Table 2 lists factors associated with the existential impact of having a life-threatening illness that can play a role in shifts in identity and self-image.

Table 2. Alterations Associated with Having a Life-Threatening Illness that Contribute to Self Image and Identity Changes

- Fear of a potential shortened life
- Sense of altered life priorities and/ or values
- Increased sense of the value of specific relationships
- Increased life meaning or purpose
- Alterations in religiosity or spirituality
- Sense of increased resilience, sense of positive personal growth or self-actualization
- Feeling of empowerment (or feeling less empowered or loss of control)
- Altered perspectives around work life; family; goals

Interventions are sometimes required to help reconstruct versions of a pre-experience identity or to draw on past memory in a way that helps to preserve a continuity between past memory, present experience and constructions of the future. Interventions can use past and current experience to recognize facets of established identity, and to incorporate new experience, by imbuing the experience with meaning and recognizing the enlarged identity made possible by survival [92]. While couple approaches may be helpful, they are limited if the woman's own shifts in identity are not fully worked out, as her "unspoken" (or even unrecognized) identity shifts can be a barrier in communicating with a partner and in her level of trust, comfort with, and interest in partners. Methods to assist women to manage this experience and to express and to "work through" these changes in order to recognize new possible selves and identities, and to communicate such shifts with partners are available. Particularly relevant are interventions geared towards open expression of these personal issues (e.g. safe environment of a closed support group; 1: 1 counselling; couple intervention) and creative therapies geared towards expression, identification of new self schemas and adjustment to loss and grief, and those thatassist a woman to establish new goals. Therapies such as art therapy, guided imagery or other mind-body or creative approaches are helpful. Group approaches, such as supportive-expressive support groups are also relevant resources to address these issues.

Clinical Implications for Assessment and Treatment

Psychosocial Assessment

As all women and their families are prone to experience various potential adjustment reactions as they confront a cancer diagnosis and its treatments, psychological screening is an important dimension of cancer care. Recent attempts to standardize and integrate psychological screening into cancer care include the recognition of psychosocial functioning as the "sixth vital sign" [10]. The integration of the notion of a "sixth vital sign" into standard of care assessments recognizes the importance of distress as a marker of well-being and its reduction as a target outcome [10].

Several tools have been developed [97] and validated to screen for psychological distress but have not been consistently incorporated into standard clinical care. Several of these scales utilize brief self-report methods. However, cancer centers can be challenged in using them in routine practice, primarily due to the lack of psychosocial personnel or resources. Screening questions as simple as "How are you doing emotionally? "or "How are you dealing with the day to day challenges of having cancer or in managing your treatments?" and "How do you feel about the changes the cancer has brought to your body?" can facilitate discussions and assist in identifying specific personal issues. Evidence suggests that even a simple visual analogue type self-rating device, referred to as a "distress thermometer" - a visual depiction of a thermometer with ratings ranging from 0- indicating "no distress" to 10 indicating "extreme distress" -is an effective screening instrument in identifying the various ranges of psychosocial need and in identifying those, who in particular require added support [18]. Cutoffs for identifying significant distress levels for these simple tools have been established [18].

In relation to the specific issues of body image and sexual functioning difficulties, little evidence exists that these problems are being properly assessed or treated [5]. A failure of health professionals to assess or raise subjects of sexual functioning, intimacy or body image changes results in a message- that body image or sexuality issues are not a medical concern within the context of other medical concerns. This leaves women feeling isolated and silenced and to discuss or to try to deal with their problems either alone, or with partners, with little added information or support. The lack of clinical intervention or acknowledgement of sexuality as aspects of one's quality of life is a consistent finding in reports of various cancer diagnoses [76,98] and is likely an important factor in relation to the reported prevalence rates of these difficulties. Specific assessment of, and interventions geared towards addressing these persistent and personal issues need to be included as part of survivor services in order to enable these women to preserve their sexuality and to restore a healthy body image and identity after a cancer diagnosis and treatment.

Support Resources and Counselling Approaches for Improving Quality of Life in Cancer

The range of problems encountered by female cancer survivors strongly suggests that interventions need to be comprehensive in nature, available to all groups of women with cancer and across the cancer continuum. The core support services need to include educational or psycho educational interventions, given that providing information is an important source of support, especially in the early stages of the cancer trajectory and during stressful experiences (e.g. diagnostic period, during treatments) [99].

Table 3. Continuum of Distress Levels

Low Level of Distress →	*Moderate Level of Distress* →	*High level of Distress*
Educational Pamphlets, CDs Didactic Teaching Internet support Psychoeducational Group Relaxation Training/ Guided Imagery Peer Counseling Peer Support Groups	Cognitive-behavioral (e.g. stress management, coping strategies for living with uncertainty, dealing with treatments) Interactive CD ROMS	Individual Psychotherapy/ Supportive counseling Professionally led support groups
	Manual & computer-based decisional aids	Family counseling
Creative Therapies (Art Therapy)	Telephone counseling and follow-up 1:1 counseling	Psychotropic Medication
Mindfulness-based Stress Reduction	Peer support (1:1; Group)	
Yoga	Mindfulness-based Stress Reduction/ Meditation	Mindfulness-based Stress Reduction/ Meditation
Creative Therapies (e.g. Art Therapy)	Couple Counseling	Couple Counseling
	Yoga Creative Therapies (e.g. Art Therapy)	

Women with cancer require different interventions based upon where they are on the distress continuum. Table 3 indicates a continuum of psychosocial distress and the type of interventions that might be helpful for various distress levels. There are several evidence-based interventions available from which to draw, including: pamphlets, CD ROMS, Peer and community supports (1:1; groups in community), professionally-led 1:1 counselling (e.g. cognitive behavioural), relaxation and meditation techniques, professionally led group support (e.g. cognitive-behavioural, supportive-expressive), couple counselling and family supports to assist in managing the impact on families and children. Information on treatments, their side effects as well as medical and psychological interventions that assist women to manage these potential symptoms should be routinely provided. Wherever possible, women should be provided with opportunity to ask questions and to clarify an understanding of potential effects of either the illness or treatments. With high levels of distress medical intervention in the form of psychotropic medication (e.g. antidepressants) can be beneficial to help women to manage, optimally in combination with supportive counselling and other support services.

There have been several trials of psychological interventions to enhance coping with and adjustment to cancer [100,101]. The vast majority of the psychosocial interventions are conducted with women with early-stage cancer and limited to that in active treatment or soon after treatment. Across diagnostic cancer groups, most of the psychosocial and psycho educational interventions have been developed for cancer patients in active or palliative treatment, many consisting of supportive and educational components, with some also including problem-solving or behavioural interventions, such as relaxation training [5]. In general, results have indicated that patients who received any intervention experience an improvement in psychosocial adaptation, irrespective of the content or whether the format was individual or group [102-105]. However, contrary to the overall report of success of interventions across disease sites, results have been more mixed with regard to breast cancer patients [101]. The negative findings in breast cancer may relate to specific problems experienced by cancer patients, such as the difficulties with sexual functioning, an altered body image and self identity, which may be more difficult to ameliorate with non-specific interventions for these issues [5]. Others suggest that the interventions have been conducted too early in survivors' clinical course [5].

Few studies (individual or group counselling) have examined impacts on body image and sexuality. One possible reason for the lack of attention to such vital dimensions of well-being is that women have inadequate information about the physical and psychological effects of the cancer diagnosis and treatment [75]. Furthermore, health care professionals, patients and partners are often reluctant to discuss sexual functioning [75,105]. Among intervention studies that that did measure constructs of sexuality or body image (e.g. couple interventions) the effect sizes have been small or findings inconsistent [46,106-108]. While a couple intervention may seem most relevant, unfortunately only a smaller percentage of couples participate in interventions when offered and they tend to have less impact on body image, compared to other aspects, such as couple adjustment or sexual functioning. Furthermore, the "self identity" issues are important to address in order to maximize the benefit of a couple approach.

Group approaches have been identified as a cost-effective approach, improving quality of life and enhancing mutual support and adjustment [103,104,109,110]. Although findings have been inconsistent [109] group interventions have also been shown to enhance immune functioning and survival [104,110]. Group interventions are an ideal format in reducing isolation through the validation of meeting other women in similar situations with similar experiences. Women benefit through the expression and working through of emotions that several models encourage and through the vicarious learning of active coping techniques used by other group members or encouraged by group leaders. In addition, group interventions can easily incorporate creative or behavioural therapies (e.g. guided imagery, mindfulness-based stress reduction, art therapy) to assist women to manage their stress and anxiety and to get in touch with their inner emotional experience. Group interventions can lead to increased insight, facilitate adjustment to losses and to assist women to negotiate the changes they are experiencing in order for them to feel a sense of continuity and survivorship as they move forward.

Group interventions should be developed and provided keeping in mind that homogenous and universal coping themes and stressors are required in order to maximize the benefits and to establish optimal mutual understanding among women, thereby reducing the potential for dropouts [99,111]. For example, conducting a support group of breast cancer patients is best provided separately for women with newly diagnosed breast cancer and those with metastatic disease. While there are shared issues of concern (e.g. existential issues; coping with treatments) between both sub groups, there are unique and separate highly relevant issues among each group (e.g. heightened fear and anxiety concerning treatments among newly diagnosed breast cancer; altered self image and a more imminent need to focus on the existential issues such as fears associated with dying from breast cancer, pain management and relational issues among metastatic breast cancer patients). Other examples include combining disease sites or older and younger groups of women. While it is possible to conduct mixed groups of cancer patients or those that include both younger and older women, group leaders need to be aware of potential challenges and allow for sub-group unique themes to emerge, yet maintain the most focus on homogenous and universal themes among subgroups in order to promote group cohesion and to keep it personally relevant to all the women. Groups tend to be more easily facilitated when women can relate to universal themes and feel that the focus of the group is personally relevant [99,111].

Further research is needed on specific interventions that involve patients from the time of treatment completion to address specific adjustment problems that remain untreated or worsen. Studies suggest that by intervening earlier in the post-treatment phase, problems may be alleviated, or even prevented, thereby facilitating long-term adjustment. Further research is also needed on innovative treatment approaches, using rigorous research methods and comparative trials to determine who is best suited for a specific approach. Finally, there is a need for studies on interventions offered for women with other cancers (e.g. gynecological, lung) to build further upon the existing empirical evidence, given that the majority of intervention studies have been conducted in breast cancer.

CONCLUSION

In summary, the diagnosis of cancer is challenging with psychosocial impacts on women and their families at all stages of cancer, including at the time of diagnosis, during treatments and recovery, during periods of recurrence, advanced disease and throughout survivorship. While the majority of women adapt and experience improvements in mood within the first 2 to 3 years following their diagnoses, there can be persistent difficulties that significantly impact quality of life. And, a subset of women continue to experience significant levels of distress and impairments on their quality of life over the long term. Self and body images alterations and impacts on sexual functioning can extend over the long-term and need to be better addressed through standard care. Psychological screening should be integrated within cancer care programs in order to identify women who may benefit from psychological or added supportive treatments. Education on potential changes and the management of side effects of treatments or disease impacts should be provided, along with opportunities for women to ask questions or to express concerns. There are a number of empirically-based treatments that can be provided to address the psychosocial impact of cancer during treatment and all phases of survivorship. However, future work is needed on the testing of innovative treatments during survivorship, on comparative trials of interventions and for populations of women with other types of cancers, in addition to the work already undertaken for breast cancer.

REFERENCES

[1] Canadian Cancer Society. (2005). *Canadian Cancer Statistics 2005* (On-line).

[2] Ganz PA. 1990. Current issues in cancer rehabilitation. Cancer, 65(3 Suppl):742-51.

[3] Moyer, A. Psychosocial outcomes of breast-conserving surgery versus mastectomy: A meta-analytic review. *Health Psychol*, 1997 16, 284-298.

[4] Levy, SM; Haynes, LT; Herberman, RB; Lee, J; McFeeley, S; Kirkwood, J. (1992). Mastectomy versus breast conservation surgery: mental health effects at long-term follow-up. *Health Psychol*, 11(6), 349-54.

[5] Kornblith, AB; Ligibel, J. Psychosocial and sexual functioning of survivors of breast cancer. *Seminars in Oncology*, 2003 30, 799-810.

[6] Kornblith, AB; Herndon, JE; Weiss, RB; et al.. Long-term adjustment of survivors of early stage breast cancer carcinoma 20 years after adjuvant chemotherapy. *Cancer*, 2003 98, 679-689.

[7] Norton, T; Manne, S; Rubin, S; Carlson; J; Hernandez, E; Edelson, M; Rosenblum, N; Warshal, D; and Bergman; C. Prevalence and predictors of psychological distress among women with ovarian cancer, *J. of Clinical Oncology*, 2004 22(5), 919-926.

[8] Zabora, J; BrintzenhofeSzoc, K; Curbow, B; Hooker, C; Piantadosi, S. The prevalence of psychological distress by cancer site. *Psycho-Oncology*, 2001 10(1), 19-28.

[9] Carlson, LE; Bultz, BC. Efficacy and medical costs offset of psychosocial interventions in cancer care: Making the case for economic analyses. *Psycho-Oncology*, 2004 13(2); 837-849.

[10] Bultz, BD; and Carlson, LE. Emotional distress: the sixth vital sign-future directions in cancer care, 2006 15, 93-95.

[11] Bodurka-Bevers, D; Basen-Engquist, K; Carmack, CL; et al. Depression, anxiety, and quality of life in patients with epithelial ovarian cancer, *Gynecolog Oncology*, 2000 78, 302-308.

[12] Kornblith, AB; Thaler, HT; Wong, G; et al. Quality of life of women with ovarian cancer. *Gynecol Oncology*, 1995 59, 231-242.

[13] Potash, M; Breibart, W. Affective disorders in advanced cancer. *Hematol Oncology Clinic of North America*, 2002 16(3), 671-700.

[14] Cordova, MJ; Andrykowski, MA; Kenady, DE; McGrath, PC; Sloan, DA; Redd, WH. Frequency and correlates of posttraumatic-stress-disorder-like symptoms after treatment for breast cancer. *J Consult Clin Psychol*, 1995 63, 981-986.

[15] Kennard, BD; Smith, SM; Olvera, R; et al. Nonadherence in adloescent oncology patients: preliinary data on psychological risk factors and relationships to outcome. *J. of Clincal Psych Medical Settings*, 2004 11, 39-39.

[16] Von Essen, L; Larsson, G; Oberg, K; Sjoden, PO. "Satisfaction with care": Associations with health-related quality of life and psychosocial function among Swedish patients with endocrine gastrointestinal tumours. *Eur J Cancer Care*, 2002 11, 91-99.

[17] Skarstein, J; Aass, N; Fossa, SD; Skovlund, E; Dahl, AA. Anxiety and depression in cancer patients: relation between the hospital anxiety and depression scale and the European Organization for Research and Treatment of Cancer Core Quality of Life Questionnaire. *J Psychosomatic Research*, 2000 49. 27-34.

[18] Jacobson, PB; Donovan, KA; Trask, PC; Fleishman, SB; Zabora, J; Baker, F; Holland, J. Screening for psychologic distress in ambulatory cancer patients: A multicenter evaluation of the distress thermometer. *Cancer*, 2005 103(7), 1494-1502.

[19] Devins, G; Bezjak, A; Mah, K; Loblaw, A; Gotowiec, A. Context moderates illness-induced lifestyle disruptions across life domains: A test of the illness intrusiveness theoretical framework in six common cancers.*Psycho-Oncology* (in press), 2005.

[20] Arman, M; Rehnsfeldt, A. The hidden suffering among breast cancer patients: A qualitative metasynthesis. *Qualitative Health Research, 2003 13*(4), 510-527.

[21] Lee, V; Cohen, R; Edgar, L; Laizner, A; Gagnon, A. Clarifying "meaning" in the context of cancer research: A systematic literature review. *Palliative and Supportive Care*, 2004 2, 291-303.

[22] Chochinov, H; Hack, T; McClement, S; Kristjanson, L; Harlos, M. Dignity in the terminally ill: A developing empirical model. *Social Science and Medicine,* 2002 54(2002), 433-443.

[23] Cohen, M; Ley, CD. Bone marrow transplantation: The battle for hope in the face of fear. *Oncology Nursing Forum,* 2000 27(3), 473-480.

[24] Farrell, C; Heaven, C; Beaver, K; Maguire, P. Identifying concerns of women undergoing chemotherapy. *Patient Education and Counseling*, 2005 56, 72-77.

[25] Landmark, B; Strandmark, M; Wahl, A. Living with newly diagnosed breast cancer: the meaning of existential issues. *Cancer Nursing*, 2001 24(3), 220-226.

[26] Kelly, B; Burnett, P; Pelusi, D; Badger, S; Varghese, F;Robertson, M. Association between clinician factors and a patient's wish to hasten death: terminally ill cancer patients and their doctors. *Psychosomatics,* 2004 45(4); 311-318.

[27] Mak, Y. Voices of the terminally ill: Uncovering the meaning of desire for euthanasia. *Palliative Medicine,* 2005 19, 340-350.

[28] Griffiths, C; Norton, L; Wagstaff, G; Brunas-Wagstaff, J. Existential concerns in late stage cancer. *European Journal of Oncology Nursing,* 2002 6(4), 243-246.

[29] Raffa, RB; Duong, PV; Finney, J; Garber, DA; Lam, LM; Mathew, SS; Plaskett, KC; Shah, M; Jen Weng, HF. Is "chemo-fog"/"chemo-brain" caused by cancer chemotherapy? *J. of Clinical Pharmacy and Therapeutics*, 2006 31, 129-138.

[30] Falleti, MG; Sanflippo, An; Maruff, P; Weih, L; Philips, KA. The nature and severity of cognitive impairment associated with adjuvant chemotherapy in women with breast cancer: A meta-analysis of the current literature. Brain and Cognitition, 2005 59, 60-70.

[31] Richer, M; Ezer, H. Living in it, living with it, and moving on: Dimensions of meaning during chemotherapy. *Oncology Nursing Forum*.2002 29(1),113-119.

[32] Friedrichsen, M; Strang, P; Carlsson, M. Breaking bad news in the transition from curative to palliative cancer care- patient's view of the doctor giving the information. *Supportive Care in Cancer,* 2000 8, 472-478.

[33] Kirk, P; Kirk, I; Kristjanson, J. What do patients receiving palliative care for cancer and their families want to be told? A Canadian and Australian qualitative study. *British Medical Journal,* 2004 328, 1343-1347.

[34] Yalom. *Existential Psychotherapy*. New York, N.Y.: BasicBooks, A Member of the Perseus Books Group, 1980.

[35] Brogdon, CF. Women and cancer, Journal of Intraven Nursing, 1988 21(6), 344-355.

[36] Mystakidou, K; Parpa, E; Katsouda, E; Galanos, A; Lambros, V. The role of physical and psychological symptoms in desire for death: A study of terminally ill cancer patients. *Psycho-oncology, in press, 2005*

[37] Klemm P, Miller MA, Fernsler J. 2000. Demands of illness in people treated for colorectal cancer. Oncol Nurs Forum. 27(4):633-9.

[38] Fang, CY; Manne, SL;Pape, SJ. Functional impairment, marital quality, and patient psychological distress as predictors of psychological distress among cancer patients' spouses, *Health Psychology*, 2001 20, 452-457.

[39] Given, CW; Stommel, M; Given, B; et al. The influence of cancer patients' symptoms and functional states on patients' depression and family caregivers' reaction to depression. *Health Psychology*, 1993 12, 277-285.

[40] Avis, NE; Crawford, S; Manuel, J. Psychosocial problems among younger women with breast cancer. *Psycho Oncology*, 2004 13(5), 295–308.

[41] Mor, V; Allen, S; Malin M. The pschosocial impact of cancer on older versus younger patients and their families. *Cancer*, 1994 74, 2118-2127.

[42] Morris, T; Greer, HS; White, P. Psychological and social adjustment to mastectomy: A two-year follow-up study. *Cancer*, 1997 40, 2381-2387.

[43] Maunsell, E; Brisson, J; Deschenes, L. Psychological distress after initial treatment of breast cancer: Assessment of potential risk. *Cancer*, 1992 70(1), 120-125.

[44] Helgeson, VS; Cohen, S. Social support and adjustment ot cancer: Reconsciling descriptive, correlational and intervention research. *Health Psychology*, 1996 15, 135-148.

[45] Leszcz, M; Goodwin, P. The rationale and foundations of group psychotherapy for women with metastatic breast cancer. *International Journal of Group Psychotherapy,* 1998 48(2), 245-273.

[46] Scott, JL; Halford, WK; Ward, BG. United We Stand? The effects of a Couple-Coping Intervention on Adjustment to Early Stage Breast or Gynecological Cancer. *Journal of Consulting and Clinical Psychology*, 2004 72(6), 1122-1135.

[47] Peters-Golden; H. Breast cancer: Varied perceptions of social support in the illness experience. *Social Science and Medicine,* 1982 16, 483-491.

[48] Lugton J. (1997)The nature of social support as experienced by women treated for breast cancer.J Adv Nurs. Jun;25(6):1184-91

[49] Moore, R; Butow, P. *Culture and oncology: Impact of context effects*. New York: Kluwer Academic, Plenum Publishers. 2004.

[50] Jones, S; Mitchell, T. The psycho-social effects of chemotherapy toxicity- a patient perspective: short report. *European Journal of Oncology Nursing*, 2003 7(4), 259-260.

[51] Antoni, MH; Lehman, JM; Kilbourn, KM; et al. Cognitive-behavioral stress management intervention decreases the prevalence of depression and enhances benefit finding among women under treatment for early stage breast cancer. *Health Psychol*, 2001 20, 20-32.

[52] Carver, CS; Meyer, B; Antoni, MH. Responsiveness to threats and incentives, expectancy of recurrence, and distress and disengagement: Moderator effects in women with early stage breast cancer, *Jounral of Consulting and Clinical Psychology*, 2000 68, 965-975.

[53] Sorlie, T; Sexton, HC. Predictors of the process of coping in surgical patients. *Personality and individual differences*, 2001 30, 947-960.

[54] Coyne, JC; Gottlieb, BH. The mismeasure of coping by checklist. *Journal of Personality*, 1996 64, 959-991.

[55] Carver, DS; Pozo, C; Harris, SD; Noriega, V; Scheier, MF; Robinson, DS; et al. How coping mediates the effect of optimism on distress: A study of women with early stage breast cacner. *Journal of Personality and Social Psychology*, 1993 65, 375-390.

[56] McCaul, KD; Sandgren, AK; King, B; O'Donnell, S; Branstetter, A; Forman, G. Coping and adjustment to breast cncer. *Psycho-Oncology*, 1999 8, 230-236.

[57] Bloom, JR; Stewart, S; Chang, S; Banks, P. Then and now: Quality of life of young breast cancer survivors. *Psycho-Oncology*, 2004 13, 147-160.

[58] Sahlberg-Blom, E; Ternestedt, B; Johansson, J. Is good 'quality of life' possible at the end of life? An explorative study of the experiences of a group of cancer patients in two different care cultures. *Journal of Clinical Nursing*, 2001 10, 550-562.

[59] Ferrell, BR; Grant, MM; Funk, B; Otis-Green, S; Garcia, N. Quality of life in breast cancer survivors as identified by focus groups. *Psycho-Oncology*, 1997 6(1), 13-23.

[60] Ganz, PA; Coscarelli, A; Fred, C; Kahn, B; Polinksy, ML; Petersen, L. Breast cancer survivors: Psychosocial concerns and quality of life. *Breast Cancer Research and Treatment*, 1996 38(2), 183-199.

[61] Dorval, M; Maunsell, E; Deschenes, L; et al. Long-term quality of life after breast cancer: Comparison of 8-year survivors with population controls. *J Clin Oncol* 1998 16, 487-494.

[62] Gotay, C; Muraoka, MY. Quality of life in long-term survivors of adult-onset cancers. *J. of the National Cancer Institute*, 1998 90(9), 656-666.

[63] Halttunen, A; Hietanen, P; Jallinoja, P; Lonnqvist, J. Getting free of breast cancer. An eight-year perspective of the relapse-free patients.*ACta Oncol*, 1992 31, 307-310.

[64] Cull, A; Cowie, VJ; Farquharson, DIM; Livingstone, MRB; Smart, GE; Elton, RA. Early stage cervical cancer: psychosocial and sexual outcomes of treatment. *British J. of Cancer*, 1993 68, 1216-20.

[65] Corney, RH; Everett, H; Howells, A; Crowther, ME. Psychosocial adjustment following major gynecological surgery for carcinoma of the cervix and vulva. *J. of Psychosomatic Research*, 1992 36, 561-8.

[66] De Groot, JM; Mah, K; Fyles, A; Winton, S; Greenwood, S; DePetrillo, AD; Devins, G. The psychosocial impact of cervical cancer among affected women and their partners, International. *J. of Gynecol Cancer*, 2005 15, 918-925.

[67] Holland, JC; Kash, KM; Passik, S; et al. A brief spiritual beliefs inventory for use in quality of life research in life-threatening illness. *Psycho-Oncology*, 1998 7, 460-469.

[68] Foley, K; Farmer, D; Petronis, V; Smith, R; McGraw, S. A qualitative exploration of the cancer experience among long-term survivors: Comparisons by cancer type, ethnicity, gender, and age. *Psycho-oncology,* 2006 15(3), 248-258.

[69] Fehring, R; Miller, J; Shaw, C. Spiritual well-being, religiosity, hope, depression, and other mood states in elderly people with cancer. *Oncology Nursing Forum,* 1997 24(4), 663-671

[70] McClain, Rosenfeld, and Breitbart (2003). Effect of spiritual well-being on end-of-life despair in terminally ill cancer patients. Lancet, 361 (9369), 1603-1607

[71] Blinderman, C; Cherny, N. Existential issues do not necessarily result in existential suffering: Lessons from cancer patients in Israel. *Palliative Medicine,* 2005 19, 371-380.

[72] Kemeny, MM; Wellisch, DK; Schain, WS. Psychosocial outcome in a randomized surgical trial for treatment of primary breast cancer. *Cancer*, 1988 62(6), 1231-7.

[73] Brandberg, Y; Malm, M; Blomqvist, L. A prospective and randomized study, "SVEA," comparing effects of three methods for delayed breast cancer reconstruction on quality of life, patient-defined problem areas of life, and cosmetic result. *Plast Reconst Surg* 2000 105, 66-74.

[74] Schover, LR; Yetman, RJ; Tuason, LJ; et al. Partial mastectomy and breast reconstruction: A comparison of their effects on psychosocial adjustment, body image, and sexuality. *Cancer* 1995 75, 54-64.

[75] Burbie, G; Polinsky, M. Intimacy and sexuality after cancer treatment: Restoring a sense of wholeness. *J. of Psychosocial Oncology*, 1992 10(1), 19-33.

[76] Butler, L; Banfield, V; Sveinson, T; Allen, K. Conceptualizing sexual health in cancer care. *Western J. of Nursing Research*, 1998 1, 1-13.

[77] Omne-Ponten, M; Holmberg, L; Sjoden, PO. Psychosocial adjustment among women with breast cancer stages I and II: Six year follow-up of consecutive patients. *J Clin Oncol*, 1994 12, 1778-1782.

[78] Hoskins, CN. Breast cancer treatment-related patters in side effects, psychological distress, and perceived health status. *Oncol Nurs Forum*, 1997 24, 1575-1583.

[79] Margolis, G; Goodman, RL; Rubin, A. Psychological effects of breast-conserving cancer treatment and mastectomy. *Psychosomatics* 1990 31, 33-39.

[80] Polinsky, ML. Functional status of long-term breast cancer survivors: Demonstrating chronicity. *Health Soc Work*, 1994 19, 165-173.

[81] Meyer, L; Aspegren, K. Long-term psychological sequelae of mastectomy and breast conserving treatment for breast cancer. *Acta Oncol*, 1989 28:13-18.

[82] Rowland, JH; Desmond, KA; Meyerowitz, BE; et al. Role of breast reconstruction surgery in physical and emotional outcomes among breast cancer survivors. *J Natl Cancer Inst*, 2000 92, 1422-1429.

[83] Germino B, Fife B & Funk S. Cancer and the partner relationship: What is its meaning? *Seminars in Oncology Nursing*, 1995 11(1), 43-50.

[84] Anderson, BL; Cyranowski, JM. Women's Sexual Self-Schema. *Journal of Social Psychology and Personality*, 1994 67, 1079-1100.

[85] Johnson, B. Older adults and sexuality: A multidimensional perspective. *J. of Gerontological Nursing*, 1996 22(2), 6-15.

[86] Dobkin, P; Bradley, I. Assessment of sexual dysfunction in oncology patients: Review, critique, and suggestions. *J. of Psychosocial Oncology*, 1991 9(1), 43-74.

[87] Ganz, PA; Rowland, JH; Desmond, K; Meyerowitz, BE; Wyatt, GE. Life After Breast Cancer: Understanding Women's Health-Related Quality of Life and Sexual Functioning. *Journal of Clinical Oncology*, 1998 16(2), 501-514.

[88] Ganz PA. 1999. The status of cancer rehabilitation in the late 1990s. Mayo Clinic proceedings, 74(9):939-40.

[89] Wellisch DK, DiMatteo R, Silverstein M, Landsverk J, Hoffman R, Waisman J, Handel N, Waisman-Smith E, Schain W.(1989) : Psychosocial outcomes of breast cancer therapies: Lumpectomy versus mastectomy. Psychosomatics, 30:365-373.

[90] McCorkle, R; Pasacreta, J; Tzuh, Tang; S. Psychological issues in ovarian cancer. *Hoistic Nursing Practice*, 2003 17(6), 300-308.

[91] Berglund, G; Nystedt, M; Bolund, C; et al. Effect of endocrine treatment on sexuality in premenopausal breast cancer patients: A prospective randomized sudy. *J. Clinicall Oncology*, 2001 19, 2788-2796.

[92] Little, PM; Jordens, C; Syers, E. Survivorship and discourses of identity. *Psycho-oncology*, 2002 11, 170-178.

[93] Glover, JI. I: *The Philosophy and Psychology of Personal Identity*. Penguin Books. London: 1989.

[94] Harré, R; Gillett, G. *The Discursive Mind. Thousand Oaks*, CA: Sage Publications; 1994.

[95] Chamberlain, Wilmoth M. The Aftermath of Breast Cancer: An Altered Sexual Self. *Cancer Nursing*, 2001 24(4), 278-2861.

[96] Sundquist and Yee. Sexuality and body image after cancer. *Australian Family Physician*, 2003 32(1-2), 1922.

[97] Carlson, LE; Bultz, BD. Cancer distress screening: Needs, methods and models. *J. Psychosomatic Research*, 2003 55, 403-409.

[98] Lalos, 1995. Lalos A, Jacobsson L, Lalos O, Stendahl U. (1995). Experiences of the male partner in cervical and endometrial cancer--a prospective interview study. J Psychosom Obstet Gynaecol. 1995 Sep; 16(3):153-65.

[99] Spira, J. Understanding and Developing Psychotherapy Groups for Medically Ill Patients. In: Spira, JL (Ed). *Group Therapy for Medically Ill Patients*. New York: The Guilford Press; 1997, 3-51.

[100] Andersen, BL. Biobehavioral outcomes following psychological interventions for cancer patients. *Journal of Consulting and Clinical Psychology*, 2002 70, 590-610.

[101] Newell, SA; Sanson-Fisher, RW; Savolainen, NJ. Systematic review of psychological therapies for cancer patients: Overview and recommendations for future research. *Journal of the National Cancer Institute*, 2002 94, 558-584.

[102] Andersen, 1992. Andersen, BL (1992). Psychological interventions for cancer patients to enhance the quality of life. J. Consult and Clinical Psychology

[103] Fawzy, FI; Fawzy, NW;, Hyun, CS; Elashoff, R; Guthrie, D; Fahey, JL;Morton, DL. Malignant melanoma. Effects of an early structured psychiatric intervention, coping, and affective state on recurrence and survival 6 years later. *Archives of General Psychiatry*, 1993 50(9), 681-689.

[104] Meyer, T; Mark, M. Effects of psychosocial interventions with adult cancer patients: A meta-analysis of randomised experiments. *Health Psych*, 1995 14, 101-108.

[105] Ganz, 1990. Ganz PA. 1990. Clinical trials. Concerns of the patient and the public. Cancer, 65(10 Suppl): 2394-9. Review

[106] Christensen, DN. "Postmastectomy couple counselling: An outcome study of a structured treatment protocol." *Journal of Sex and Marital Therapy*, 1983 9, 266-275.

[107] Greer, S; Moorey, S; Baruch, JDR; Watson, M; Robertson, B, Mason, A. Adjuvant psychological therapy for patients with cancer: A prospective randomised trial. *British Medical Journal*, 1992 304, 675-680.

[108] Helgeson, VS; Cohen, S; Schulz, R; Yasko, J. Education and peer discussion group interventions and adjustment to breast cancer. *Archives of General Psychiatry*, 1999 56, 340-347.

[109] Goodwin, P; Leszcz, M; Ennis, M; Koopmans, J; Vincent, L; Guther, H;Drysdale, E; Hundleby, M; Chochinov, H; Navarro, M; Speca, M; Hunter, J. The Effect of Group Psychosocial Support on Survival in Metastatic Breast Cancer. *The New England Journal of Medicine*, 2001 345(24), 1719 - 1726.

[110] Spiegel, D; Bloom, JR; Kraemer, HC; Gottheil, E. Effect of psychosocial treatment on survival of patients with metastatic breast cancer. *Lancet*, 1989 2, 888–891.

[111] Yalom, I; Leszcz, M. *The theory and practice of group psychotherapy* (5th Ed). New York: Basic Books; 2005.

In: Women and Cancer
Editor: Laurie Elit, pp. 203-226
ISBN: 978-1-60021-494-3

Chapter II

IDENTITY CHALLENGES AND SUPPORTIVE CARE NEEDS: A RESPONSE FROM A SOCIAL WORK PERSPECTIVE

Heather J. Hair[1] and Linda Learn[2,*]
[1]Wilfrid Laurier University, Waterloo, Ontario, Canada;
[2]Juravinski Cancer Centre, Hamilton, Ontario, Canada.

ABSTRACT

When a woman learns she has cancer, she is confronted with the implications of the diagnosis, decisions about the treatment plan, and the often rigorous and physically demanding medical regimes. Following treatment, the identity of "cancer survivor" will be added to her life along with the 50% possibility of premature death. Cancer challenges a woman's roles in a patriarchal society, in which she is viewed as caretaker, nurturer and provider. Thus, a woman's ability to live well following a diagnosis of cancer is influenced not only by her understanding and beliefs about the disease, but by her self-perceptions about her multiple roles and how well a system of care meets her many needs. The ability of medical systems to provide equitable cancer care is challenged by the diversity and vulnerability of a woman's various identities and social situations. As a member of a cancer treatment team, social workers are trained from an ecosystemic perspective to assess the biopsychosocial needs of this vulnerable population. Personalised treatment plans are developed that consider a woman's identity and relational challenges in the face of cancer and lower both systemic and internal barriers to equitable care. Therefore, social workers provide a particular understanding of the unique and complex supportive care needs of their patients with the result of improved medical care and decreased costs to the medical system. The purpose of this chapter is to assess the identity challenges of women diagnosed with cancer and to address their

* Correspondence concerning this article should be addressed to Linda Learn, Juravinski Cancer Centre, 699 Concession Street Hamilton, Ontario, Canada L8V 5C2. Phone 905 387-9495; Email: linda.learn@hrcc.on.ca.

supportive care needs. In order to accomplish this, we have three primary aims. First, we investigate how a cancer diagnosis can influence and infiltrate a woman's various identities and roles that have been constructed through the multiple relationships in her life. In this discussion we also consider the various supportive care needs that surface when a woman's self-perception and role responsibilities are confronted by cancer. Secondly, we propose how the perspective and practices of social work are uniquely qualified to address and provide for a woman's supportive care needs. Finally, we explore current gaps in oncological psychosocial interventions and suggest directions for future program development and research.

INTRODUCTION

When a woman learns she has cancer, her ideas about herself and her place in her self-described world are harshly and unequivocally challenged and changed. The multiple implications of the diagnosis, decisions during treatment planning, and the often rigorous and physically demanding medical interventions inevitably transform a woman's conceptualization of herself [1,2,3]. The most obvious difference follows treatment as she gains the title of "cancer survivor" along with the knowledge that she has a 50% possibility of premature death [3,4]. Less obvious but no less significant is how a cancer diagnosis and the treatment process can shatter the certainty of self-identities and transform a woman's relationship with others [5].

The ability of medical systems to provide equitable cancer care is challenged by the diversity and vulnerability of a woman's various identities and social situations. To date, the cancer care literature has paid little attention to the psychosocial needs of women diagnosed with cancer [6]. Nevertheless, mental health has been closely correlated with recovery rates and positive responses to treatment [7]. Given that mental health for woman is associated with identity self-perceptions and relationship satisfaction [8,9,10] it is imperative that cancer care consistently embrace a holistic approach.

As members of a cancer treatment team, social workers are trained from an ecosystemic perspective to assess and address the biopsychosocial needs of persons with life threatening illness. Social workers have the skills to develop personalised treatment plans that take into consideration women's multiple identities and relational challenges in the face of cancer [11,12]. Therefore, social workers provide a particular understanding of the unique and complex supportive care needs of their patients that contributes to improved medical care and decreased costs to the medical system.

The purpose of this chapter is to assess the identity challenges of women with cancer and advocate how oncology teams can best address women's supportive care needs. In order to accomplish this, we have two primary goals. First, we investigate how having cancer can influence and infiltrate a woman's various identities and roles that have been constructed through the multiple relationships in her life. In this discussion we consider the various supportive care needs that surface when a woman's self-perception and role responsibilities are confronted by cancer. Secondly, we suggest ways in which the perspective and practices of social work are uniquely qualified to address and provide for a woman's supportive care needs.

We begin this chapter by identifying aspects of ourselves that we believe have influenced and informed our current perspectives and ideas on this complex topic. Secondly, we review the theoretical lenses through which we have viewed and critiqued the literature. Next, we present our criteria for literature and research selection. This information leads into the two main areas of discussion: Our exploration of the impact of cancer on women's identity and relationships begins with a brief discussion about the general role of women in patriarchal society. This forms the context for our analysis of how learning to live with cancer can affect women's identity, relations, and supportive care needs, particularly for those women marginalized according to the intersection of socio-political constructions such as race, gender, class, ethnicity, or faith identification. Our second area of focus is psychosocial interventions, where we highlight the unique contributions of social work. We conclude with suggestions for future program development and research.

SITUATING THE AUTHORS WITH THE SUBJECT

The exploration of women's identities and the intrusion of cancer are simultaneously of personal and professional interest to us. Consequently, the process of determining what to include in this chapter and how to shape that content has been influenced by our own relationships with the subject. In order to be sensitive to the variety of women's identities, the isolation and social exclusion that a life-threatening illness can present, and the psychosocial needs that result, it behoves us to examine our own potential sociopolitical "blind spots." Therefore, we believe it is important to highlight particular aspects of ourselves that are significant for our topic.

Certain parts of our identities are similar. We are both White, English-speaking, Canadian born, able-bodied women. Out of working class backgrounds we have both been able to pursue post-secondary education in mental health disciplines. To date neither of us has been touched with cancer, although we have known the ravages of the disease through the experiences of family members and friends.

Linda's unique identity includes a husband and three grown sons. Concurrent with her multiple roles as partner and mother, she has had a long and varied career as a social worker, particularly in the field of violence against women, followed by a change to the field of oncology. Currently as a social worker assigned to the Breast and Gynecological Oncology Disease Site teams at a large Canadian Cancer Centre, she provides counselling services for women who come to the Centre at various stages in their cancer care journey. She has been struck by the many stories of women – stories of resilience, strength and beauty along side stories of despair, systemic marginalization, loneliness, isolation and poverty. It is with the accumulation of these stories in mind that she took on this project in an effort to explore the impact of cancer on women in a larger context than the size, grade, and stage of a tumour.

After 25 years in various mental health positions in social services, Heather has recently drawn benefits from a single, childless life and taken time out from full-time employment and returned to university for a PhD in Social Work and a new career in academe. A privilege of this journey has been the opportunities to reflect and share learnings with many people who have enriched her life beyond measure. Her interest in this chapter is the opportunity to explore how certain voices, experiences and ideas are privileged, how personal strengths encounter terrible adversity, and how truths are determined from many different stories.

Thus, although these are our words, they are the outcome of many experiences and ideas woven together. Many of our experiences are supported and affirmed by dominant narratives of success and entitlement. Cancer, however, is not partial to race, ethnicity, sexual orientation, ableness, faith, education or age. Through acknowledging our relatively privileged experiences we are better able to remain vigilant that women with all their various identities are recognized and served well. It is our hope that the knowledge we co-create will be beneficial to other health practitioners and women in their relationships with themselves and others along their path with cancer.

Our Conceptual Framework for Viewing and Critiquing the Literature

Our understanding and critique of the literature has been filtered through two conceptual lenses. First, we understand knowledge to be an integration or the weaving together of "a nature that we have not made and a society that we are free to change" [13]. From this viewpoint, society can be conceived as a gathering of ideas that are co-created between people. Through these personal and societal interactions particular knowledge comes to dominate socio-cultural understandings and practices [14,15].

Secondly, relations between people means there are relations of power [16,17,18]. Hence, when certain ideas gain notable social eminence a discourse or paradigm of knowledge is created which gains acceptance as truth about what can be said and thought, who can speak and practice, and with what authority within a given place and time [14,17]. The outcome is that certain knowledge becomes either preferred or subjugated [16]. Thus, the social acknowledgement and value given to relationships, women's roles, education, and professional status influences which voices are heard and which are silenced.

Scientific procedures, medical diagnoses and interventions, and the status granted to the people who claim expertise in these areas are examples of dominant discourses or paradigms with privileged authority world-wide. When women have an illness or are in need of medical attention these particular discourses significantly influence what knowledge is socially privileged about women, gender relations, health, wellness, and how knowledge is created and disseminated [10]. Moreover, when medical care is needed, these accepted sociocultural dominant discourses determine who can participate in the creation of diagnosis and treatment.

The conceptualization of dialogically created discourse and relations of power challenge medical practioners in general and social workers specifically to recognize not only the physiological needs of women with cancer but emotional needs, relational needs, and their strengths and resiliencies. Furthermore, these perspectives challenge helping professionals to be mindful of the influential presence of various social constructions such as race, class, language, gender, age, and mental/physical ability on their understanding of illness and recovery. Our engagement with the following literature, chosen in the light of our selected conceptual framework, reflects our commitment to equitable, collaborative services for women with cancer that honour their multiple identities and respectfully provides for their social care needs.

Selecting Literature and Research

For our investigation, published literature and research were identified through library searches using Cambridge Scientific Abstracts (PsycINFO, Social Services Abstracts, Sociological Abstracts, ERIC), Social Work Abstracts, PubMed (Medline), and the CINHAHL database. Selection was limited to articles or books in English published between 1990 and 2005. The title and/or abstract clearly identified a focus on women's identity and/or role plus oncology and/or social work, and/or a psychosocial treatment focus. We discovered that overall there is a paucity of literature and research concerning the impact of cancer on women's roles and identity, and their supportive care needs.

To better understand the implications for the Canadian context, we endeavoured to discover the social and/or geographic location of the authors. The majority of authors appeared to be in the United States or Britain. However, there is notable representation from Israel, the Netherlands, and Australia. Interestingly, the literature seemed virtually silent about the development and place of social work with oncology in Canada. Among various countries, however, social work has many developmental and conceptual similarities, reflecting the ongoing influence of colonialism and Western ideas [6]. Thus, we have determined that the literature is applicable to the Canadian context.

Finally, along with documentation, we sought to gain first-hand narratives about life with cancer. We are grateful that Grace, a cancer survivor, agreed to be interviewed and allowed excerpts of our conversation to be included in this chapter. Her confidentiality has been protected through the use of a pseudonym.

A Conceptualization of Women's Identity within Current Social Discourse

In line with our conceptual framework, we propose that self-identity and how we create meaning for and understanding of each other and ourselves is predominantly gathered through relationships and expressed through language [19,20,21]. In other words, our identity is woven out of our interactions with others, and the words used to give meaning to those interactions, as well as the dominant discourses of society. This idea of a socially constructed self has been considered a fitting notion from which to develop theoretical understandings of the unique qualities of women's ways of being in the world.

Investigators into women's self-identity have proposed that a woman's sense of self becomes organized and developed around being able to make and maintain relationships [9,10,22,23]. These reciprocal relationships include cognitive and emotional connections as well as shared experiences that together shape a woman's identity [23]. Furthermore, the centrality of connection profoundly informs how women can approach personal crises and relational conflicts [22]. Not surprisingly, understanding and acknowledging the importance of relationships to and for women is essential for helping professionals interested in supporting women's growth and development.

Acknowledging interpersonal relationships as recognized shapers of women's identity has given "voice" to women's unique experiences and challenged dominant psychosocial discourses [9,22]. A relational self-development perspective is in sharp contrast to the traditional Western notion that a mentally healthy identity develops through differentiation from others and is characterized by autonomy, independence and self-reliance [8,23]. This dominant identity discourse recognizes qualities for success that are not honouring or inclusive of women's psychology. Moreover, women's relationships are rarely valued or sought out as signs of personal resiliency and strength. Consequently, for generations the social status and corresponding socially sanctioned power of women in the public spheres of life has been negligible [9]. Women are systematically marginalized and silenced further if they do not correspond to the dominant image of being White, English speaking, healthy, able-bodied, financially independent, educated, heterosexual, and married with children [8,18,24].

Although socially unrewarded, women's relational values and abilities have been repeatedly reinforced as essential to the integrity of our social fabric. Across various racial and ethnic groups women are traditionally "carriers" of different aspects of human experience including the psychosocial and emotional development and growth of others [8,9]. McGoldrick [8] has pointed out that

> Women's lives [have] always involved a weaving together of many strands, attending to multiple tasks, sounds, and images at once. They created the "nest" that was home for everyone else; they provided the food, the nurturance, and the care for all from the youngest to the oldest; they created the family rituals, bought the presents, made birthdays and Thanksgivings happen. They nursed the sick, washed and mourned the dead, and attended to the needs of other mourners. (p. 106)

These roles of women, however, have rarely received acknowledgement as integral elements of a healthy and vibrant society. There is typically little social reward for the needed insights, skills, and commitment to successfully navigate the multiple needs of others and their attendant responsibilities and tasks. For many women, attempting to care for self, including taking needed time away from the duties of relational commitments, has been viewed as selfish and potentially destructive to relationships [9]. Thus, when illness assaults a woman, effective interventions will depend on helping professionals recognizing the relational facets of a woman's life and self-identity as a potential source of challenge and strength.

The Impact of Having Cancer on Women's Identity and Relations

Nothing ever prepares us for the really bad things in life, and loss is an encompassing life theme. Losses are a part of life – we lose loved ones, we lose jobs, we lose chances, and we lose dreams [2].

At some point, it is likely that cancer will touch every Canadian directly or through a family member, friend, or work colleague. Across Canada, approximately 38% of women will be diagnosed with cancer during their lifetimes. Breast cancer is the most common cancer particularly for younger women, followed by colorectal and lung cancers [4]. Surviving the life-threatening experience of cancer can carry a dark shadow of uncertainty and fear of re-occurrence that persists long after physical recovery has occurred [1,2,25,26]. Such apprehensions about health, relationships, and future planning can easily be understood given that current mortality rates estimate that 1out of every 4 women will die from cancer [4].

The progression of cancer and women's changing identity and relations are a co-constructive process. The shock at discovery unfolds into a variety of responses and needs throughout treatment, creating significant shifts in a woman's self-understanding and her interpersonal relationships which can potentially continue for the rest of her life. The trajectory of the illness has been punctuated by medically recognized transition points. Traditionally, these are the time of diagnosis, the period of active treatment, and for five years post-treatment [27]. We have chosen to use these pivotal moments to discuss the identity transformations of women with cancer. In particular, we focus on women's supportive care needs, which could benefit from effective psychosocial interventions.

Along with the above mentioned transition points, we believe that there is considerable value for oncology professionals to consider the power of cancer before diagnosis is confirmed. Therefore, although there is a lack of literature or research that discusses women's experiences prior to diagnosis, we begin with the *potential* of what cancer can do to a woman's identity and her relationships before she enters the diagnostic and treatment world of oncology.

Waiting for Diagnosis

The impact of an encounter with cancer on a woman's identity begins with the worry, fears, and wonderings about what medical tests will reveal [3,25]. For some women finding a lump or noticing unexplained pain or body changes has finally prodded them to persistently voice their observations to their physician [28]. For these women, medical examination validates their knowledge of their own bodies even as fear and worry increase [26]. Alternatively, there are other women who do not experience physical symptoms of an illness that could actually help to confirm the need for subsequent tests [29]. A lack of symptoms or a previous experience of having physical findings discounted by a physician prior to medical investigation can create a cognitive dissonance for a woman and shake her trust and reliance on her own self-awareness. For too many women, waiting for medical test results means acknowledging that what is going on in her body waits to be explained and named by dominant Western medical scientific discourse and nomenclature, which can easily reinforce her lack of socially valued knowledge and/or position [28,31].

During the days and weeks prior to formal diagnosis, the spectre of cancer can infiltrate daily responsibilities and persistently demand cognitive and emotional attention. For example, the thought that something has been growing in her body without her knowledge and control, can precipitate the first intimations of unexpected self-betrayal [29]. However, a woman's multiple roles as caretaker, mother, employee, and partner can insist that self-reflection and pre-occupation with "what-ifs" are a pastime she cannot afford. The struggle to stay other-focused and to resist suspicion can effectively silence any wish to share concerns with family members or friends. Actually, given the various relational expectations she experiences, it would not be uncommon for a woman to recruit denial and minimization in order to resist being overwhelmed by the potential horror of a cancer discovery. Finally, a woman's socially endorsed identities as sexual partner, child-bearer, nurturer, and caretaker can already be threatened, particularly if the potential malignancy is located in her breasts or reproductive organs [30]. Thus the distraction of uncertainty can unsettle interpersonal relationships and a woman's ability to successfully fulfill her various roles.

At the Time of Diagnosis

There is consistent agreement that no matter how much women try to contain worry or consider the meanings about upcoming test results, shock is a prevalent and predominant response to the devastating news of having cancer [1,26,32,33,34]. A woman who has survived breast cancer recalls the meeting following the exploratory biopsy when the surgeon told her she had a malignant tumour:

Shocked. I was shocked. There was numbness, a feeling of unreality. Everything stopped. There was nothing else – no one else was in the room just me, even though there were other people in the room. It was like someone kicked me in the gut...I don't think I'll ever forget that moment. (Grace, personal communication, February 11, 2006)

A woman's emotional responses to a cancer diagnosis are constructed from dominant socio-cultural beliefs. These beliefs proclaim cancer is a silent, invisible killer that has somehow infiltrated the intimate depths of self with the sole intention of painfully consuming the host. As confirmation, medical discourse provides scientific evidence that the malignant tissue is really part of a woman's body that, although growing out of control, can be medically treated through intrusive and invasive interventions [1,29,30]. Thus, a woman finds out that within her most basic identity relationship – with physical self – a gross betrayal has been made by an element of her own cellular system that potentially leaves her without self-control or the means to help herself [1].

The profound disruption to a woman's perception of her physical self and the transfer of authorative knowledge to oncology personnel can fracture a woman's constructed identity, her confidence in her own knowledge, and her relational place in her world. Under this threat to her life, a woman can be compelled to evaluate who she is within the context of her many interpersonal relations [5,29,31]. As Colyer [1] has noted a "diagnosis of cancer may not in itself be a death sentence, but it raises the spectre of death and thus brings life more sharply in focus, often prompting examination of who we are and what we are doing with our lives" (p. 498).

When a woman discovers she has cancer, often the first of many challenges is deciding who to tell and how to find words to describe the traumatic experience as it unfolds. The significance of disclosure was investigated by Kulik and Kronfeld [33] as part of their quantitative investigation of 60 women and their adjustment to breast cancer. The researchers concluded that better psychosocial adjustment occurred for women who could talk about their illness within intimate relationships such as family members. Most importantly, given the reciprocal co-creation process of identity, a significant aspect of disclosure and the subsequent discussions will be the responses received. How a woman might perceive the potential impact and response from family members was identified as significant in the research of Hirshman and Bourjolly [34]. The investigators document that for some women there is no space in their self-identified familial roles to potentially "burden" or worry their family members. Consequently, there are women who will refrain from or delay telling others.

Whether or not a woman tells others of her diagnosis, during the days that follow she is likely to find herself struggling to know what effect her illness and any treatment will have on the significant individuals in her life [5]. Possible questions can include: How can she continue to fulfill her role as partner, mother, caregiver, and employee? What can she do about the guilt and shame that accompanies her thoughts and feelings focused on herself rather than on others? How can she continue to make future plans, even for tomorrow, when living them out has suddenly become questionable and potentially meaningless?

Ironically, although many of her questions are about relations with others, a woman's speculation, worry, and fears are often keep to herself. Finding words to break through the trauma of discovery is difficult at best. Unfortunately, the prevalent, deeply held social stigma that surrounds cancer encourages a lack of understanding and indeed avoidance by others [29,30,31]. At a time when connection could be beneficial, women can find themselves feeling isolated, alienated and silenced [1].

During Active Treatment

A positive diagnosis of malignancy catapults a woman into the world of oncology, medical terminology, and treatment protocols. According to the research of Langellier and Sullivan [31] concerning women's experiences of breast cancer, the diagnosis and treatment of cancer "results in a traumatized body, subjected not only to the fragmenting and objectifying language of medicine and the dread of cancer but also to the violence of treatments" (p. 81). Pain, muscle weakness, physical exhaustion, nausea, and hair loss are only some of the physical outcomes described by women who have undergone the treatment regimes of cancer that include invasive surgeries, radiation and chemotherapies [5,26,31].

The biomedical objectification of the body and its diseased parts [29,31] helps oncology specialists remain focused on the physical survival of the woman. The intention of each element of medical intervention is to at least halt the progression of the disease and, at best, to eradicate all the malignant cell tissue to prevent further recurrence [4]. Furthermore, an important aspect of medical care is the attention to pain management and, as much as possible, the compassionate relief of physical discomfort [4]. Conversely, during difficult treatments little or no attention is given by medical personnel to the lived experiences of cancer and the intervention process or a woman's relational needs and altering identity. During our interview, Grace (personal communication, February 11, 2006) described how she came to understand this aspect of her cancer treatment experience:

> I don't think they [the medical professionals] want to know about feelings. The only way you can effectively treat a person without getting emotionally attached and burnt-out in a matter of months is to have distinct boundaries. And one of those boundaries is not dealing with how people are feeling. There needs to be someone available but I don't think it will be the medical profession. The medical profession needs to recognize that there may be a need to talk – they don't ask so they don't know. My doctor didn't ask me.

For many women, meetings with various doctors, surgeons, nurses, and technical staff are often full of new and unfamiliar information. Moreover, during conversations with medical personnel there is rarely any time or space permitted for a woman to articulate what it means to her to have cancer, discuss her understanding and acceptance of Western oncology interventions, and/or explore any awareness she may have of alternative or complementary healing practices [6]. To disregard a woman's speculations or knowledge can become a direct affront to her intellectual capabilities as well as her spiritual, ethnic, and/or racial identities [26,34,35,36,37,38,39,40].

For example, the research of Bourjolly [36] identified that religious faith was statistically significant for Black women participants as a way of understanding and coping with their cancer. The results of her research prompted Bourjolly to query

> "if God is seen as a healer….how does this belief impact on a person's involvement with the health care system, particularly her relationship with physicians and other professionals?" (p. 33).

The researcher concluded that potentially valuable resources typically utilized by a particular ethnic or racially identified group of women will be overlooked unless there are intentional inquiries by oncology team members.

The potential for treatment success for Aboriginal women can be extrapolated from a preliminary investigation by Levin and Herbert [39] of the experiences of urban Aboriginals with Canadian health care services. Key informants identified that medical professionals routinely are ignorant of or do not understand the relevance of Aboriginal worldviews, spirituality, and/or relational and cultural practices for healing. Awareness of these identity elements is essential for informed inquiries into the unique qualities of each First Nations woman with cancer, no matter where she lives. Thus, the lack of appropriately informed conversations with an oncology team member could result in apparent non-compliance by women expected to engage in cancer treatments that they view as culturally irrelevant or disrespectful [39].

Beyond the walls of consultation appointments and meetings with medical doctors and staff, a woman's life and her relational perceptions of self and others are rapidly changing. Notably, most women will have no idea of the upcoming formidable challenges to their own sense of self and the ripple effects throughout their social world. The internally whispered threat that cancer will alter a woman's ability to maintain the relationships that are intimately woven into her self-identity will now become fully realized. Once the news has been shared, a woman soon discovers that taken-for-granted self-perceptions and accompanying tasks crumble in the wake of cancer treatments. In particular her roles as nurturer, caregiver, sexual partner, and employee can be radically impacted [5,25,29,34,37,41]. Moreover, when the affected tissue is part of a woman's breast or reproductive organs, the injury to these symbolically important body parts can significantly alter her personal perceptions of her own womanhood, femininity, and sexuality [1,26,30,31,42,43].

The research results of Sormanti and colleagues [5] have indicated that a life-threatening illness such as cancer can generate considerable internal dissonance for a woman. For example, if a woman holds that part of her identity construction is to primarily care for the needs of others even at the expense of her own, then self-care, including compliance with post-surgical care and ongoing treatment, will be difficult. Sormanti and her colleagues propose the possibility that having cancer "may be a catalyst for a woman to move beyond the dichotomy of responsibility to others vs. responsibility to oneself " (p. 93). However, navigating such a new found self-conceptualization can be difficult challenge without adequate support. The qualitative investigation by Hirschman and Bourjolly [34] into how 33 women experienced tangible supports provides further evidence that it can be difficult for women with cancer to adjust to identity and role changes. In particular, the researchers discovered that the women's narratives repeatedly told of their struggle to adequately care for self when caring for others, including the various duties necessary to maintain a home.

Since a woman's identity transformations are not voluntarily initiated they can jeopardize her sense of accomplishments and validity while impacting her ability to effectively interact with others [41]. For example, the pragmatics of recovery from surgery and the subsequent weeks of scheduled treatments invade and disrupt the many precious, ritualized moments of a woman's day. Employment life can become disrupted and potentially create financial loss and distress for a woman and her dependents [25,29]. The caregiving tasks of a family usually routinely carried out by the mother before cancer treatment will likely need to be reallocated amongst family members [5]. The research of Fitch and colleagues [25] does provide hopeful results that for some women, "the diagnosis and treatment of cancer facilitate or allow for new ways of being a woman or living as a woman to emerge." (p. 59). For example, the results of their Canadian wide survey of 315 women's experiences of living with ovarian cancer found that 6 times the number of women indicated that after the cancer was found there was a positive impact verses a negative impact on their close relationships. The researchers speculated that the family life of the women might have changed in supportive ways such as the renegotiation of roles and the attendant responsibilities.

In order for women to be able to re-create their preferred identities with the important people in their life, family members and friends also must find ways to navigate and cope with the new and frightening changes that come with cancer [44,45]. According to Davis-Ali and colleagues [32] the shift in identity roles can be sabotaged by the assumption that the partners of women do not wish or need to be actively involved in the cancer treatment. In contrast, their quantitative research determined that partners experience emotional and physical distress equal to that of patients. Therefore, during treatment planning and implementation it behoves oncology teams to intentionally include the significant others invested in the lives of women with cancer [43,44].

Surviving Through the First Five Years

For many women, regular visits to a hospital or clinic for radiation and/or chemotherapy eventually come to an end and an oncologist or medical doctor declares that there is no apparent sign of cancer [3]. Often at this stage in her cancer experience a woman is introduced to follow-up care, such as a mammogram every six months or ongoing daily medications for the next five years. Nevertheless, the weeks and months of intense treatments are over and the assumption for women seems to be that pre-cancer identities and role continuity will resume. Life is supposed to move on as it was before cancer [3,26,45].

In contrast, the limited research about post-treatment experiences confirms that surviving the trauma of cancer leaves indelible imprints upon the identities and relationships of women [3,27]. According to Langellier and Sullivan [31], participant narratives "of how women incorporated cancer into their lives and identities suggest ongoing stories-in-progress that negotiate the changing relations among body, self, and others" (p. 91). For many women, their relationship with their own bodies has already undergone significant changes from the sense of betrayal at diagnosis to one of strangeness and disconnection post-treatment. Permanent physical alterations such as the loss of a breast, scar tissue, a colostomy bag, premature menopause, and the inability to have children profoundly alter a woman's sense of self long after medical treatment ends [3,26,43]. Moreover, even if her body appears unchanged, a woman's cognitions, perceptions, and affect have just collectively managed to navigate the harsh landscape of diagnosis and treatment and now must somehow transition into a life supposedly without cancer.

In spite of the extreme experience, the strong attraction for a woman to disregard her own needs and distance herself from the frightening and painful memories can help her return to her pre-cancer relations with others. Not surprisingly, the significant persons in a woman's life are also eager to put the cancer behind them and return to familiar interactions [3,32,45] . However, no matter how successful identity roles are re-initiated, for a number of women the years following cancer treatment will continue to be tainted with the knowledge that the cancer could return [46]. Moreover, for many women feelings of dislocation, fear, anger, guilt, and grief can persist – feelings that are not easily attended to or understood by family members or friends [3,26,43]. At a time when a woman might need supportive care, contact with medical personnel has typically ended, aside from widely spaced follow-up visits. Thus, after the period of intense treatments the social isolation and the impact on a woman's self-identity can be profound [46].

In their research concerning the identity transformations of survivors of cancer, Little and colleagues [3] have noted that the extreme experience of cancer takes time to be integrated into everyday post-treatment life. Survivorship from cancer needs to be conceptualized as more than the absence of illness. As Little and colleagues suggest, for women surviving cancer is a life lived in a context of new knowledge. Its task is the assimilation of that knowledge into the dynamic evolution of identity in a way that recognizes both the continuity of identity and the powerful forces of change inherent in extreme experience. (p. 176-177)

Concluding Comments

Women's narratives and the accompanying empirical research demonstrate that the trauma of having cancer significantly impacts a woman's socially dominant identities and the dynamics of her relational world. In order for women post-treatment to have lives characterized by resiliency and hope, better attention needs to be paid to the lived experience of cancer throughout the trajectory of the illness. Thus, the transformative journey of identity is best understood in the context of women's multiple roles and their shared experiences with the significant persons in their lives. Clearly, oncology team members have a responsibility to provide psychosocial interventions that can help enhance and enrich the lives of women who strive to move beyond the oppressive hand of cancer.

Psychosocial Interventions and the Contribution of Social Work

The importance and efficacy of psychosocial interventions to help address a variety of supportive care needs of women with cancer has been thoroughly reviewed and substantiated [6,47,48,49]. According to Holland [6] the "scientific base for psychosocial oncology is now secure with a body of knowledge, textbooks and journals which have led to the development of evidence–based clinical practice guidelines for psychosocial services in several countries" (p. 445). Nevertheless, in spite of empirical evidence, there remains a significant gap in the availability and utilization of psychosocial interventions as an integrated part of oncology treatment [6,25,48,50]. Thus, at a national level, the Canadian Cancer Society [4] has provided strong endorsement that supportive care resources need to be an expected part of interdisciplinary health services. Moreover, to help Canadian women with cancer achieve rewarding and productive lives, suitable psychosocial interventions need to be available throughout the trajectory of the illness from diagnosis to the years of adjustment post-treatment [4,25,43].

The developers and investigators of psychosocial interventions primarily come from psychiatry, psychology, social work, and nursing [6]. The distinct perspective of each of these disciplines shapes the focus and entry point of treatment as well as who should participate. In particular, as a member of an oncology team, the perspectives and practices of social work are uniquely qualified to address and provide comprehensive, supportive care for women challenged by identity transitions and relational changes.

A Conceptualization of Social Work

Social work is a practice-focussed discipline committed to the relationship between the individual and society viewed from a person-in-environment or ecological perspective, or systems approach [51,52,53]. The purpose of social work is to work collaboratively with community partners toward "the liberation of the dispossessed and vulnerable" [54] individual, family, and group with an eye for social justice and change [51,53,55]. This intention of social work – to seek out the voices that have been silenced – marks the discipline as value-driven not value-neutral [31,54,55,57].

Social workers respond to systemic complexities such as poverty, homelessness, violence, and prejudice that interact with and influence mental well-being. A person-in-environment perspective informs social workers as they provide "counselling, therapy and referrals to other supportive social services… [and] respond to other social needs such as unemployment, racism and poverty" [58].

To summarize, in 2000 the International Federation of Social Workers [59] adopted a new definition of social work that although comprehensive is not meant to be exhaustive. The following excerpt is pertinent to our discussion:

> The social work profession promotes social change, problem solving in human relationships and the empowerment and liberation of people to enhance well-being. Utilising theories of human behaviour and social systems, social work intervenes at the points where people interact with their environments. Principles of human rights and social justice are fundamental to social work….Social work utilises a variety of skills, techniques, and activities consistent with its holistic focus on persons and their environments. Social work interventions range from primarily person-focused psychosocial processes to involvement in social policy, planning and development. These include counselling, clinical social work, group work, social pedagogical work, and family treatment and therapy as well as efforts to help people obtain services and resources in the community. (p. 1)

Thus, social workers can conceptualize the various identities and relations of women impacted by cancer from a distinct holistic view of persons, problems, and context. As well, social workers have the skills to actively engage women and the significant people in their lives to collaboratively shape a future of hope with change [5,11,12,60,61].

Social Work: Providing Effective Oncology Psychosocial Interventions

Supportive care or psychosocial interventions developed and implemented by social workers generally take four forms: individual counselling, psycho-education, cognitive-behavioural training, and a variety of support groups [62,63]. Professionally led, manualized support groups have been particularly successful and popular [45,46,48,49]. However, in their research review of professionally directed psychosocial interventions, Cwikel and Behar [48] found that individual and group treatment seemed to be equally effective for increasing women's sense of hope and personal agency while minimizing experiences of loneliness, isolation, and alienation. Therefore, interventions should be tailored to best meet the needs of individual women as well as utilizing the strengths of supportive care social workers [49].

For many women, however, contact with a social worker is not included as a part of treatment. As already noted above, psychosocial interventions are not an accepted and integrated part of Canadian oncology interventions and after-care, even though such practice is endorsed by the Canadian Association of Psychosocial Oncology [64]. Depending on where a woman has to go for treatment, available services might not include those of a social worker. Alternatively, where social workers are part of an oncology team, the offer for supportive care might not be made by the medical staff or the services are not well explained [65]. As we have already noted, during our interview with Grace we learned that neither her surgeon nor her oncologist described to her the supportive care services available through the regional Cancer Centre. Thus, in Canada, many women will likely not engage with social work services. Alternatively, in Australia [66] and the United States [67] clinical guidelines for supportive care services and distress management for cancer patients have firmly established the role for and participation of social work.

Given that psychosocial interventions as a part of cancer treatments can be beneficial for all women with cancer as well as their loved ones [5,32,46,48,50,68], a reconfiguration of Canadian treatment protocols and standards of practice is warranted. Clearly, a multidisciplinary team approach is needed to address the complexity of the cancer experience [25,61]. As Davis-Ali and colleagues [32] have pointed out, "cancer cells may exclusively invade the *body* of the cancer patient, but the cancer experience clearly invades the *lives* of both the patient and the spouse" (p. 62, italics in original). As a member of the team, the social worker brings the voices of women and their loved ones to medical team members and advocates for a holistic approach to medical care [69,70]. The following are suggested practices for social workers as part of a multidisciplinary team serving women with cancer.

At the Time of Diagnosis

During the initial meeting with a surgeon or oncologist, at the very least information about supportive care services could be shared. A pamphlet describing the available services and staff is one option. Ideally, for each woman a meeting with a social worker would be arranged as a regular part of treatment planning. Each woman would be encouraged but would not be obligated to bring a partner, family member or friend who will be accompanying her on her journey with cancer. The routine scheduling of such a meeting could help dispel for medical professionals as well as women and their loved ones any socially reinforced minimization, fears or stigma about talking to someone about so-called mental health or relational concerns that can accompany a diagnosis of cancer [6].

During these early days of the cancer journey, following the initial meeting any further supportive care with a social worker would be voluntary for women and their loved ones. Meetings could effectively focus on providing a safe, private place for a woman and her partner/family member/friend to begin adjusting to the discovery of cancer. The meeting format could be for individual, couple, family, or groups [48]. Except for planned psychoeducational or support groups, a woman would determine who would attend meetings with her.

A significant aspect for the social worker would be to inquire about a woman's understanding of her identities, not only in relation to significant others but also those facets of herself that could be potentially challenged by a cancer diagnosis or that could be reservoirs of resiliency and strength. Pertinent for discussion would be instrumental issues such as alternative income sources, medication coverage, and home and child care needs, which are integral to a woman's ability to care for her family. A social worker's social awareness and a systemic perspective would inform exploratory questions about a woman's understanding of her faith life, her ethnicity, social status, racial and/or sexual identity [35,36,37,39,40,71]. Similar attention could be given to the significant person the woman chose to include in the meeting(s) since both are participants in the cancer experience [32,44,72].

It would be important for the social worker to inquire about the quality of a woman's relationships and discuss the upcoming potential changes to a woman's roles and relations as her treatment progresses [5,33,34,48,73,74]. The research of Sormanti and colleagues [5] has demonstrated that relational exploration during the initial stages of treatment planning could help to normalize and prepare a woman and her family, particularly as to how her role as caregiver could be altered and create significant ripples throughout family life.

[Relational changes] would be an important issue to assess during the early meetings with the cancer patient's family. Talking about this issue allows the family to prepare for the woman's diminished ability to be a caregiver and to begin securing additional resources that can be of help with routine activities such as house cleaning and childcare. The family may experience a sense of loss when the wife/mother is no longer able to participate in these activities. Discussion about this will help family members to anticipate losses and will provide them with a sense of control during a time when people feel quite helpless and vulnerable [5].

Thus, at the time of diagnosis, a social worker can provide a valuable opportunity for a woman to find her "voice," strengthen her sense of identity and her relationships, as well as begin preparation for the treatment days to come.

During Active Treatment

As the cancer experience unfolds into the arduous, often painful period of active treatment, any supportive care planning can be particularly challenging. Not surprisingly, post-operative recovery and subsequent treatments discourage many women from attending further appointments outside of necessary medical visits [75]. However, many women indicate that talking to someone during this time is desirable [25]. Therefore, social workers need to be flexible and creative in order to have easily available and effective services.

If, however, the oncology treatment team has valued supportive care services and has put in place the opportunity for contact during the diagnostic phase, then ongoing contact with the social worker can be potentially rewarding for women and their significant relations. The relationship can be helpful for ongoing support, information, and for reflection on the woman's changing identities and roles. As well, the social worker can be available to help a woman and her partner/family member/friend understand traditional treatment options, and explore their ideas and considerations about complementary, alternative, or culturally compatible ways of healing. The social worker can also provide advocacy for women for any questions or concerns that need to be addressed by medical personnel [60].

Social workers are particularly skilled in the development and facilitation of and advocacy for groups tailored to meet the particular needs of the participants [48,74]. During the active treatment phase, groups for women with cancer can have a variety of purposes such as psychoeducation, support, leisure, relaxation, or stress management [5,25,33,62,74,76].

In their review of 40 intervention studies, Cwikel and Behar [48] determined that psychosocial services, including individual and group formats during the cancer treatment phase, achieved the most effective results compared to those offered at other transition points of the illness. The researchers note, however, that this period of the cancer journey has also been the focus of the most research using high quality designs. Nevertheless, their data does provide persuasive empirical evidence that a variety of supportive care services need to be available for women during active treatment.

Along with offering professionally organized supportive care services, social workers can be instrumental in consulting with and/or advocating for community support groups voluntarily run by women survivors of cancer. International groups such as Gilda's Club [77], national organizations such as the Canadian Cancer Society [4], as well as Canadian urban organizations such as Southern Ontario's Willow [78], Wellwood [79], and Wellspring [80] have detailed websites and a variety of supportive programs for women including services available via virtual access. Not surprisingly, many women, especially from rural areas, are not able to physically join already established groups due to distance and/or diverse cultural differences [61]. In these circumstances, social workers, particularly of regional cancer sites, can be instrumental in advocating for and facilitating the development of professionally led and/or self-help groups suitable for rural or remote areas, while being sensitive to significant components of women's identities such as spiritual beliefs, ethnicity, race, and/or sexual orientation [37,40,61].

Surviving Through the First Five Years

Prior to the cessation of treatment, social workers can provide valuable information to help prepare women and their significant relations for the possible psychosocial adjustments that lie ahead [46]. For many women their own strengths, resiliencies and resourcefulness combined with any preparatory information can be enough to move them forward and successfully re-adjust. If needed, these women are able to self-initiate contact with cancer resources in their own communities or through Internet access. In recent years, women survivors of breast cancer have gained tremendous strength in numbers as well as national and local community support. Various self-initiated activities have become available for personal enjoyment and support such as belonging to running clubs or participating on Dragonboat teams such as Knot A Breast, Ontario.

However, as we have previously discussed, the transition for women to life apparently absent from cancer can be fraught with continued identity and relational challenges, along with the fear of recurrence [1]. Research has indicated that for women and their loved ones, the practice of little or no contact with health care professionals following the end of treatment can be difficult [46,68]. Unfortunately, there is a notable absence of any organized psychosocial interventions typically available by oncology teams once treatment is completed [43,46,68]. Consequently, the time following treatment is an area in need of further development by social workers and their fellow oncology team members.

Shining a light on the shadows. During the last few years, through her social work position at the Juravinski Cancer Centre in Hamilton, Ontario, Linda Learn participated on a multidisciplinary committee consisting of a medical oncologist (head of the supportive care department), an advanced practice nurse (chairperson of the breast disease site team), a dietitian, and symptom management nurse. Subsequently, Linda became the primary investigator of a post-treatment psychosocial pilot project for women titled, *Out of the Shadows – Challenging Post Treatment Monsters* [81].

Initially, topics of interest were generated from 160 women who completed a needs assessment questionnaire. These areas were included in the wellness focused educational program that was designed to meet the information needs of women who completed medical treatment for early stage breast cancer. The thematic focus of the six session program was psychosocial wellness and patient self-empowerment through the dissemination and exchange of information. The Mission Statement notes that "information is power – evidenced based knowledge provides tools to challenge cancer's influence on physical and emotional health" (p. 2). Analysis of respondent data from the first completed round of sessions demonstrated strong support for the program. According to results,

> The sessions themselves seemed to empower some of the attendees: to feel more secure about what they were experiencing; to feel more comfortable about asking direct questions to their health providers; to proactively seek help from other individuals or "ask their questions again." (p. 6)

Although the *Out of the Shadows* post-treatment group was not specifically focused on identity or relational changes, research results indicate that these aspects of women were positively, albeit indirectly, affected. Thus, the potential is clearly present that post-treatment groups could provide a valuable opportunity for women as well as their partners/family members/friends.

Concluding Comments

Cancer does not spare any part of a woman's life. The silent explosion of cells deep within her body ripples out and traumatically interfaces with her ideas of self and her relationships with others. The resulting counter-attack from health professionals needs wise planning and intentional organization. As a member of the team, social workers offer a systemic perspective that expands interventions to (a) include a woman's identity and roles, (b) provide space for her to reclaim her power and voice, and (c) invite her loved ones into the treatment process. Thus, each member of an oncology team can bring a unique and needed perspective to the war against cancer.

Conclusion and Recommendations

Cancer silently, mysteriously, and with deadly abandon penetrates into the lives of women. Medical diagnosis makes the invisible visible and brings the cellular mutiny into an existence that has to be confronted. The naming of the trouble within her body immediately re-shapes a woman's ideas and knowledge about herself and her identities in relation to others. A woman's roles such as child-bearer, nurturer, caretaker, sexual partner, employee, and friend, along with her corresponding relationships, become altered with the discovery of the cancer and the medical interventions used to control, if not eliminate the disease. Following the intense weeks and months of treatment, a woman and her loved ones most often only want back what the cancer has taken. But life will not be the same again.

Multidisciplinary oncology teams are needed to adequately address the complex, multifaceted needs of women with cancer. It is not enough to focus on the biological invasion. Attention to women's identities and relationships is essential to ensure adherence to treatment and to achieve the best opportunity for a well-adjusted post-treatment period. The systemic, person-in-environment perspective and skills of social workers make a unique contribution towards the recovery of women and their loved ones from cancer. In Canada, the routine offering of supportive care by social workers on multidisciplinary oncology teams will increase as (a) the stigma of mental health and relational issues are dispelled by all medical personnel, and (b) the psychosocial needs of all women afflicted with cancer are considered worthy of specialized care.

In turn, social workers have a responsibility to the social work profession, medical colleagues, and patients to clearly and respectfully articulate what aspects of a woman's life with cancer are appropriate for social work intervention and how social work participation can compliment medical treatments and enhance the wellbeing of patients. Furthermore, social workers are encouraged to substantiate the effectiveness of social work involvement by investing in research development. As DeCoster [82] has stated, "Health care social work, today, requires efficient and effective interventions, guided by convenient, pragmatic and conceptually stable knowledge" (p. 20). The outcomes of current social work research are weakened by insufficient funding, small sample sizes, inconsistency of measurement, lack of clear questions, and differences between therapeutic approaches [47,48,49]. Equally important, social work studies need to reflect the discipline's commitment to include the voices and experiences of women often marginalized according to the intersection of socio-political constructs such as gender, race, ethnicity, class, language, or spiritual beliefs.

The hard work of medical professionals invested in the prevention, treatment, and the eradication of cancer can be strengthened by an equitable partnership with social workers and their supportive care knowledge and initiatives. Together, with the voices of women and their loved ones, the fight against cancer can remain strong.

REFERENCES

[1] Colyer, H. Women's experience of living with cancer. *Journal of Advanced Nursing,* 1996 23, 496-501.

[2] Leigh, SA; Clark, EJ. Psychosocial aspects of cancer survivorship. In: Berger, A, Portenoy, RK, Weissman, DE (Eds.). *Principles and practice of supportive oncology*. Philadelphia, PA: Lippincott-Raven; 1998; 1034-1040.

[3] Little, M; Paul, K; Jorden, CF; Sayers, E. Survivorship and discourses of identity. *Psycho-Oncology*, 2002 11, 170-178.

[4] Canadian Cancer Society/National Cancer Institute of Canada (2005). *Canadian cancer statistics* 2005. Toronto, ON: Author. Retrieved February 10, 2006, from www.cancer.ca

[5] Sormanti, M; Kayser, K; Strainchamps, E. A relational perspective of women coping with cancer: A preliminary study. *Social Work in Health Care,* 1997 25(1/2), 89-106.

[6] Holland, J.C. IPOS Sutherland memorial lecture: An international perspective on the development of psychosocial oncology: Overcoming cultural and attitudinal barriers to improve psychosocial care. *Psycho-Oncology,* 2004 13, 445-459.

[7] Cordova, MJ; Cunningham, LC; Carlson, CR; Andrykowski, MA. Social constraints, cognitive processing, and adjustment to breast cancer. *Journal of Consulting and Clinical Psychology,* 2001 69, 706-711.

[8] McGoldrick, M. Women through the family life cycle. In Carter, B, McGoldrick, M (Eds.), *The expanded family life cycle: Individual, family and social perspectives* (3rd Ed.). Boston, MA: Allyn & Bacon; 2005; 106-123.

[9] Miller, JB. *Toward a new psychology of women* (2nd Ed.). Boston, MA: Beacon Press; 1986. Miller, JB. Women and power: Reflections ten years later. 1991. In: Goodrich, TJ (Ed.), *Women and power: Perspectives for family therapy*. New York: W. W. Norton & Co; 16-47

[10] McGoldrick, M; Carter, B. Self in context: The individual life cycle in systemic perspective. In: Carter,B; McGoldrick, M (Eds.). *The expanded family life cycle: Individual, family and social perspectives* (3rd Ed.). Boston, MA: Allyn & Bacon; 2005; 27-46.

[11] Davis, C. Psychosocial needs of women with breast cancer: How can social workers make a difference? *Health and Social Work,* 2004 29(4), 330-334.

[12] Smith, ED; Walsh-Burke, K;Crusan, C. Principles of training social workers in oncology. In Holland, JC (Ed.), *Psycho-Oncology*. New York: Oxford Press; 1998; 1061-1068

[13] Latour, B. *We have never been modern* (Porter, C, Trans.). Cambridge, MA: Harvard University Press; 1993 (Original work published 1991).

[14] Foucault, M. *The archaeology of knowledge* (Sheridan Smith, AM, Trans.).Great Britain: Tavistock Publications Limited; 1972 (Original work published 1969).

[15] Rorty, R. *Philosophy and the mirror of nature*. Princeton, NJ: Princeton University Press; 1979.

[16] Foucault, M. Two lectures. In Gordon, C (Ed.), *Power/knowledge: Selected interviews & other writings 1972-1977 by Michel Foucault.* New York: Pantheon Books; 1980; 78-92.

[17] Kuhn, TS. *The structure of scientific revolutions,* (3rd ed.). Chicago: University of Chicago Press; 1996.

[18] Webb-Watson, L. The sociology of power. In Goodrich, TJ (Ed.), *Women and power: Perspectives for family therapy.* New York: W. W. Norton & Co; 1991; 48-60.

[19] Burr, V. *An introduction to social constructionism.* New York: Routledge; 1995.

[20] Gergen, KJ. *The saturated self: Dilemmas of identity in contemporary life.* New York: Basic Books; 1991.

[21] Rorty, R. *Philosophy and social hope.* London, UK: Penguin Books; 1999.

[22] Gilligan, C. *In a different voice: Psychological theory and women's development.* Cambridge, MA: Harvard University Press; 1982.

[23] Surry, JL. The self-in-relation: A theory of women's development. In: Jordan, JV; Kaplan, AG; Miller, JB; Stiver, IP; Surry, JL, (Eds.). *Women's growth in connection: Writings from the Stone Center.* New York: Guilford Press; 1991; 51-66.

[24] Adleman, J; Enguidanos, G., (Eds.). *Racism in the lives of women: Testimony, theory, and guides to antiracist practice.* New York: Harrington Park Press; 1995.

[25] Fitch, MI; Gray, RE; DePetrillo, D; Franssen, E; Howell, D. Canadian women's perspectives on ovarian cancer. *Cancer Prevention and Control,* 1999 3, 52-60.

[26] Schaefer, KM; Ladd, EC; Lammers, SE; Echenberg, RJ. In your skin you are different: Women living with ovarian cancer during childbearing years. *Qualitative Health Research,* 1999 9(2), 227-241.

[27] Tomich, PL; Helgeson, VS. Five years later: A cross-sectional comparison of breast cancer survivors with healthy women. *Psycho-Oncology,* 2002 11, 154-169.

[28] Shaffer, ER. Breast cancer and the evolving health care system: Why health care reform is a breast cancer issue. In: Ferguson, AS; Ferguson, SJ, (Eds.), *Breast cancer: Society shapes an epidemic.*New York: Palgrave; 2000; 89-118.

[29] Petersen, S; Benishek, LA. Social construction of illness: Addressing the impact of cancer on women in therapy. In: Kaschak,E, (Ed.). *Minding the body: Psychotherapy in cases of chronic and life-threatening illness.* New York: Haworth Press; 2001; 75-100.

[30] Rosenbaum, ME; Roos, GM. Women's experiences of breast cancer. In: Kasper, AS; Ferguson, SJ, (Eds.). *Breast Cancer: Society shapes an epidemic.* New York: Palgrave; 2000; 153-181.

[31] Langellier, KM;Sullivan, CF. Breast talk in breast cancer narratives. *Qualitative Health Research,* 1998 8(1), 76-92.

[32] Davis-Ali, SH; Chesler, MA; Chesney, BK. Recognizing cancer as a family disease: Worries and support reported by patients and spouses. *Social Work in Health Care,* 1993 19(2), 45-65.

[33] Kulik, L; Kronfeld, M. Adjustment to breast cancer: The contribution of resources and causal attributions regarding the illness. *Social Work in Health Care,* 2005 41(2), 37-57.

[34] Hirschman, KB; Bourjolly, JN. How do tangible supports impact the breast cancer experience? *Social Work in Health Care,* 2005 41(1), 17-32.

[35] Barn, R; Sidhu, K. Understanding the interconnections between ethnicity, gender, social class and health: Experiences of minority ethnic women in Britain. *Social Work Health Care,* 2004 39(1/2), 11-27.

[36] Bourjolly, JN. Differences in religiousness among black and white women with breast cancer. *Social Work in Health Care,* 1998 28(1), 21.

[37] Bourjolly, JN; Kerson, T; Nuamah, IF. A comparison of social functioning among black and white women with breast cancer. *Social Work in Health Care,* 1999 28(3), 1-20.

[38] Im, EO; Meleis, AI. Women's work and symptoms during midlife: Korean immigrant women. In: Meleis, AI, (Ed.). *Women's work, health and quality of life.* NY: Haworth Press; 2001; 83-103.

[39] Levin, R; Herbert, M. The experience of urban aboriginals with health care services in Canada: Implications for social work practice. *Social Work in Health Care,* 2004 39(1/2), 165-179.

[40] Lowe, JI; Barg, FK; Bernstein, MW. Educating African-Americans about cancer prevention and detection: A review of the literature. *Social Work in Health Care,* 1995 21(4), 17-36.

[41] Ferrell, BR; Smith, SL; Ervin, KS; Itano, J; Melancon, C. A qualitative analysis of social concerns of women with ovarian cancer. *Psycho-Oncology,* 2003 12, 647-663.

[42] Avis, NE; Crawford, S; Manuel, J. Psychosocial problems among younger women with breast cancer. *Psycho-Oncology,* 2004 13, 295-308.

[43] Juraskova, I; Butow, P; Robertson, R; Sharpe, L; McLeod, C; Hacker, N. Post-treatment sexual adjustment following cervical and endometrial cancer: A qualitative insight. *Psycho-Oncology,* 2003 12, 267-279.

[44] Edwards, B; Clarke, V. The psychological impact of a cancer diagnosis on families: The influence of family functioning and patients' illness characteristics on depression and anxiety. *Psycho-Oncology,* 2004 13, 562-576.

[45] Lethborg; CE; Kissane, D; Burns, WI. It's not the easy part: the experience of significant others of women with early stage breast cancer, at treatment completion. *Social Work in Health Care,* 2003 37(1), 63-85.

[46] Arnold, EM. The cessation of cancer treatment as a crisis. *Social Work in Health Care,* 1999 29(2), 21-38.

[47] Cwikel, JG; Behar, LC. Organizing social work services with adult cancer patients: Integrating empirical research. *Social Work in Health Care,* 1999 28(3), 55-76.

[48] Cwikel, JG; Behar, LC. Social work with adult cancer patients: A vote-count review of intervention research. *Social Work in Health Care,* 1999 29(2), 39-67.

[49] Lillquist, PP; Abramson, JS. Separating the apples and oranges in the fruit cocktail: The mixed results of psychosocial interventions on cancer survival. *Social Work in Health Care,* 2002 36(2), 65-79

[50] Kash, KM; Mago, R; Kunkel, EJ. Psychosocial oncology: Supportive care for the cancer patient. *Seminars in Oncology,* 2004 32, 211-218.

[51] Parton, N. Some thoughts on the relationship between theory and practice in and for social work. *British Journal of Social Work,* 2000 30, 449-463.

[52] Payne, M. *What is professional social work?* Birmingham, UK: Venture Press; 1996.

[53] Shulman, L. *The skills of helping individuals, families, groups, and communities,* (3rd ed.). Itasca, IL: F.E. Peacock Publishers; 1992.

[54] Saleebey, D. Culture, theory, and narrative: The intersection of meanings in practice. *Social Work,* 1994 39(4), 351-359.

[55] Bisman, C. Social work values: The moral core of the profession. *British Journal of Social Work,* 2004 34(1), 109-123.

[56] Lundy, C. *Social work and social justice: A structural approach to practice.* Peterborough, ON: Broadview Press, Ltd; 2004.

[57] Reamer, FG. Social work values and ethics. In: Reamer, FG (Ed.). *The foundations of social work knowledge.* New York: Columbia University Press; 1994; 195-230.

[58] Human Resources Development Canada (2004, October 27). *National occupational classification: 4152 – Social workers.* Retrieved February 20, 2006, from http://www23.hrdc-drhc.gc.ca/2001/e/groups/4152.shtml

[59] International Federation of Social Workers (2000). *Definition of social work.* Retrieved February 17, 2006, retrieved from, http://www.ifsw.org/en/p38000208.html

[60] Bricker-Jenkins, M. Feminist practice and breast cancer: "The patriarchy has claimed my right breast..." *Social Work in Health Care,* 1994 19(3/4), 17-42.

[61] Davis, C; Williams, P; Redman, S; White, K; King, E. Assessing the practical and psychosocial needs of rural women with early breast cancer in Australia. *Social Work in Health Care,* 2003 36(3), 25-36.

[62] Carlson, LE; Bultz, BD. Efficacy vs.cost of psychosocial: An evidence-based call for action. *Oncology Exchange,* 2002 1(2), 34-51.

[63] Fawzy, FI. Psychosocial interventions for patients with cancer: What works and what doesn't. *European Journal of Cancer,* 1999 *35*, 1559-1564.

[64] Canadian Association of Psychosocial Oncology (1999). *National psychosocial oncology standards for Canada.* Retrieved February 20, 2006, from www.capo.ca/eng/finalstandards.asp

[65] Gregorian, C. A career in hospital social work: Do you have what it takes? *Social Work in Health Care,* 2005 40(3), 1-14.

[66] National Breast Cancer Centre and National Cancer Control Initiative (2003). *Clinical practice guidelines for the psychosocial care of adults with cancer.* National Breast Cancer Centre, Camperdown, NSW, Australia: Author. Retrieved February 20, 2006, from http://www.nhmrc.gov.au/publications/synopses/cp90syn.htm

[67] National Comprehensive Cancer Network (2005). *Distress management: Version 1.2005.* Retrieved February 20, 2006, from http://www.nccn.org/professionals/physician_gls/PDF/distress.pdf

[68] Lethborg, CE; Kissane, D. It doesn't end on the last day of treatment: A psychoeducational intervention for women after adjuvant treatment for early stage breast cancer. *Journal of Psychosocial Oncology,* 2003 21(3), 25-41.

[69] Gurowka, KJ; Lightman, ES. Supportive and unsupportive interactions as perceived by cancer patients. *Social Work in Health Care,* 1995 21(4), 71-88.

[70] Kitchen, A; Brook, J. Social work at the heart of the medical team. *Social Work in Health Care,* 2005 40(4), 1-18.

[71] Lesbians and Breast Cancer Project Team. *Coming Out About Lesbians and Cancer.* Toronto: Ontario Breast Cancer Community Research Initiative; 2004.

[72] DeGroot, JM; Mah, K; Fyles, A; Winton, S; Greenwood, S; DePetrillo, AD; et al. The psychosocial impact of cervical cancer among affected women and their partners. *International Journal of Gynaecological Cancer,* 2005 15, 918-925.

[73] Kayser, K; Sormanti, M. A follow-up study of women with cancer: Their psychosocial well-being and close relationships. *Social Work in Health Care,* 2002 35(1/2), 391-406.

[74] Parrish, MM; Satariano, WA; Freisthler, B; Feinberg, LF; Adams, S. Older women with breast cancer: Caregiving and the risk of depression-An exploratory analysis. *Social Work in Health Care,* 2005 40(4), 41-59.

[75] Donnelly, JM; Kornblith, AB; Fleishman, S; Zuckerman, E; Raptis, G; Hudis, CA; et al. A pilot study of interpersonal psychotherapy by telephone with cancer patients and their partners. *Psycho-Oncology,* 2000 9, 44-56.

[76] Shannon, CS; Bourque, D. Overlooked and underutilized: The critical role of leisure interventions in facilitating social support throughout breast cancer treatment and recovery. *Social Work in Health Care,* 2005 42(1), 73-92.

[77] Gilda's Club (2005). *About us.* Retrieved February 20, 2006, from http://www.gildasclub.org

[78] Willow (2004). *Willow breast cancer support & resource services.* Retrieved February 20, 2006, from http://www.willow.org/

[79] Wellwood (2006). *Wellwood: Helping people live well with cancer.* Retrieved February 20, 2006, from http://www.wellwood.on.ca/

[80] Wellspring (2006). *Wellspring: A network of support centres for people with cancer and their love ones.* Retrieved February 20, 2006, from *http://www.wellspring.ca/home.html*

[81] Learn, L; Biggs, K; Gage, C; Tozer, R; Wiernikowski, J. *Out of the shadows – challenging post-treatment monsters.* 2005, Unpublished manuscript.

[82] DeCoster, VA. Health care social work treatment of patient and family emotion: A synthesis and comparison across patient populations and practice settings. *Social Work in Health Care,* 2002 30(4), 7-24.

In: Women and Cancer
Editor: Laurie Elit, pp. 227-234
ISBN: 978-1-60021-494-3

Chapter III

SEXUALITY AND CANCER

John Lamont [*]
Department of Obstetrics and Gynecology, McMaster University, Hamilton, Canada.

ABSTRACT

Objective: To review the importance of discussing sexuality with women at the time of treatment planning, and during the follow-up phase of managing gynecologic cancers.

Methods: Components of the sexual history, various barriers to discussing sexual function (ie., lack of knowledge) are reviewed using gynecologic cancers as an example. The interaction between quality of life and illness on sexual function is explored. Management strategies are discussed.

Conclusion: There may be sensitivities about broaching this topic for both the patient and the health care team. Usually the health care team can manage most of the issues; however, referral to sexual medicine may be required in complex situations.

INTRODUCTION

The domains of female sexuality and gynaecologic cancer at first glance seem to overlap very little. A diagnosis of cancer in women evokes a response of alarm and a desire to hasten the treatment in order to decrease morbidity and to enhance survival for the woman. The patient and the oncology team share a quest for the patient's survival. On the other hand, sexuality in the context of a cancer diagnosis evokes a sense of unease. The oncology team recognizes the importance of quality of life issues in the patient's total care, but where is it appropriate to fit in the question of sexuality? The oncology team may lack knowledge,

[*] Correspondence concerning this article should be addressed to John Lamont MD, Henderson Hospital, 711 Concession Street Hamilton, Ontario, Canada L8V 1C3. Phone 905 574-8606; Fax: 905 575-2587; E-mail: lamont@mcmaster.ca

comfort or skill in identifying where sexual rehabilitation fits into the patient's priority list as they move from diagnosis, through treatment, to recovery [1].

An issue requiring acknowledgement is the fact that both the oncology team and the patient may share a sexual socialization that avoids frank discussion and openness so that routine history taking and treatment for sexual concerns may be shunted to the bottom of the priority list for care. Most oncology patients feel they do not get enough information from their physician or the oncology team about the impact of their disease and its treatment on their sexual function. Unfortunately this message is not clearly communicated to the oncologist because the patients hope that the physician or the nurse will take the initiative in discussing these matters [2]. Patients are generally quite comfortable discussing sexual and emotional issues with a physician or nurse.

Sexuality is rarely an item for discussion at the time of diagnosis. Once a treatment plan is initiated, the patient and the oncology team start to consider quality of life issues including sexuality. Since most cancer victims become survivors, the impact of the diagnosis and treatment on sexuality is an area of growing interest for professionals and concern for patients. When the patient is able to assess how "normal" life can be after completion of her treatment there are a number of important factors to discuss. These factors include general knowledge about sexuality, psychosocial issues in the patient's past and present life, assessment of pre-diagnosis sexual morbidity, sexual problems generally experienced by oncology patients, and the effects of specific cancers and their treatment on the patient and her partner during diagnosis, treatment and recovery.

Research has shown that in gynaecologic cancer, *levels of communication* between health care professionals and the women with cancer is still low [3]. Stead states that reasons for not discussing sexual issues in this study included, "it is not my responsibility", embarrassment, lack of knowledge and experience, and lack of resources to provide support if needed. A further reason for the lack of communication about sexual issues is the lack of research evidence to support the discussion. A recent study shows that for women with gynaecologic cancer, the maintenance of a positive self-image and feelings of sexuality is one of the central issues of importance in the provision of quality health care and in contributing to the quality of their daily living.

As a society, we equate sexual activity with coital activity because of the importance of coital function in reproduction. These traditional attitudes are further supported by sex roles where women are socialized to accommodate their partner's sexual needs and men are socialized to feel entitled to coital activity in a committed relationship. The professional providing supportive care for the oncology patient may harbour some of these *traditional attitudes*. There are many barriers to taking a sexual history (see Table I) [4]. Care of these women requires sensitive inquiry by professionals who are comfortable discussing sexuality, and who have knowledge of sexual physiology, options for sensual and sexual pleasure, and what affects aging, socialization and relationship dynamics can have on a woman's sexual function. Other issues of importance in history taking include establishing a sense of privacy and confidentiality, avoiding assumptions or judgements, avoiding jargon or technical terms, and being aware of cultural differences.

Table I. Barriers to taking a sexual history

• lack of time • fear of intruding or offending patient • belief that cancer survivors may be too ill, or • are not interested in sex
• belief that disfigured bodies are not sexually • attractive
• fear of boundary transgressions and • medicolegal implications
• lack of adequate training and/or skills in • this area
• cultural issues – gay patient, single patient, • different cultural beliefs about illness and • disease
• age and gender of patient – young patient, • old patient
• presence of a third party (partner, parent) • fear of opening a "Pandora's box" – previous • sexual assault, difficult relationship

Other issues to be considered in assessing the patient are her *life stresses* and losses prior to or coincidental with the development of her cancer. The onset of her cancer symptoms prior to diagnosis may be important in that she may have already experienced a change in her sexual function due to these symptoms such as abnormal vaginal bleeding, pelvic pain, dyspareunia or fatigue. Sexual complaints are usually not viewed as heralding the onset of a cancer, however, loss of sexual desire, low arousal and pain have been reported as early complaints in women later diagnosed with cervical or endometrial cancer [5].

It's likely that the patient who has cherished her sexual relationship, enjoyed her sexual response, experimented with a variety of routes to pleasure and orgasm, will seek a prompt resumption of physical intimacy as an important and early part of the rehabilitation process as soon as she feels well.

On the one hand, those individuals who have suffered from sexual inhibition, abuse or monotonous and repetitious sexual interaction and have had a lifetime of accommodating their partner, may find that their cancer or its treatment an excuse to limit their sexual activity or give it up all together [6]. On the other hand, the partner's attitudes and behaviours are of vital importance in rehabilitation. Continued evidence of love and affection along with an expectation of continued sexual intimacy and an eagerness to maintain intimate physical contact will greatly assist the woman in her recovery.

Quality of Life

Sexual functioning is the most enduringly compromised quality of life issue after treatment for gynaecologic cancer, affecting from 50-80% of patients [5,7]. Any treatment of gynaecologic cancer can disrupt a woman's quality of life. Quality of life refers to a multi-dimensional concept of the impact of a medical problem and its treatment on physical, emotional and social well being [2]. Cancer treatment may involve loss of sexually responsive tissue, alteration of physiologic sexual response, loss of hormonal support of these tissues, loss of fertility, and alteration of body image. Emotional reactions to the diagnosis and treatment of a gynaecologic cancer can result in negative affect including dysphoria, anger, anxiety, fear and anhedonia. Quality of life issues are rarely identified at the time of diagnosis, but evolve as the patient moves from diagnosis to treatment and rehabilitation [8]. The complexity of the treatment and its consequences result in an accumulative affect on quality of life as the treatment progresses. Quality of life improves as the patient develops confidence in her survival as the symptoms of her treatment begin to subside. A major factor in her recovery involves the quality of a woman's social support and primary relationships including the doctor/patient relationship.

Effect of Illness on Sexuality

A review of the literature describes a universal deterioration in female cancer patients from pre-treatment to post-treatment level of sexual functioning. It is apparent that most cancer survivors attempt to maintain a sex life, but the prognosis of that sex life depends on a number of variables including the magnitude of their treatment, the age of the patient, the variety of treatments used with the individual patient, the pre-treatment level of interest and function, and the quality of the relationship prior to diagnosis as well as the presence or absence of partner issues related to the diagnosis and treatment of the cancer [9].

Negative affect can be generated during any part of the illness. This negative affect combined with preoccupation with the illness and fatigue from the emotional and physical strain of treatment; result in a loss of erotic focus for the patient with a resulting decrease in sexual interest and receptivity. Other psychological mechanisms that influence erotic focus have to do with threats to sexual identity and self-esteem, loss of personal control over bodily functions, loss of intimacy and a loss of reproductive function. For young women with severe illness and extensive treatment, role change in the family and loss of economic stability for the family may also result in significant stress. The extent of the impact of treatment on sexual function is additive. If more than one modality of treatment is used, it is additive in the sense that loss of functioning tissue, loss of hormonal support for those tissues, and psychologic mechanisms have a compounding effect on eliminating erotic focus, decreasing desire and impairing physiologic sexual function.

An assessment of sexual morbidity is best understood by knowing the pre-morbid level of sexual interest and function and acknowledging the patient's losses, both symbolic and functional, as a result of her disease and treatment. Depending on age, socialization and reproductive history, the loss of pelvic structures, the loss of menstrual function, the loss of fertility and the loss of sexually responsive tissue and its hormonal support may have profoundly different effects on individual women. Self-esteem and self-image are equally important to a 35-year-old patient with cancer of the cervix and a 75-year-old patient with cancer of the ovary. However, issues of personal priority regarding interpersonal and sexual relationships may be quite different, depending on the woman's social, sexual and family status. The more profound a woman's loss through her treatment, the more important and profound is the grieving process. Acknowledgement of her loss may be helpful in initiating recovery of her esteem and the development of a new body image.

Reports on sexual rehabilitation dating back to the 1950's agree that close to 100% of female cancer patients treated with radical surgery who were previously sexually responsive and enjoyed sex (with an accepting and sexually interested partner) have the same ability to respond sexually after treatment [1].

The Effect of Treatment on Sexual Function

Sexual function is a total body response under the influence of the autonomic nervous system [15]. For this to occur requires relaxation accompanied by a neurovascular-vasocongestive response under the dominant influence of the parasympathetic nervous system. The linear components of sexual response include desire or receptivity, arousal, and orgasm. Desire or receptivity is influenced by the presence of an erotic focus and to some degree, circulating free testosterone. The diagnosis of a gynaecologic cancer results in a variety of negative affective states including fear, anxiety and preoccupation, which in effect replaces any erotic focus and results in a loss of desire and receptivity to sexual invitation. Treatment on the other hand, has direct and indirect effects on sexually responsive tissue in the pelvis. Direct impairment of sexual function relates to the loss of sexually functioning tissue through surgical removal or radiation impairment. Indirect impairment relates to loss of ovarian function through radiation or chemotherapy with resulting loss of menstrual function, premature menopause, loss of fertility and loss of hormonal support for the sexually sensitive tissues.

Each treatment modality may have a specific impact on sexual function. Radiation, surgery or chemotherapy can interfere with the normal pelvic response from parasympathetic stimulation, impairing pelvic vasocongestion and delaying physiologic response. Surgery involves the loss of sexually responsive tissue and shortening of the vagina. The degree of surgery may result in significant loss of the autonomic nervous system's supply to the pelvis, whereas pelvic scarring and vaginal shortening may result in dyspareunia. Surgery can also have an impact on body image by the presence of scar tissue on the abdomen or vulva, which may equally impact on erotic focus through a women's sense of mutilation. Despite these changes and even with radical pelvic surgery, partial preservation of the autonomic nervous system in the motivated patient, may still preserve sexual response. During rehabilitation some couples may discover new erogenous zones and new routes to arousal and orgasm, resulting in a return of sexual response through effective stimulation.

Radiation of the pelvic tissue results in a loss of elasticity of the internal genital tissues and blood vessels and atrophy of the vaginal epithelium from loss of gonadal hormone production. The vagina may be shortened by scarring and vaginal lubrication made more difficult due to the radiation resulting in dyspareunia. Radiation for carcinoma of the cervix causes anatomic distortion and alteration of vaginal function in more than 80% of cases studied [11]. A definite inverse relationship has been demonstrated between the degree of pelvic fixation and the degree of post-treatment sexual satisfaction. Some oncologists recommend dilatation of the vagina in the early post-treatment phase of radiation to maintain full depth of the vagina. The importance of maintaining the physical space in the vagina through dilatation or early intercourse comes at a time when the patient and/or her partner may experience dysphoria and an unfortunate loss of sexual appetite. Sixty per cent of both male and female partners report an increased need for physical contact, but 100% of females and 90% of males report decreased interest in intercourse at the time the diagnosis of cervical cancer is made [10].

Chemotherapy often results in specific physical effects including gastrointestinal symptoms, loss of gonadal hormone production, loss of body hair, and extreme fatigue. These symptoms of chemotherapy usually result in a marked decrease in interest in physical and sexual contact. The nature of administration of chemotherapy also contributes to the patient focusing on her poor health and uncertain future. Repetitive doses of cancer treatment drugs tend to stimulate the patients rumination on her disease and the accompanying "ill feeling" re-emphasizes her uncertain future. A general withdrawal from the relationship can be expected which grows worse with the prolonged treatment and the increased number of treatments required for some cancers. The patient herself may find it hard to believe that her partner still finds her attractive. In this emotional state, she may in fact be repulsed by any physical advance her partner might make.

Despite the increasing success in treating gynaecologic cancer, there are a few articles in the literature describing the "psychological terrain" of the woman who has completed treatment and who is free of evidence of disease over a continued period of time [9]. Our oncology team may feel unprepared for this new role and better suited for diagnosis and treatment of the disease itself. However, from the patient's point of view, these psychologic concerns are an essential sequelae of gynaecologic cancer treatment and therefore, an essential component of oncology practice.

Psychosocial Support of the Terminal Patient

When cancer treatment for gynaecologic malignancies is not effective, psychosocial support continues to be important [1]. The patient continues to look for support from her cancer treatment team and desperately hopes that she will not be abandoned. As the patient acknowledges her terminal condition, her need for sexual outlet may decrease but her need for physical contact and emotional support will stay the same or increase. Leber found that a major change after onset of illness was a decreased desire for sexual intercourse accompanied by an increased desire for physical closeness of other kinds, such as simple proximity, holding hands, embracing and kissing [12]. This phenomenon suggested that comforting and reassurance were needed more than before and that sexual stimulation and release were needed less. Few patients report an increased interest in sexual intercourse, but over half wished for more physical closeness after the illness began.

Conclusion

In conclusion, the gynaecologic cancer patient requires special and specific input into the psychosocial and sexual aspects of her disease. Through diagnosis, treatment and follow-up, psychosexual morbidity of any kind can be experienced. To provide total patient care, the oncology team needs to know what emotional reaction may result from cancer treatment of genital tract malignancy. Each patient deserves information and reassurance about the effect or lack of effect of specific treatments on her sexual response, sexual interest, and sexual relationship. Cancer treatment does not eliminate sexual interest or sexual function in a previously sexually responsive woman, especially if she has an interested educated partner who is optimistic about continuing a pleasurable intimate physical relationship with her. Sexually responsive tissue can be affected by any of the treatment modalities and alter coital function. Optimistic sexual rehabilitation encourages the patient and her partner to explore a range of options to intercourse. A variety of resources are needed by the oncology team, including the option for sexual and relationship therapy for the patient in order to offer her a holistic approach to her disease.

As an oncology team, we need to broaden our assessment of the patient and her partner with regard to their pre-morbid sexual function, their attitudes and information about pelvic cancer and sexuality. Careful prospective evaluation needs to assess the effect of the diagnosis of cancer, the disease itself, and the various modes of treatment. With increasing information for both the professional and the patient, a fear of cancer and performance anxiety about sexual function will be put in their proper perspective. Only then can a woman with pelvic cancer obtain maximum benefit from her treatment and rehabilitation.

References

[1] Lamont, J; DePetrillo, D. Psychosexual Impact of Gynecologic Cancer (Chapt. 68). In: Harper; Row. *Gynecology and Obstetrics*.1980.

[2] Sun, CC; Frumovitz, M; Bodurka, DC. Quality of Life and Gynecologic Malignancies. *Current Oncology Reports*, 2005 7, 459-465.

[3] Stead, ML. Sexual Function After Treatment for Gynecologic Malignancy. *Current Opinion in Oncology*, 2004 16, 492-495.

[4] Sundquist, K; Yee, L. Sexuality and Body Image After Cancer. *Australian Family Physician, Jan/Feb* 2003 32, 19-32.

[5] Anderson, B; Elliott, ML. Female Cancer Survivors: Appreciating their sexual concerns. *The Canadian Journal of Human Sexuality*, 1994 3(2) Summer, 107-122.

[6] Clifford, D; Rutter, M; Selby, J. *"The Impact of Illness on Sexuality" in Caring for Sexuality in Health and in Illness*. Diane Wells, Ed., 212-216

[7] Taylor, CLC; Basen-Engquist, K; Shinn, EH; Bodurka, DC. Predictors of Sexual Functioning in Ovarian Cancer Patients. *J. of Clin. Oncology*, 2004 22:5, 881-889.8.

[8] Tabano, M; Condosta, D; Coons, M. Symptoms Affecting Quality of Life in Women with Gynecologic Cancer. *Seminars in Oncology Nursing*, 2002 18(3), 223-230.

[9] Auchincloss, SS. After Treatment: Psychosocial Issues in Gynecologic Cancer Survivorship. *Cancer*, 1995 76(10), 2117-2124.

[10] Wilmoth, MC; Spinelli, AS. Sexual Implications of Gynecologic Cancer Treatments. *JOGNN*, 2000 29(4), 413-421.

[11] Schultz, WCM; Van De Wiel, HBM; Hahn, DEE; Van Driel, MF. Sexuality and Cancer in Women. *Annual Review of Sex Research*, 1992 3, 151-199.

[12] Leiber, L; et al: The Communication of Affection Between Cancer Patients and TheirSpouses. *Psychosom Med*, 1976 38, 379.

Section 6: Cancer and the Reproductive Spectrum of a Woman's Life

In: Women and Cancer
Editor: Laurie Elit, pp. 237-257
ISBN: 978-1-60021-494-3

Chapter I

FERTILITY AND THE MANAGEMENT OF CANCER

***Janice S. Kwon*[1,*] *and Allison M. Case*[2]**

[1]Department of Gynecologic Oncology, MD Anderson Cancer Center, Houston, Texas;
[2]Department of Obstetrics, Gynecology and Reproductive Sciences, University of Saskatchewan, Canada.

ABSTRACT

Objective: In an era where cancer is more and more often to be cured, strategies to preserve fertility in premenopausal women are becoming increasingly important.

Methods and Results: The impact of radiation and/or chemotherapy on ovarian function are reviewed. Both strategies are dependent on the age of the patient and dose of the agent. Strategies to preserve ovarian function such as GnRH agonists are discussed. Cryopreservations of embyos or ovarian tissue reimplantation are becoming options for those willing to pay. Fertility sparing surgical management such as radical trachelectomy for cervical cancer are becoming more widely available.

Conclusions: It is important to evaluate outcomes when challenging current cancer treatment strategies. It is important to ensure that fertility-sparing options are not just feasible but actually safe for the patient and her potential offspring.

INTRODUCTION

Over the last half century, there has been an increase in the cure rates of young women with early stage malignancies [1]. There has been a trend away from the Halstead phenomenon of radical treatment for managing cancer, with more emphasis on optimizing quality of life and preserving fertility. A number of innovative approaches are now available

* Correspondence concerning this article should be addressed to Janice Kwon MD, Department of Gynecologic Oncology, Division of Surgery, MD Anderson Cancer Center, PO Box 301439, Houston, Texas, 77230-1439. Tel: 713.745.4243. Fax: 713.792.7586..Email:jskwon@mdanderson.org

to minimize the negative impact of cancer treatment on fertility, including hormonal manipulation, cryopreservation of embryos or ovarian tissue, and alternatives to definitive surgery for malignancy.

The Effects of Radiation on Fertility

Ionizing radiation interacts with intracellular water to create highly reactive free radicals that interfere with a cell's ability to reproduce. We have learned about the effects of ionizing radiation in women from several historical sources [2-5].

- Young women with Hodgkin's disease were routinely treated with up to 3,500 rads to the pelvis, which uniformly resulted in amenorrhea and infertility.
- Pelvic radiation was once administered as treatment for menorrhagia. While this strategy effectively controlled the condition, the majority of women who received radiotherapy likely became menopausal. Of those who did become pregnant after treatment, most pregnancies ended in spontaneous abortion, probably due to chromosomal abnormalities or adverse effects on the endometrium interfering with implantation.
- Radiotherapy to the pituitary and pelvis was once prescribed as treatment for infertility. The dose of radiation to the pituitary and pelvis was significantly less than in the menorrhagia study, and as a result 39% of women were able to conceive. It became apparent that there had to be a threshold dose of radiation to the ovaries below which ablation of reproductive function did not occur.

It is now well recognized that the effects of radiation on female reproductive function are both age- and dose-dependent [5]. A total dose in excess of 1500 cGy (rads) appears to be sufficient to cause permanent infertility as a result of irreversible ovarian failure [6]. A woman who is diagnosed with a locally advanced cervical cancer is generally treated with a combination of chemotherapy and pelvic radiation as primary treatment. The total dose of pelvic radiation required is 8,500 cGy (85 Gy), which is far in excess of the threshold for ovarian failure. Therefore even though this woman does not undergo a hysterectomy and she may be of reproductive age, she is rendered infertile and menopausal as a result of her cancer treatment. When pelvic radiation is offered in an adjuvant setting after primary surgery for early stage cervical or endometrial cancer, the total dose often exceeds 4,500 rads or 45 Gy, and even these doses are in excess of the ovarian failure threshold. Therefore, radiotherapy to the pelvis as primary or adjuvant treatment for gynecologic cancers will induce ovarian failure in virtually all women who still have their adnexae at the time they are treated for these malignancies.

Transposition of the Ovaries

To minimize radiation exposure and the risk of ovarian failure, surgical transposition of ovaries out of the pelvis has been recommended prior to pelvic radiotherapy [7,8]. The ovaries can be transposed high in the paracolic gutter above the pelvic brim, just beneath the lower pole of the kidney [9]. The procedure can be done laparoscopically or at the time of laparotomy for malignancy in which adjuvant pelvic radiotherapy is anticipated [7-14]. Despite its technical feasibility, ovarian transposition does not necessarily protect ovarian function following pelvic radiotherapy because of the inevitability of radiation scatter [15-20]. Table 1 summarizes the rates of ovarian failure following adjuvant radiotherapy following radical hysterectomy and ovarian transposition for cervical cancer. In general, the mean age at which menopause occurs after radical hysterectomy, ovarian transposition, and pelvic radiotherapy appears to be at least a decade earlier than that expected in the general population. As devascularization injury to the ovary with hysterectomy results in menopause approximately five years before expected in the general population [21], it is possible that exposure to pelvic radiation after this initial devascularization may be sufficient to induce ovarian failure in the majority of women undergoing the procedure. Also, the rate of symptomatic ovarian cysts requiring medical or surgical intervention (oophorectomy) following transposition is significant—as high as 25% [17,18]. Even if ovarian function is preserved after transposition and pelvic radiotherapy, it is unlikely that fertility can be preserved in those who still have a uterus. Radiotherapy can adversely affect local uterine vasculature with subsequent impairment of implantation if conception should occur [22].

Table 1. Outcomes after ovarian transposition (at radical hysterectomy for cervical cancer)

Author	Mean age at surgery (in years)	Ovarian failure (without radiation)	Mean age of ovarian failure (without radiation), in years	Ovarian failure (with pelvic radiation)	Mean age of menopause (with radiation), in years
Feeney [18]	33.5	3/104 (2.9%)	NR	14/28 (50%) at 24 months	NR
Buekers [19]	32.6	1/61 (2%)	47.2	10/17 (59%) at 12 months	36.6
Chambers [18]	NR	1/24 (4%)	NR	4/14 (29%) at 35 months	38.5
Anderson [17]	31	9/58 (16%)	40	20/24 (83%) at 13 months	33
Van Eijkeren [19]	NR	2/36 (5.5%)	46	5/18 (28%)	35

NR = Not Reported

The Effects of Chemotherapy on Reproductive Function

As with radiation, the effects of chemotherapy on reproductive function are both age- and dose-dependent [23,24]. Toxicities to ovarian function range widely, depending on the drug's mechanism of action. Alkylating agents are among the more toxic as they result in DNA cross-links with single and double-strand breaks that inhibit synthesis of DNA, RNA, and proteins [25]. These drugs, such as cyclophosphamide and busulfan, act in a cell cycle *non-specific* manner.

Cyclophosphamide has an important role in current treatment protocols, especially for breast cancer [26]. The dose of cyclophosphamide resulting in ovarian failure is age-dependent [28], with a cumulative dose of 20.4 g required to induce ovarian failure in a woman 20-29 years old, versus a cumulative dose of 5.2 g in a woman over 40. To put this in perspective, an average size woman with a body surface area of 1.7 m^2 receiving six cycles of CMF (cylophosphamide, methotrexate, 5-fluorouracil) or CEF (epirubicin replacing methotrexate) for breast cancer would receive a total of 11-15 g of cyclophosphamide chemotherapy [29]. Therefore, many women treated with CMF or CEF, especially those in their 30s and 40s, are rendered infertile and menopausal at the completion of treatment [27,28]. Busulfan, an alkylating agent used in high dose chemotherapy regimens prior to autologous bone marrow transplantation, has also been shown to have a detrimental effect to fertility, even in young prepubertal or adolescent girls [29].

Certain chemotherapeutic drugs are known to be *minimally toxic* to ovarian function. These are the cell cycle-*specific* drugs such as anti-metabolites (methotrexate, 5-FU), plant alkaloids (vincristine, vinblastine, etoposide), and antibiotics (actinomycin-D, doxorubicin, bleomycin) [25]. In contrast, these drugs are highly toxic to testicular function because of the constant cell division in spermatogenesis. The literature on the use of these drugs in treating women with gestational trophoblastic disease and ovarian germ cell tumors suggests that reproductive function is not impaired [30-38]. Although cisplatin is an alkylating-like agent, it has been incorporated into chemotherapy protocols for ovarian germ cell tumors without significant impact on ovarian function [32,36].

Hormonal Manipulation to Minimize Effects of Radiation and Chemotherapy

It is well recognized that the ovary of a prepubertal girl has a higher threshold to radiation and chemotherapy than the ovary of a woman of reproductive age [2,28,41]. This may be the consequence of a higher number of oocytes and no meiotic activity in the prepubertal ovary. One method of preventing ovarian failure from cancer treatment may be the use of hormonal manipulation to suppress ovulation as a method of "saving" oocytes, by rendering the ovary quiescent as in its prepubertal state.

Use of Oral Contraceptives

Ovarian suppression during chemotherapy using oral contraceptives has resulted in variable outcomes. One study involved six women between the ages of 18 and 32 who used oral contraceptives during MVPP chemotherapy (nitrogen mustard, vinblastine, procarbazine, and prednisone) for Hodgkin's disease [39]. Five of the six resumed normal menses following treatment, and one eventually conceived. Ovarian biopsies revealed preservation of follicles in these women, in contrast to historical controls who did not use oral contraceptives. In contrast, a different outcome was reported in a cohort of women aged 13 to 45 (median age 23) who also received MVPP chemotherapy for Hodgkin's disease [40]. Only nine patients used the oral contraceptive pill during chemotherapy, but four developed amenorrhea and three developed oligomenorrhea, suggesting that these patients had not been protected from chemotherapy-induced ovarian damage. Among women who received chemotherapy comprised of ifosfamide (alkylating agent), methotrexate, adriamycin, and cisplatin for osteosarcoma of the extremities, there was no difference in ovarian failure rate among postpubertal women who used oral contraceptives compared to the control group [41].

Gonadotropin-releasing Hormone Agonists

More consistent results have been reported with the use of gonadotropin-releasing hormone (GnRH) agonists. Several studies have reported successful preservation of ovarian function with GnRH agonists (with or without GnRH antagonists) [42-45]. In one study, a cohort of 44 women aged 15 to 40 received monthly depot injections of a GnRH agonist prior to starting chemotherapy for lymphoma, leukemia, or autoimmune diseases, for a maximum of six months [42]. A control group of 55 women received similar chemotherapy without a GnRH agonist. All but one of the women in the GnRH group resumed spontaneous ovulation and menses within six months of completing treatment, compared to only 40% of the controls. Similar results come from another study of five women aged 14 to 20 [43]. They received monthly intramuscular injections of a GnRH agonist (leuprolide acetate 3.75 mg) soon after starting multiagent chemotherapy prior to bone marrow transplantation for Hodgkin's disease or acute myeloblastic leukemia. All five treated with the GnRH agonist had resumed menses 45 to 120 days after completing chemotherapy. A second treatment group of seven women, aged 14 to 18, received high-dose chemotherapy and radiation for Hodgkin's disease, followed by monthly intramuscular injections of a GnRH agonist for a maximum of six months. Five of the seven women resumed normal menses. In comparison, four controls between the ages of 17 and 20 all developed secondary amenorrhea and required long-term hormone replacement therapy. A second control group included five girls between the ages of 3 and 7.5 who received multiagent chemotherapy. These girls were followed for 18 years, and all had spontaneous menarche between the ages of 12 and 17.9. It is possible that prepubertal girls are spared the potential deleterious effects of chemotherapy because of the endocrine "quiescence" of their ovaries during treatment. Postpubertal women are spared the detrimental effects of chemotherapy because a similar endocrine state is induced with administration of GnRH agonists.

During treatment with a GnRH agonist, initial stimulation is followed by suppression of gonadotropin release, decreased secretion of estrogens, progestogens, and androgens, and finally cellular apoptosis and follicular atresia [46]. As a result, oocyte maturation is inhibited and involution occurs, thereby avoiding the deleterious effects of chemotherapy on the dividing cell [47]. In contrast to oral contraceptives, GnRH agonists revert the ovary to its prepubertal state, which may explain its effectiveness in protecting ovarian function.

Cryopreservation of Embryos or Ovarian Tissue

Preservation of reproductive function may be achieved by cryopreservation of embryos, or more recently, cryopreservation of ovarian tissue with subsequent grafting as a xenotransplant or autotransplant.

Embryo cryopreservation is highly successful and can be considered prior to radiation or chemotherapy. However, there are a number of disadvantages of embryo cryopreservation, including:

- expense (the cost of fertility drugs, investigations, and technical services can run as high as $10,000 USD per cycle) [48]
- the risk of ovarian hyperstimulation syndrome, which is potentially life-threatening [49],
- the need for hormones that may be contraindicated in certain malignancies (e.g. breast cancer),
- delay in initiating definitive treatment with chemotherapy or radiation in order to facilitate the entire process of embryo cryopreservation.
- the fact that this method is impossible for young women who do not have a partner and are unwilling to use donor sperm.

While cryopreservation of sperm is well-documented and is the optimal method of preserving reproductive potential in men, cryopreservation of oocytes is not yet a universal option for young women. Oocytes are much more sensitive than sperm to the freeze-thaw process [50]. However, in the last five years there have been an increasing number of reports of successful pregnancies resulting from cryopreserved oocytes [51-55].

Cryopreservation of ovarian tissue has also become a very promising alternative [56-58]. Thawed ovarian tissue can then be grafted as a xenograft into another host, such as in an immunodeficient SCID mouse [59,60]. Successful grafts have occurred on the renal capsule of the SCID mouse, presumably because the rich blood supply of the capsule enhances the viability of the graft, rendering it less likely to be rejected [61]. However, xenotransplantation carries the unresolved ethical dilemma of animal-to-human tissue transfer, and the possibility of transfer of unknown infectious agents from animal to human.

More recently, ovarian tissue has been grafted back into the donor as an autotransplant. This graft can be heterotopic (remote location, i.e., subcutaneous tissue in the abdomen or forearm) [62-65] or orthotopic (original location, i.e., adnexal area). The concept of heterotopic transplant is appealing for patients who require radiotherapy to the pelvis, such as women with locally advanced cervical cancer. When ovarian tissue is grafted to an area (e.g., forearm) that is remote from the primary tumor site (e.g., pelvis), the establishment of blood supply to support the graft is less likely to be impaired in the area where there has been no exposure to radiotherapy. Orthotopic autotransplantation re-establishes native blood supply to the graft (i.e., ovarian vessels supply the ovarian tissue graft). There are several reports describing successful orthotopic reimplantation of cryopreserved ovarian tissue after cancer treatment, including a live birth after multiagent chemotherapy for Hodgkin's lymphoma [58,66-68]. The concept of orthotopic transplant is appealing because the ovarian tissue graft can potentially resume function as it did prior to being harvested before cancer treatment. The live birth that was reported after orthotopic transplantation of ovarian tissue had occurred by spontaneous conception without ovarian stimulation or in vitro fertilization (IVF) [67]. A heterotopic transplant would require oocyte retrieval with subsequent IVF or intracytoplasmic sperm injection (ICSI).

Many legal and ethical issues surrounding ovarian cryopreservation and transplantation need to be resolved. An unknown risk is the possibility of undetected microscopic tumor cells in cryopreserved ovarian tissue, and the subsequent reintroduction of tumor cells after transplantation of this tissue following completion of cancer treatment. It has been demonstrated that ovarian tissue with cancer cells have the capacity to transfer cancer to the graft recipient, resulting in death from disease [69]. Furthermore, as the technique of ovarian cryopreservation is refined and ovarian tissue banking becomes a reality, a decision will need to be made about the applicability of this technology. Will it be reserved for cancer patients alone, or will there be a role for cryopreservation in women who wish to delay their childbearing for reasons related to personal or career circumstances? Additional experience with autotransplantation of cryopreserved ovarian tissue is required before this technique can be introduced universally into clinical practice.

Conservative Management of Gynecologic Malignancies

The standard treatment for most gynecologic cancers involves surgery, which renders a woman infertile. Treatment of ovarian, endometrial, and early cervical cancer consists of some type of hysterectomy, with or without bilateral salpingo-oophorectomy. Women with locally advanced cervical cancer receive pelvic radiotherapy with weekly chemotherapy as primary treatment instead of surgery. All of these treatment regimens eliminate reproductive potential and may subject the women to long-term consequences of ovarian failure. Over the last few decades, there has been an evolution in the treatment of early-stage gynecologic malignancies, as well as advanced ovarian germ cell tumors.

Early Cervical Cancer: Trachelectomy

The standard treatment for women with early-stage cervical cancer (excluding microinvasive cancer) remains radical hysterectomy with pelvic lymphadenectomy or radical radiotherapy with concomitant platinum-based chemotherapy [70]. However, neither treatment is ideal for the young woman who wishes to preserve her fertility. Within the past decade, radical trachelectomy has been proposed as a fertility-sparing treatment for a select group of women with early-stage cervical cancer for whom a radical hysterectomy with pelvic lymphadenectomy would usually be recommended [71-77]. A radical trachelectomy is defined as removal of the cervix and surrounding parametria, without removal of the uterus or ovaries. The rationale for this procedure is based on prior knowledge of cervical cancer spread patterns. Cervical cancer tends to spread laterally into the parametria, inferiorly to the upper vagina, and very rarely spreads superiorly into the uterus [78]. Therefore, the cervix and surrounding parametria can be resected from the lower uterine segment (i.e., trachelectomy), leaving the rest of the uterus intact, without compromising survival. A summary of studies describing radical trachelectomy and pelvic lymphadenectomy is presented in Table 2. Pelvic lymphadenectomy is usually carried out first to confirm the absence of metastatic nodes. The radical trachelectomy can be completed vaginally or abdominally. After the cervix and parametria have been removed, a permanent cerclage is placed at the lower uterine segment to prevent subsequent early pregnancy loss. While cerclage placement does not necessarily result in the need for reproductive technologies to conceive, it does mandate Cesarean section for delivery.

Table 2. Outcomes after radical trachelectomy for early-stage cervical cancer

Author	# patients	Median follow-up (months)	Recurrences	# conceptions / # attempting to conceive (# live births)
Shepherd [77]	30	NR	0	8/13 (9)
Dargent [75]	47	52	2	13/16 (10)
Roy and Plante [73]	30	25	1	6/6 (4)
Covens [74]	32	29	1	4/13 (3)
Rodriguez [76]	3	NR	0	1/3 (1)
Burnett [108]	21	31.5	0	3/3 (1)
Schlaerth [109]	12	47.6 (mean)	0	4/2 (2)
Ungar [110]	30	47	0	3/5 (2)

NR = Not Reported

Overall, survival after trachelectomy appears comparable to that after standard radical hysterectomy [73-75,77]. While the benefits of trachelectomy are obvious—less blood loss, reduced hospital stay, and uterine preservation, there are potential complications that may arise, including posteroperative infection leading to tubo-ovarian abscess, or cervical stenosis, both of which can lead to subsequent infertility [79,80]. Only a very specific group of women with early cervical cancers are considered eligible for this procedure. A tumor width of 2 cm has been suggested as a threshold size for eligibility [74,75,77]. The presence of lymphovascular space invasion or the diagnosis of adenocarcinoma is not necessarily a contraindication to this procedure [74]. However, patients who undergo this procedure still need to be followed very carefully. There have been reports of central pelvic and ovarian recurrences with a Stage IB1 cervical adenocarcinoma following radical trachelectomy [81,82].

A cone biopsy with pelvic lymphadenectomy may seem like another reasonable alternative to radical surgery or radiotherapy for early invasive cervical cancer. However, in one reported series there was discontinuous spread of tumor in three of four cases of extracervical disease [75]. Simple conization may miss tumor emboli in the parametria or lateral portion of the cervix and thus does not appear to be an appropriate treatment for cervical cancer except for microinvasive carcinoma [83].

Endometrial Cancer: Progestin Therapy

The conventional treatment for endometrial cancer is total hysterectomy and bilateral salpingo-oophorectomy. Endometrial cancer is uncommon in premenopausal women, and therefore preservation of fertility is generally not an important issue. However, young women with obesity, non-insulin dependent diabetes, and polycystic ovaries are at increased risk for endometrial cancer because of chronic anovulation and prolonged exposure to endogenous estrogens unopposed by progesterone [84-88], and many of these women still wish to preserve their fertility.

The use of progestins as an alternative fertility-sparing method to treat endometrial cancer has been described in several series (Table 3). Most reports describe the use of high dose oral medroxyprogesterone acetate. One report describes a complete response using the progesterone-containing intrauterine device [89]. The majority of subjects in these studies had Grade 1 endometrioid carcinoma. There are only two case reports describing progestin treatment of Grade 2 endometrial carcinoma [90,91]. Those with evidence of myometrial invasion or a concomitant ovarian cancer are less likely to respond to progestin therapy [92-94].

There is no consensus on the ideal progestational agent or dose to use for young women with endometrial cancer who wish to preserve their fertility. After a woman has responded to progestin therapy, it has been suggested that she continue to use low-dose progestins or oral contraceptives to prevent cancer recurrence until she is ready to attempt conception [95]. Surveillance every three months with dilatation and curettage or endometrial biopsy is recommended [96,97], with emphasis on the need for prompt, definitive surgical management with any evidence of recurrent cancer, and complete hysterectomy and bilateral salpingo-oophorectomy after childbearing has been completed.

Table 3. Fertility-sparing treatment of endometrial cancer

Author	# patients	*Treatment*	Response rate	Recurrence rate among initial responders	Median follow-up (months)	# conceptions / # attempting to conceive (# live births)
Bokhman [91]	19	17α HPC, 500 mg x 3 months	15/19 (79%)	NR	NR	NR
Kim [96]	21	Various regimens, including MA 160 mg/d x 3 months	13/21 (62%)	3/13	NR	3/13 (6)
Randall & Kurman [97]	12	MA 40-160 mg/d x 2-18 months	9/12 (75%)	0/9	40	3/10 (5)
Sardi [111]	4	MPA 200-500 mg/d x 3-9 months	3/4 (75%)	0	35.7	2/4 (3)
Duska [112]	12	NR	10/12 (83%)	NR	54	4/10 (5)
Gottlieb [113]	13	MA 160 mg/d, MPA 200-600 mg/d, HPC 2-3 g/week, NA 5 mg/d	13/13 (100%)	6/13 (median 40 months)	82	5/3 (9)
Jobo [114]	2	MPA 600 mg/d x 22-29 weeks	2	0/2	31, 60	2/2 (2)
Pinto [115]	1	MA 160 /d x 3 months	1	0	NR	1/1 (1)
Vinker [116]	1	MPA 400 mg/d x 10 weeks	0 (TAH BSO, staging)	0 (persistence at surgery, required adjuvant RT)	48	0
Kaku [117]	12	MPA 200-800 mg/d, 2-14 months	9	2	24	2/2 (1)
Imai [118]	15	MPA (median 29 weeks)	8	3/8	59	2/2 (3)
Wang [119]	9	MA 160 mg/d +/- Tamoxifen 30 mg/d	8	2	69	3/2 (3, incl. twins)
Ogawa [120]	1	MPA 400 mg/d x 12 weeks	1	NR	NR	1/1 (1)
Mitsushita [121]	1	MPA 400 mg/d x 4 months, then 600 mg/d x 8 months	0	1 (persistence at 6 month hysterectomy)	NR	1/1 (1)
Montz [89]	12	Progestin-IUD	6/8 at 1 year	0	12	NR
Niwa [92]	12	MPA 400-600 mg/d x 6-10 months	12/12 within 10 months	8/9 by 30 months	30	7/10 (5)
Yang [93]	6	MPA	4/6	2/4	48.8	(2)
Ota [94]	12	MPA 600 mg/d	4/12	8/12	NR	(2)

NR = Not Reported

MA = Megestrol acetate

MPA = Medroxyprogesterone acetate

HPC = Hydroxyprogesterone caproate

NA = Norethisterone acetate

RT = radiotherapy

Ovarian Cancer: Conservative Surgery

Malignant ovarian germ cell tumors characteristically arise in children and adolescents. Conservative surgery is now the accepted standard of treatment; this includes a unilateral salpingo-oophorectomy and staging procedure [32-35,38]. The uterus and contralateral ovary remain intact. Conservative surgery is acceptable for malignant germ cell tumors for several reasons. First, germ cell tumors almost always present as a unilateral adnexal mass, the only exception being dysgerminoma with a bilaterality rate of up to 15% [98]. Second, recurrences of malignant germ cell tumors rarely develop in the uterus or contralateral ovary [38], therefore removing these at initial surgery do not have any impact on the risk of recurrent disease. Finally, malignant germ cell tumors are curable with multiagent chemotherapy, even in the setting of metastatic disease [38,99,100]. For all these reasons, conservative surgery is feasible in malignant germ cell tumors without risk of compromise in survival.

Table 4. Fertility-sparing surgery for epithelial ovarian cancer

Author	# patients	# patients receiving adjuvant therapy	Recurrences	Median time to recurrence (months)	Median follow-up (months)	# conceptions / # attempting to conceive (# live births)
Zanetta [122]	56	3 (platinum x 6)	5/56 (9%)	12	84	20/NR (17)
Colombo [123]	56	16 (platinum)	3/56 (5%)	13	75	17/17 (16)
Duska [124]	5	NR	0	-	NR	2/5 (2)
Raspagliesi [105]	10	1 (radiation); 7(chemotherapy)	0	-	70	3/5 (2)
Schilder [125]	52 (Stage IA: 42, IC: 10)	Stage IA: 11 (PT, PC, M), IC: 8 (PT, PC, M)	5 (Stage IA: 4, IC: 1)	13	68	32/17 (26)
Morice [126]	25 (Stage IA: 19, IC: 1, Stage II: 2, unstaged: 3	Stage IA: 1, IB: 4, chemotherapy and EBR in 1	7 (5 on remaining ovary)	15	47	4/4 (3)

NR = Not Reported
EBR = External beam radiotherapy
PT = Platinum and Taxol (paclitaxel)
PC = Platinum and cyclophosphamide
M = Melphalan

Epithelial ovarian cancer is rare in the reproductive age group. Most women with epithelial ovarian cancer present with advanced stage disease for which the standard surgery consists of hysterectomy, bilateral salpingo-oophorectomy, and debulking of tumor. For young women who present with early stage disease that appears to be confined to one ovary, conservative surgery has been offered, which usually consists of unilateral salpingo-oophorectomy and staging (omentectomy, peritoneal biopsies, pelvic and para-aortic node dissection). Far more common in the reproductive age group is the diagnosis of borderline epithelial tumors. However, many of these women can be managed successfully with conservative surgery, even in the presence of non-invasive implants beyond the ovary [101-103]. Conservative surgery for these women may consist of ovarian cystectomy instead of oophorectomy, although it is recognized that the involvement of tumor along the resection margin as well as the presence of more than one borderline cyst are risk factors for recurrent borderline tumor [104].

The outcomes of conservative surgery for early-stage ovarian cancer are summarized in Table 4. These studies suggest that in a highly select group of young patients with early-stage ovarian cancer, conservative surgery may be considered [105]. Ovarian cancer during pregnancy has been reported [106,107], including surgery and chemotherapy before delivery. Outcomes of these cases appear to be similar to those of non-pregnant women.

Where do we Go from Here?

Our current understanding of the reproductive sequelae of radiation and chemotherapy has enabled us to tailor cancer treatment to optimize fertility and hormonal preservation without compromising survival. Treatment of Hodgkin's disease has evolved such that contemporary multiagent chemotherapy regimens using cell-cycle specific drugs are far less likely to result in permanent infertility compared to historical regimens. Some strategies are theoretically appealing but much less promising, such as ovarian transposition prior to radiotherapy or suppressing ovarian function during chemotherapy with oral contraceptives. However, we have come a long way in the treatment of gynecologic malignancies. In selected women with early-stage cancers, we can offer fertility-sparing surgery without compromising survival. There is exciting research on ovarian cryopreservation and transplantation, which may allow many more women to preserve their fertility despite cancer treatment. However, there are many unresolved ethical issues surrounding the use of innovative technologies. We need to keep raising questions about the safety of all fertility-sparing treatment strategies. It is most important to keep scrutinizing and evaluating outcomes while challenging existing dogma and practices so that we "first, do no harm" as we proceed through this evolution in cancer care.

References

[1] Edwards, BK; Howe, HL; Ries, LA; Thun, MJ; Rosenberg, HM; Yancik, R; Wingo, PA; Jemal, A; Feigal EG. Annual report to the nation on the status of cancer, 1973-1999, featuring implications of age and aging on U.S. cancer burden. *Cancer*, 2002 May 15 94(10), 2766-92.

[2] Rowley, MJ; Leach, DR; Warner, GA; Heller, CG. Effect of graded doses of ionizing radiation on the human testis. *Radiat Res*, 1974 Sep 59(3), 665-78.

[3] Kaplan, II. The treatment of female sterility with X-ray therapy directed to the pituitary and ovaries. *American Journal of Obstetrics and Gynecology*, 1958 76, 447-53.

[4] Dickson, RJ. The late results of radium treatment for benign uterine haemorrhage. *British Journal of Radiology*, 1969 42, 582-94.

[5] Ash, P. The influence of radiation on fertility in man. *Br.J.Radiol*, 1980 Apr 53(628), 271-8.

[6] Schuck, A; Hamelmann, V; Bramswig, JH; Konemann, S; Rube, C; Hesselmann, S; Riesenbeck, D; Horst, E; Bolling, T; Paulussen, M; et al. Ovarian function following pelvic irradiation in prepubertal and pubertal girls and young adult women. *Strahlenther Onkol*, 2005 Aug 181(8), 534-9.

[7] Morice, P; Castaigne, D; Haie-Meder, C; Pautier, P; El Hassan, J; Duvillard, P; Gerbaulet, A; Michel, G. Laparoscopic ovarian transposition for pelvic malignancies: indications and functional outcomes. *Fertil Steril*, 1998 Nov 70(5), 956-60.

[8] Classe, JM; Mahe, M; Moreau, P; Rapp, MJ; Maisonneuve, H; Lemevel, A; Bourdin, S; Harousseau, JL; Cuilliere, JC. Ovarian transposition by laparoscopy before radiotherapy in the treatment of Hodgkin's disease. *Cancer*, 1998 Oct 1 83(7), 1420-4.

[9] Clough, KB; Goffinet, F; Labib, A; Renolleau, C; Campana, F; de la, RA; Durand, JC. Laparoscopic unilateral ovarian transposition prior to irradiation: prospective study of 20 cases. *Cancer*, 1996 Jun 15 77(12), 2638-45.

[10] Tulandi, T; Al Took, S. Laparoscopic ovarian suspension before irradiation. *Fertil Steril*, 1998 Aug 70(2), 381-3.

[11] Howard, FM. Laparoscopic lateral ovarian transposition before radiation treatment of Hodgkin disease. *J Am AssocGynecol Laparosc*, 1997 Nov 4(5), 601-4.

[12] Treissman, MJ; Miller, D; McComb, PF. Laparoscopic lateral ovarian transposition. *Fertil Steril*, 1996 Jun 65(6), 1229-31.

[13] Covens, AL; van der Putten, HW; Fyles, AW; Leung, PM; O'Brien, PF; Murphy, KJ; DePetrillo, AD. Laparoscopic ovarian transposition. *Eur J Gynaecol Oncol*, 1996 17(3), 177-82.

[14] Williams, RS; Littell, RD; Mendenhall, NP. Laparoscopic oophoropexy and ovarian function in the treatment of Hodgkin disease. *Cancer*, 1999 Nov 15 86(10), 2138-42.

[15] Feeney, DD; Moore, DH; Look, KY; Stehman, FB; Sutton, GP. The fate of the ovaries after radical hysterectomy and ovarian transposition. *Gynecol Oncol*, 1995 Jan 56(1), 3-7.

[16] Buekers, TE; Anderson, B; Sorosky, JI; Buller, RE. Ovarian function after surgical treatment for cervical cancer. *Gynecol Oncol*, 2001 Jan 80(1), 85-8.

[17] Anderson, B; LaPolla, J; Turner, D; Chapman, G; Buller, R. Ovarian transposition in cervical cancer. *Gynecol Oncol*, 1993 May 49(2), 206-14.

[18] Chambers, SK; Chambers, JT; Kier, R; Peschel, RE. Sequelae of lateral ovarian transposition in irradiated cervical cancer patients. *Int J Radiat Oncol Biol Phys*, 1991 Jun 20(6), 1305-8.

[19] Van Eijkeren, MA; Van DW I; El Sharouni, SY; Heintz, AP. Benefits and side effects of lateral ovarian transposition (LOT) performed during radical hysterectomy and pelvic lymphadenectomy for early stage cervical cancer. *Int J Gynecol Cancer*, 1999 Sep 9(5), 396-400.

[20] Ishii, K; Aoki, Y; Takakuwa, K; Tanaka, K. Ovarian function after radical hysterectomy with ovarian preservation for cervical cancer. *J Reprod Med*, 2001 Apr 46(4), 347-52.

[21] Siddle, N; Sarrel, P; Whitehead, M. The effect of hysterectomy on the age at ovarian failure: identification of a subgroup of women with premature loss of ovarian function and literature review. *Fertil Steril*, 1987 Jan 47(1), 94-100.

[22] Critchley, HO. Factors of importance for implantation and problems after treatment for childhood cancer. *Med Pediatr Oncol*, 1999 Jul 33(1), 9-14.

[23] Miller, JJ III; Williams, GF; Leissring, JC. Multiple late complications of therapy with cyclophosphamide, including ovarian destruction. *Am J Med* 1971 Apr 50(4), 530-5.

[24] Rose, DP; Davis, TE. Ovarian function in patients receiving adjuvant chemotherapy for breast cancer. *Lancet,* 1977 Jun 4 1(8023), 1174-6.

[25] Young, RC; Markman, M. Chemotherapy. In: Berek, JS; Hacker, NF; editors. *Practical Gynecologic Oncology. 3 ed.* Lippincott Williams & Williams; 2000, 83-117.

[26] Hartman, AR; Fleming, GF; Dillon, JJ. Meta-analysis of adjuvant cyclophosphamide/methotrexate/5-fluorouracil chemotherapy in postmenopausal women with estrogen receptor-positive, node-positive breast cancer. *ClinBreast Cancer*, 2001 Jul 2(2), 138-43.

[27] Reichman, BS; Green, KB. Breast cancer in young women: effect of chemotherapy on ovarian function, fertility, and birth defects. *J Natl Cancer Inst, Monogr* 1994 16, 125-9.

[28] Reyno, LM; Levine, MN; Skingley, P; Arnold, A; Abu, ZH. Chemotherapy induced amenorrhoea in a randomised trial of adjuvant chemotherapy duration in breast cancer. *Eur J Cancer*, 1992 29A(1), 21-3.

[29] Teinturier, C; Hartmann, O; Valteau-Couanet, D; Benhamou, E; Bougneres, PF. Ovarian function after autologous bone marrow transplantation in childhood: high-dose busulfan is a major cause of ovarian failure. *Bone Marrow Transplant*, 1998 Nov 22(10), 989-94.

[30] Berkowitz, RS; Goldstein, DP. Gestational trophoblastic disease. *Cancer*, 1995 Nov 15, 76(10 Suppl), 2079-85.

[31] Newlands, ES; Paradinas, FJ; Fisher, RA. Recent advances in gestational trophoblastic disease. *Hematol Oncol ClinNorth Am*, 1999 Feb 13(1), 225-44.

[32] Zanetta, G; Bonazzi, C; Cantu, M; Binidagger, S; Locatelli, A; Bratina G; Mangioni, C. Survival and reproductive function after treatment of malignant germ cell ovarian tumors. *J Clin Oncol*, 2001 Feb 15 19(4), 1015-20.

[33] Perrin, LC; Low, J; Nicklin, JL; Ward, BG; Crandon, AJ. Fertility and ovarian function after conservative surgery for germ cell tumours of the ovary. *Aust N Z J Obstet Gynaecol*, 1999 May 39(2), 243-5.

[34] Low, JJ; Perrin, LC; Crandon, AJ; Hacker, NF. Conservative surgery to preserve ovarian function in patients with malignant ovarian germ cell tumors. A review of 74 cases. *Cancer*, 2000 Jul 15 89(2), 391-8.

[35] Kanazawa, K; Suzuki, T; Sakumoto, K. Treatment of malignant ovarian germ cell tumors with preservation of fertility: reproductive performance after persistent remission. *Am J Clin Oncol*, 2000 Jun 23(3), 244-8.

[36] Brewer, M; Gershenson, DM; Herzog, CE; Mitchell, MF; Silva, EG; Wharton, JT. Outcome and reproductive function after chemotherapy for ovarian dysgerminoma. *J Clin Oncol*, 1999 Sep 17(9), 2670-5.

[37] Adewole, LF; Rustin, GJ; Newlands, ES; Dent, J; Bagshawe, KD. Fertility in patients with gestational trophoblastic tumors treated with etoposide. *Eur J Cancer, ClinOncol*, 1986 Dec 22(12), 1479-82.

[38] Ezzat, A; Raja, M; Bakri, Y; Subhi, J; Memon, M; Schwartz, P; Stuart, R. Malignant ovarian germ cell tumours -- a survival and prognostic analysis. *Acta Oncol*, 1999 38(4), 455-60.

[39] Chapman, RM; Sutcliffe, SB. Protection of ovarian function by oral contraceptives in women receiving chemotherapy for Hodgkin's disease. *Blood*, 1981 Oct 58(4), 849-51.

[40] Whitehead, E; Shalet, SM; Blackledge, G; Todd, I; Crowther, D; Beardwell, CG. The effect of combination chemotherapy on ovarian function in women treated for Hodgkin's disease. *Cancer*, 1983 Sep 15 52(6), 988-93.

[41] Longhi, A; Pignotti, E; Versari, M; Asta, S; Bacci, G. Effect of oral contraceptive on ovarian function in young females undergoing neoadjuvant chemotherapy treatment for osteosarcoma. *Oncol Rep*, 2003 Jan 10(1), 151-5.

[42] Blumenfeld, Z. Ovarian rescue/protection from chemotherapeutic agents. *J Soc Gynecol Investig*, 2001 Jan 8(1 Suppl Proceedings), S60-S64.

[43] Pereyra, PB; Mendez Ribas, JM; Milone, G; Fernandez, I; Kvicala, R; Mila, T; Di Noto, A; Contreras, OO; Pavlovsky, S. Use of GnRH analogs for functional protection of the ovary and preservation of fertility during cancer treatment in adolescents: a preliminary report, *Gynecol Oncol* 2001, Jun 81(3), 391-7.

[44] Franke, HR; Smit, WM; Vermes, I. Gonadal protection by a gonadotropin-releasing hormone agonist depot in young women with Hodgkin's disease undergoing chemotherapy. *Gynecol Endocrinol*, 2005 May 20(5), 274-8.

[45] Del, ML; Catzeddu, T; Boni, L; Bell, C; Sertoli, MR; Bighin, C; Clavarezza, M; Testa, D; Venturini, M. Prevention of chemotherapy-induced menopause by temporary ovarian suppression with goserelin in young, early breast cancer patients. *Ann Oncol*, 2006 Jan 17(1), 74-8.

[46] Palter, SF; Olive, DL. Reproductive Physiology. In: Berek, JS; Adashi, EY; Hillard, PA; editors. *Novak's Gynecology. 12 ed.* Baltimore: Williams & Wilkins, 1996, 149-72.

[47] Ataya, K; Moghissi, K. Chemotherapy-induced premature ovarian failure: mechanisms and prevention. *Steroids*, 1989 Dec 54(6), 607-26.

[48] Collins, J. An international survey of the health economics of IVF and ICSI. *Hum Reprod Update*, 2002 May 8(3), 265-77.

[49] McElhinney, B; McClure, N. Ovarian hyperstimulation syndrome. *Baillieres Best Pract Res Clin Obstet Gynaecol*, 2000 Feb 14(1), 103-22.

[50] Oktay, K; Newton, H; Gosden, RG. Transplantation of cryopreserved human ovarian tissue results in follicle growth initiation in SCID mice. *Fertil Steril*, 2000 Mar 73(3), 599-603.

[51] Quintans, CJ; Donaldson, MJ; Bertolino, MV; Pasqualini, RS. Birth of two babies using oocytes that were cryopreserved in a choline-based freezing medium. *Hum Reprod*, 2002 Dec 17(12), 3149-52.

[52] Chen, SU; Lien, YR; Chen, HF; Chang, LJ; Tsai, YY; Yang, YS. Observational clinical follow-up of oocyte cryopreservation using a slow-freezing method with 1,2-propanediol plus sucrose followed by ICSI. *Hum Reprod*, 2005 Jul 20(7), 1975-80.

[53] Borini, A; Bonu, MA; Coticchio, G; Bianchi, V; Cattoli, M; Flamigni, C. Pregnancies and births after oocyte cryopreservation. *Fertil Steril*, 2004 Sep 82(3), 601-5.

[54] Fosas, N; Marina, F; Torres, PJ; Jove, I; Martin, P; Perez, N; Arnedo, N; Marina, S. The births of five Spanish babies from cryopreserved donated oocytes. *Hum Reprod*; 2003 Jul 18(7), 1417-21.

[55] Boldt, J; Cline, D; McLaughlin, D. Human oocyte cryopreservation as an adjunct to IVF-embryo transfer cycles. *Hum Reprod*, 2003 Jun 18(6), 1250-5.

[56] Oktay, K; Nugent, D; Newton, H; Salha, O; Chatterjee, P; Gosden, RG. Isolation and characterization of primordial follicles from fresh and cryopreserved human ovarian tissue. *Fertil Steril*, 1997 Mar 67(3), 481-6.

[57] Oktay, K; Newton, H; Aubard, Y; Salha, O; Gosden, RG. Cryopreservation of immature human oocytes and ovarian tissue: an emerging technology? *Fertil Steril*, 1998 Jan 69(1), 1-7.

[58] Radford, JA; Lieberman, BA; Brison, DR; Smith, AR; Critchlow, JD; Russell, SA; Watson, AJ; Clayton, JA; Harris, M; Gosden, RG; et al. Orthotopic reimplantation of cryopreserved ovarian cortical strips after high-dose chemotherapy for Hodgkin's lymphoma. *Lancet*, 2001 Apr 14, 357(9263), 1172-5.

[59] Oktay, K; Newton, H; Mullan, J; Gosden, RG. Development of human primordial follicles to antral stages in SCID/hpg mice stimulated with follicle stimulating hormone. *Hum Reprod*, 1998 May 13(5), 1133-8.

[60] Weissman, A; Gotlieb, L; Colgan, T; Jurisicova, A; Greenblatt, EM; Casper, RF. Preliminary experience with subcutaneous human ovarian cortex transplantation in the NOD-SCID mouse. *Biol Reprod*; 1999 Jun 60(6), 1462-7.

[61] Gook, DA; McCully, BA; Edgar, DH; McBain, JC. Development of antral follicles in human cryopreserved ovarian tissue following xenografting. *Hum Reprod*; 2001 Mar 16(3), 417-22.

[62] Wolner-Hanssen, P; Hagglund, L; Ploman, F; Ramirez, A; Manthorpe, R; Thuring, A. Autotransplantation of cryopreserved ovarian tissue to the right forearm 4(1/2) years after autologous stem cell transplantation. *Acta Obstet Gynecol Scand*, 2005 Jul, 84(7), 695-8.

[63] Hilders, CG; Baranski, AG; Peters, L; Ramkhelawan, A; Trimbos, JB. Successful human ovarian autotransplantation to the upper arm. *Cancer*, 2004 Dec 15 101(12), 2771-8.

[64] Oktay, K; Buyuk, E; Veeck, L; Zaninovic, N; Xu, K; Takeuchi, T; Opsahl, M; Rosenwaks, Z. Embryo development after heterotopic transplantation of cryopreserved ovarian tissue. *Lancet*, 2004 Mar 13 363(9412), 837-40.

[65] Oktay, K; Economos, K; Kan, M; Rucinski, J; Veeck, L; Rosenwaks, Z. Endocrine function and oocyte retrieval after autologous transplantation of ovarian cortical strips to the forearm. *JAMA*, 2001 Sep 26 286(12), 1490-3.

[66] Schmidt, KL; Andersen, CY; Loft, A; Byskov, AG; Ernst, E; Andersen, AN. Follow-up of ovarian function post-chemotherapy following ovarian cryopreservation and transplantation. *Hum Reprod*, 2005 Dec 20(12), 3539-46.
[67] Donnez, J; Dolmans, MM; Demylle, D; Jadoul, P; Pirard, C; Squifflet, J; Martinez-Madrid, B; van, LA. Livebirth after orthotopic transplantation of cryopreserved ovarian tissue. *Lancet,* 2004 Oct 16 364(9443), 1405-10.
[68] Donnez, J; Squifflet, J; Dolmans, MM; Martinez-Madrid, B; Jadoul. P; van, LA. Orthotopic transplantation of fresh ovarian cortex: a report of two cases. *Fertil Steril*, 2005 Oct 84(4), 1018.
[69] Shaw, JM; Bowles, J; Koopman, P; Wood, EC; Trounson, AO. Fresh and cryopreserved ovarian tissue samples from donors with lymphoma transmit the cancer to graft recipients. *Hum Reprod*, 1996 Aug 11(8), 1668-73.
[70] Hacker, NF. Cervical Cancer. In: Berek, JS; Hacker, NF editors. *Practical Gynecologic Oncology. 3 ed.* Philadelphia: Lippincott Williams & Wilkins; 2000, 345-405.
[71] Smith, JR; Boyle, DC; Corless, DJ; Ungar, L; Lawson, AD; Del Priore, G; McCall, JM; Lindsay, I; Bridges, JE. Abdominal radical trachelectomy: a new surgical technique for the conservative management of cervical carcinoma. *Br J Obstet Gynaecol*, 1997 Oct 104(10), 1196-200.
[72] Shepherd, JH; Crawford, RA; Oram, DH. Radical trachelectomy: a way to preserve fertility in the treatment of early cervical cancer. *Br J Obstet Gynaecol*, 1998 Aug 105(8), 912-6.
[73] Roy, M; Plante, M. Pregnancies after radical vaginal trachelectomy for early-stage cervical cancer. *Am J Obstet Gynecol*, 1998 Dec 179(6 Pt 1), 1491-6.
[74] Covens, A; Shaw, P; Murphy, J; DePetrillo, D; Lickrish, G; Laframboise, S; Rosen, B. Is radical trachelectomy a safe alternative to radical hysterectomy for patients with stage IA-B carcinoma of the cervix? *Cancer*, 1999 Dec 1 86(11), 2273-9.
[75] Dargent, D; Martin, X; Sacchetoni, A; Mathevet, P. Laparoscopic vaginal radical trachelectomy: a treatment to preserve the fertility of cervical carcinoma patients. *Cancer*, 2000 Apr 15 88(8), 1877-82.
[76] Rodriguez, M; Guimares, O; Rose, PG. Radical abdominal trachelectomy and pelvic lymphadenectomy with uterine conservation and subsequent pregnancy in the treatment of early invasive cervical cancer. *Am J Obstet Gynecol*, 2001 Aug 185(2), 370-4.
[77] Shepherd, JH; Mould, T; Oram, DH. Radical trachelectomy in early stage carcinoma of the cervix: outcome as judged by recurrence and fertility rates. *BJOG*, 2001 Aug 108(8), 882-5.
[78] Burghardt, E; Pickel, H. Local spread and lymph node involvement in cervical cancer. *Obstet Gynecol*, 1978 Aug 52(2), 138-45.
[79] Plante, M; Renaud, MC; Francois, H; Roy, M. Vaginal radical trachelectomy: an oncologically safe fertility-preserving surgery. An updated series of 72 cases and review of the literature. *Gynecol Oncol*, 2004 Sep 94(3), 614-23.
[80] Del, PG; Ungar, L; Smith, JR. Complications after fertility-preserving radical trachelectomy. *Fertil Steril*, 2006 Jan 85(1), 227.

[81] Morice, P; Dargent, D; Haie-Meder, C; Duvillard, P; Castaigne, D. First case of a centropelvic recurrence after radical trachelectomy: literature review and implications for the preoperative selection of patients. *Gynecol Oncol*, 2004 Mar 92(3), 1002-5.

[82] Piketty, M; Barranger, E; Najat, M; Francois, P; Darai, E. Ovarian recurrence after radical trachelectomy for adenocarcinoma of the cervix. *Am J Obstet Gynecol*; 2005 Oct 193(4), 1382-3.

[83] Morris, M; Mitchell, MF; Silva, EG; Copeland, LJ; Gershenson, DM. Cervical conization as definitive therapy for early invasive squamous carcinoma of the cervix. *Gynecol.Oncol*, 1993 Nov 51(2), 193-6.

[84] Gallup, DG; Stock, RJ. Adenocarcinoma of the endometrium in women 40 years of age or younger. *Obstet Gynecol*, 1984 Sep 64(3), 417-20.

[85] Dahlgren, E; Friberg, LG; Johansson, S; Lindstrom, B; Oden, A; Samsioe, G; Janson, PO. Endometrial carcinoma; ovarian dysfunction--a risk factor in young women. Eur J *Obstet Gynecol Reprod Biol*, 1991 Sep 13 41(2), 143-50.

[86] Dennefors, BL; Knutson, F; Janson, PO; Jansson, I; Hamberger, L. Ovarian steroid production in a woman with polycystic ovary syndrome associated with endometrial cancer. *Acta Obstet Gynecol Scand*, 1985 64(5), 387-92.

[87] Jafari, K; Javaheri, G; Ruiz, G. Endometrial adenocarcinoma and the Stein-Leventhal syndrome. *Obstet Gynecol*; 1978 Jan 51(1), 97-100.

[88] McDonald, TW; Malkasian, GD; Gaffey, TA. Endometrial cancer associated with feminizing ovarian tumor and polycystic ovarian disease. *Obstet Gynecol*; 1977 Jun 49(6), 654-8.

[89] Montz, FJ; Bristow, RE; Bovicelli, A; Tomacruz, R; Kurman, RJ. Intrauterine progesterone treatment of early endometrial cancer. *Am J Obstet Gynecol*, 2002 Apr 186(4), 651-7.

[90] Zuckerman, B; Lavie, O; Neuman, M; Rabinowitz, R; Ben-Chetrit, A; Voss, E. Endometrial carcinoma Stage I-Grade II. Conservative treatment followed by healthy twin pregnancy. *Int J Gynecol, Cancer*, 1998 8 172-4.

[91] Bokhman, JV; Chepick, OF; Volkova, AT; Vishnevsky, AS. Can primary endometrial carcinoma stage I be cured without surgery and radiation therapy? *Gynecol Oncol*, 1985 Feb 20(2), 139-55.

[92] Niwa, K; Tagami, K; Lian, Z; Onogi, K; Mori, H; Tamaya, T. Outcome of fertility-preserving treatment in young women with endometrial carcinomas. *BJOG*, 2005 Mar 112(3), 317-20.

[93] Yang, YC; Wu, CC; Chen, CP; Chang, CL; Wang, KL. Reevaluating the safety of fertility-sparing hormonal therapy for early endometrial cancer. *Gynecol Oncol*, 2005 Nov 99(2), 287-93.

[94] Ota, T; Yoshida, M; Kimura, M; Kinoshita, K. Clinicopathologic study of uterine endometrial carcinoma in young women aged 40 years and younger. *Int J Gynecol Cancer*. 2005 Jul 15(4), 657-62.

[95] Renaud, MC; Plante, M. Medical treatment of endometrial carcinoma for the premenopausal woman wanting to preserve her ability to have children. *Journal of the Society of Obstetricians and Gynaecologists of Canada*, 2001 23(3), 213-9.

[96] Kim, YB; Holschneider, CH; Ghosh, K; Nieberg, RK; Montz, FJ. Progestin alone as primary treatment of endometrial carcinoma in premenopausal women. Report of seven cases and review of the literature. *Cancer*, 1997 Jan 15 79(2), 320-7.

[97] Randall, TC; Kurman, RJ. Progestin treatment of atypical hyperplasia and well-differentiated carcinoma of the endometrium in women under age 40. *Obstet.Gynecol*, 1997 Sep 90(3), 434-40.

[98] Kurman, RJ; Norris, HJ. Malignant germ cell tumors of the ovary. *Hum Pathol*, 1977 Sep 8(5), 551-64.

[99] Gershenson, DM; Morris, M; Cangir, A; Kavanagh, JJ; Stringer, CA; Edwards, CL; Silva, EG; Wharton, JT. Treatment of malignant germ cell tumors of the ovary with bleomycin, etoposide, and cisplatin. *J Clin Oncol*, 1990 Apr 8(4), 715-20.

[100] Tangir, J; Zelterman, D; Ma, W; Schwartz, PE. Reproductive function after conservative surgery and chemotherapy for malignant germ cell tumors of the ovary. *Obstet Gynecol*, 2003 Feb 101(2), 251-7.

[101] Boran, N; Cil, AP; Tulunay, G; Ozturkoglu, E; Koc, S; Bulbul, D; Kose, MF. Fertility and recurrence results of conservative surgery for borderline ovarian tumors. *Gynecol Oncol*, 2005 Jun 97(3), 845-51.

[102] Chan, JK; Lin, YG; Loizzi, V; Ghobriel, M; DiSaia, PJ; Berman, ML. Borderline ovarian tumors in reproductive-age women. Fertility-sparing surgery and outcome. *J Reprod Med*, 2003 Oct 48(10), 756-60.

[103] Donnez, J; Munschke, A; Berliere, M; Pirard, C; Jadoul, P; Smets, M; Squifflet, J. Safety of conservative management and fertility outcome in women with borderline tumors of the ovary. *Fertil Steril*, 2003 May 79(5), 1216-21.

[104] Lim-Tan, SK; Cajigas, HE; Scully, RE. Ovarian cystectomy for serous borderline tumors: a follow-up study of 35 cases. *Obstet Gynecol*, 1988 Nov 72(5), 775-81.

[105] Raspagliesi, F; Fontanelli, R; Paladini, D; di Re, EM. Conservative surgery in high-risk epithelial ovarian carcinoma. *J Am Coll Surg*, 1997 Nov 185(5), 457-60.

[106] Zhao, XY; Huang, HF; Lian, LJ; Lang, JH. Ovarian cancer in pregnancy: a clinicopathologic analysis of 22 cases and review of the literature. *Int J Gynecol Cancer*, 2006 Jan 16(1), 8-15.

[107] Ferrandina, G; Distefano, M; Testa, A; De, VR; Scambia, G. Management of an advanced ovarian cancer at 15 weeks of gestation: case report and literature review. *Gynecol Oncol*, 2005 May 97(2), 693-6.

[108] Burnett, AF; Roman, LD; O'Meara, AT; Morrow, CP. Radical vaginal trachelectomy and pelvic lymphadenectomy for preservation of fertility in early cervical carcinoma. *Gynecol.Oncol*, 2003 Mar 88(3), 419-23.

[109] Schlaerth, JB; Spirtos. NM; Schlaerth, AC. Radical trachelectomy and pelvic lymphadenectomy with uterine preservation in the treatment of cervical cancer. *Am J Obstet Gynecol*; 2003 Jan 188(1), 29-34.

[110] Ungar, L Palfalvi, L; Hogg, R; Siklos, P; Boyle, DC; Del, PG; Smith, JR. Abdominal radical trachelectomy: a fertility-preserving option for women with early cervical cancer. *BJOG*, 2005 Mar 112(3), 366-9.

[111] Sardi, J; Anchezar Henry, JP; Paniceres, G; Gomez, RN; Vighi, S. Primary hormonal treatment for early endometrial carcinoma. *Eur J Gynaecol Oncol*, 1998 19(6) 565-8.

[112] Duska, LR; Garrett, A; Rueda, BR; Haas, J; Chang, Y; Fuller, AF. Endometrial Cancer in Women 40 Years Old or Younger. *Gynecol Oncol* 2001 Nov 83(2), 388-93.

[113] Gotlieb, WH; Beiner, ME; Shalmon, B; Korach, Y; Segal, Y; Zmira, N; Koupolovic, J; Ben Baruch, G. Outcome of fertility-sparing treatment with progestins in young patients with endometrial cancer. *Obstet Gynecol*, 2003 Oct 102(4), 718-25.

[114] Jobo, T; Imai, M; Kawaguchi, M; Kenmochi, M; Kuramoto, H. Successful conservative treatment of endometrial carcinoma permitting subsequent pregnancy: report of two cases. *Eur J Gynaecol Oncol*, 2000 21(2), 119-22.

[115] Pinto, AB; Gopal, M; Herzog, TJ; Pfeifer, JD; Williams, DB. Successful in vitro fertilization pregnancy after conservative management of endometrial cancer. *Fertil Steril*, 2001 Oct 76(4), 826-9.

[116] Vinker, S; Shani, A; Open, M; Fenig, E; Dgani, R. Conservative treatment of adenocarcinoma of the endometrium in young patients. Is it appropriate? *Eur J Obstet Gynecol Reprod Biol*, 1999 Mar 83(1), 63-5.

[117] Kaku, T; Yoshikawa, H; Tsuda, H; Sakamoto, A; Fukunaga, M; Kuwabara, Y; Hataeg, M; Kodama, S; Kuzuya, K; Sato, S; et al. Conservative therapy for adenocarcinoma and atypical endometrial hyperplasia of the endometrium in young women: central pathologic review and treatment outcome. *Cancer Lett*, 2001 Jun 10 167(1), 39-48.

[118] Imai, M; Jobo, T; Sato, R; Kawaguchi, M; Kuramoto, H. Medroxyprogesterone acetate therapy for patients with adenocarcinoma of the endometrium who wish to preserve the uterus-usefulness and limitations. *Eur J Gynaecol Oncol*, 2001 22(3), 217-20.

[119] Wang, CB; Wang, CJ; Huang, HJ; Hsueh, S; Chou, HH; Soong, YK; Lai, CH. Fertility-preserving treatment in young patients with endometrial adenocarcinoma. *Cancer*, 2002 Apr 15 94(8), 2192-8.

[120] Ogawa, S; Koike, T; Shibahara, H; Ohwada, M; Suzuki, M; Araki, S; Sato, I. Assisted reproductive technologies in conjunction with conservatively treated endometrial adenocarcinoma. *A case report. Gynecol Obstet Invest*, 2001 51(3), 214-6.

[121] Mitsushita, J; Toki, T; Kato, K; Fujii, S; Konishi, I. Endometrial carcinoma remaining after term pregnancy following conservative treatment with medroxyprogesterone acetate. *Gynecol Oncol*, 2000 Oct 79(1), 129-32.

[122] Zanetta, G; Chiari, S; Rota, S; Bratina, G; Maneo, A; Torri, V; Mangioni, C. Conservative surgery for stage I ovarian carcinoma in women of childbearing age. *Br J Obstet Gynaecol*, 1997 Sep 104(9), 1030-5.

[123] Colombo, N; Chiari, S; Maggioni, A; Bocciolone, L; Torri, V; Mangioni, C. Controversial issues in the management of early epithelial ovarian cancer: conservative surgery and role of adjuvant therapy. *Gynecol Oncol*, 1994 Dec 55(3 Pt 2), S47-S51.

[124] Duska, LR; Chang, YC; Flynn, CE; Chen, AH; Goodman, A; Fuller, AF; Nikrui, N. Epithelial ovarian carcinoma in the reproductive age group. *Cancer*, 1999 Jun 15 85(12), 2623-9.

[125] Schilder, JM; Thompson, AM; DePriest, PD; Ueland, FR; Cibull, ML; Kryscio, RJ; Modesitt, SC; Lu, KH; Geisler, JP; Higgins, RV; et al. Outcome of reproductive age women with stage IA or IC invasive epithelial ovarian cancer treated with fertility-sparing therapy. *Gynecol, Oncol*, 2002 Oct 87(1), 1-7.

[126] Morice, P; Wicart-Poque, F; Rey, A; El Hassan, J; Pautier, P; Lhomme, C; de Crevosier, R; Haie-Meder, C; Duvillard, P; Castaigne, D. Results of conservative treatment in epithelial ovarian carcinoma. *Cancer*, 2001 Nov 1 92(9), 2412-8.

In: Women and Cancer
Editor: Laurie Elit, pp. 259-289

ISBN: 978-1-60021-494-3

Chapter II

MENOPAUSE AND CANCER

Jennifer M. Blake*
Department of Obstetrics and Gynecology, University of Toronto, Toronto, Canada.

ABSTRACT

Objectives: To address the many symptoms of menopause experienced by women as a result of treatment for their cancer.

Discussion: There is a relationship of premature ovarian failure with atherosclerosis and osteoporosis. Options for treating vasomotor symptoms may include environmental factors, physical activity, paced respiration, herbal and botanical, phytoestrogens, non-hormonal and hormonal therapy. Management of sleep disturbances will be reviewed. Risk factors for a depressed mood and management including conventional modalities and estrogen will be discussed. Vulvo-vaginal symptoms, joint pain and stiffness and sexuality concerns will be reviewed.

Conclusion: With increasing numbers of cancer patients living longer, quality of survivorship becomes an important issue. Menopausal symptoms are important for women and treatment options need to be made available.

INTRODUCTION

Menopause poses unique challenges for women with cancer, some may have experienced premature ovarian failure and an early menopause as a result of their cancer or its treatment, for others, with natural menopause, symptom relief that is available to other women, is not an option for them. The symptoms of menopause are not unique, and can be confused with cancer or it's treatment. This chapter will address these issues, to assist women with cancer through the menopausal transition.

* Correspondence concerning this article should be addressed to Jennifer Blake MD MSc FRCSC, Email: Jennifer.Blake@sunnybrook.ca.

Definitions

The accepted definition of menopause is 12 months of amenorrhea, in the absence of any attributable cause [1]. Many women with cancer experience ovarian failure before the age of 40, or experience an early menopause, occurring before the age of 45.

Premature Ovarian Failure

Premature ovarian failure (POF) is common amongst women of reproductive age treated for cancer. As diagnostic methods enable earlier diagnosis, and treatment permits longer survival, the number of women surviving with cancer is increasing. Estimates are that 62% of adult patients and 77% of children survive greater than 5 years post treatment [2]. Age is the most important individual risk factor; in older patients the onset of ovarian failure is more rapid, within 2-4 months, compared to 6- 16 months in younger patients, and it is much less likely to be reversible, it is permanent in 90% of women compared to approximately 50% of younger women [5]. In women with breast cancer treated, adjuvant chemotherapy with CMF (Cytoxan, Methotrexate and 5-fluorourqacil) is associated with menopause in 40% of those less than 40 years, and 70% of women over 40 years [3]. The incidence of menopause varied by type of disease and therapy. In women with lymphoma, the incidences of POF is as high as 90% of women two years post treatment for Non Hodgkin's Lymphoma and 50% in those with Hodgkin's Lymphoma [4].

Ionizing radiation can also induce menopause. With exposure to radiation, both the amount of radiation, and the age of the patient are critical. The LD 50 of the human oocyte has been estimated to be < 2 Gy [6]. The young ovary has a larger pool of oocytes, and is more tolerant of radiation; a predictive model has been developed for the immediate cessation of ovarian function from ovarian radiation. The effective sterilizing dose (ESD: dose of fractionated radiotherapy [Gy] at which premature ovarian failure occurs immediately after treatment in 97.5% of patients) has been calculated; ESD at birth is 20.3 Gy; at 10 years 18.4 Gy, at 20 years 16.5 Gy, and at 30 years 14.3 Gy. The time to ovarian failure after lesser doses of radiation has also been modeled. Young women exposed to radiation can expect an earlier cessation of ovarian function, and the same trend to increasing sensitivity with age is seen [7].

In gynecologic cancer, bilateral oopherectomy may be necessary, with surgical menopause an inevitable consequence. In women with simple hysterectomy, the age of menopause has been reported to be younger, occurring at a mean age of 49.5 years ($p<0.001$) [8] Women with hysterectomy and ovarian conservation report more severe menopausal symptoms than women with spontaneous menopause [9]. Women post-hysterectomy with ovarian conservation appear to be at higher risk of ovarian failure [10].

The ovarian histology in therapy induced ovarian failure has the same appearance as in natural menopause with depletion of primordial follicles. FSH levels are elevated, and estradiol levels low to low-normal. Unlike physiologic menopause, there is the potential with POF of spontaneous ovulation, many years after the onset of amenorrhea. The likelihood of spontaneous ovulation is greater in younger patients, but in all cases is unpredictable, and can occur even where ovarian biopsy indicates depletion of follicles [11,12].

Clinical Impact of Premature Ovarian Failure

Women undergoing an abrupt and premature menopausal transition experience increased severity of menopausal symptoms [13,14,15] and have specific health risks in consequence of early onset menopause. In young women experiencing surgical menopause there is the immediate issue of loss of fertility, with the added stress of severe menopausal symptoms and loss of libido.

Loss of fertility will have a profound impact on health and quality of life. It is more likely to have an adverse impact in women who have reproductive regret or in cultures that place a high value on fertility. Fertility options such as ovum donation or surrogacy may be helpful.

Bilateral oopherectomy results in an abrupt fall of estradiol to menopausal levels, without the gradual decline that characterizes natural menopause. Androgen levels in surgical oopherectomy are particularly low, only 37% of the levels in naturally menopausal women [16,17]. Testosterone levels gradually decline from mid reproductive life, with the post-menopausal ovary producing more testosterone than the pre-menopausal ovary. The abrupt and profound loss of testosterone in surgical or induced menopause results in significant symptoms, including profound loss of libido, and is particularly distressing in younger women. Young women are far more likely to be distressed by low libido or sexual function score. In a study of American women aged 20-65, 25% reported marked distress about their sexuality; younger women were more troubled than their older counterparts by a lack of sexual interest, $p=0.01$ [18].

Crandall found menopausal symptoms to be more severe in breast cancer patients who experience a menopausal transition during treatment [19]. A persistent increase in hot flash severity was noted. Adjustment for tamoxifen use did not alter the symptoms reported. Concerns about menopausal symptoms emerge once the focus on active treatment has passed. A qualitative study of 27 women post-chemotherapy for breast cancer [20] documented the progression of concerns. . Initially concerns with cancer and its treatment overshadow any concerns about menopause, but as women move beyond that phase to survivorship, the reality of menopause and its difficulties emerged. Concerns were related both to typical symptoms, but also to the equating of menopause with premature aging, an interpretation that was felt irrespective of age. Women further felt that their oncologists tended to dismiss their concerns. Menopause appears to be a particularly laden term to describe the induced ovarian failure experienced by young women. Symptom management will be discussed later in this chapter.

Early onset of menopause impacts adversely on overall health. In an epidemiologic study of nearly 38,000 Norwegian women with natural menopause, the age of menopause was found to be inversely related to mortality, with increased mortality for every year of earlier onset [21]. Women with premature menopause are also at risk for degenerative diseases, notably osteoporosis and atherosclerosis.

Premature Ovarian Failure and Atherosclerosis

Premature atherosclerosis has long been suspected by the increased risk in postmenopausal women, and the ten-year apparent gap between the onset of CHD in women when compared to men. The Framingham study provided early evidence that women who were post menopausal had a higher risk for heart disease than did age matched pre-menopausal women, although there was no increase in metabolic risk factors [22]. In the Nurses' Health Study, there was no increase in risk in age matched women who had undergone natural menopause, but in women who had undergone bilateral oopherectomy and who had never taken estrogens after menopause they saw an increased risk of CHD (RR=2.2, 95% CI 1.2-4.2) [23]. In a population study of Dutch women, each year of advancement of menopausal; age was associated with a 2% increase in cardiovascular mortality [24]. Hormone replacement in younger menopausal women may reduce this resk. A recent meta-analysis of randomized trials of hormone therapy concluded that for women younger than 60 years of age there was a total reduction in cardiac events, odds ratio of 0.68 (95% CI 0.48-0.96)[25].

There is explanatory evidence that atherosclerosis is accelerated from the time of menopause, with changes noted over time from the onset of menopause in the intima media thickness of the coronary vessels [26] and evidence of an increase in carotid atherosclerosis [27]. The various lines of research evidence that point to early benefit and later harm associated with hormone therapy have been the subject of a recent review [28].

Premature Ovarian Failure and Osteoporosis

Osteoporosis and decreased bone density are also described in women with premature menopause, but appear as a particular risk factor for women with chemotherapy induced ovarian failure in cancer [29,30,31,32]. There are multiple reasons for this. There is a well known effect of hypo-estrogenism on bone metabolism, with rapid loss of bone density following menopause, and an increase in bone density with decreased risk of fracture associated with hormone replacement. For women with cancer, there are additional risk factors. There is an impact from chemotherapeutic drugs, and especially steroid use. Prolonged bed rest is a known risk factor for bone density loss, and will affect many women who have had a prolonged illness or treatment. Women who are fatigued and feeling unwell are less likely to be engaging in exercise, increasing risk of both bone loss and fracture. Adult survivors of pediatric cancer have been found to be at increased risk of osteopenia and osteoporosis, directly related to the number of courses of chemotherapy they received [33].Finally, women with breast cancer appear to be at particular risk of osteoporosis [34,35]. In an longitudinal study, Kanis found the incidence of fracture over three years follow-up from diagnosis, to be increased nearly five fold in the cancer population. In women with soft tissue recurrence this increase rose to approximately 20 fold. When fracture risk was adjusted for age, duration of follow-up and prevalent fracture, the risk was 4.7 (95% CI, 2.3-9.9; $P < 0.0001$) in women newly diagnosed with breast cancer and 22.7 (95% CI, 9.1-57.1; $P<0.0001$) in the women with recurrent breast cancer [36].

Over and above the risks associated with chemotherapy agents and steroids, women with breast cancer frequently receive anti estrogen treatment in the form of selective estrogen receptor modulators, or aromatase inhibitors. Aromatase inhibitors have a direct adverse effect upon bone metabolism, but the clinical significance of this is not clear. In the ATAC study women treated with aromatase inhibitor had higher risk of osteoporosis and fracture than those treated with tamoxifen [37] with an incidence of 7.7 % in tamoxifen, vs 11% after 5 years, in women treated with anastrozole, translating into fracture rates per 1000 woman-years of 22·6 for anastrozole and 15·6 for tamoxifen (hazard ratio 1·44, 95% CI 1·21–1·68, $p<0·0001$). Fracture rates were not increased at the hip, although these were infrequent, and are more typically a fracture of the elderly. Vertebral fractures were increased ($p<0.03$).

Goss *et al* did not find an increase in fractures after 5 years of letrozole [38] Studies comparing aromatase inhibitors are clinically relevant, as tamoxifen has been the standard of hormonal therapy, but tamoxifen appears to reduce bone density in pre-menopausal women, but may be slightly beneficial in older post menopausal women [39].

Premature Ovarian Failure: Summary

Women with induced ovarian failure therapy experience loss of fertility, increased severity of menopausal symptoms, as well as specific health risks with respect to cardiovascular disease and osteoporosis. Women should be advised of their likelihood of ovarian failure, based on their age, risk factors and planned treatment, and the time-frame within which they may expect it. As there is an understandable focus on disease treatment, information about consequences may not be fully understood, but an openness to future discussions will have been established.

Loss of fertility will be particularly hard for women somen; consultation with infertility specialists to outline options in advance of treatment may be beneficial.

Baseline screening for risk factors for cardiac disease and osteoporosis, and testing including lipids and bone density testing establish a foundation for counseling and preventive care [40,41]. With survival increasing for women with cancer, and screening programmes enabling earlier diagnosis, preparation and planning for long-term survival are recommended. The American Society of Clinical Oncology noted, “Most women with newly diagnosed breast cancer are at risk of osteoporosis due to either their age or their breast cancer treatment. Oncology professionals, especially medical oncologists, need to take an expanded role in the routine and regular assessment of these women’s bone health” [42]. In addition to appropriate dietary and exercise advice, there is a role for bis-phosphonates in prevention of osteoporosis in women at high risk of fracture.

Cardiovascular disease does appear to be accelerated in women with early menopause, for women in whom hormone therapy is not contraindicated, an early discussion with respect to the role of hormone therapy in premature ovarian failure is important, as women with this condition are likely to inappropriately apply the findings of the Women’s Health Initiative study to their situation. Using the term premature ovarian failure may help to reduce confusion with physiologic menopause.

Menopausal Symptoms in Women with Cancer

Impact and Quality of Life in Cancer Survivors

Women with cancer and natural menopause may experience more severe symptoms and require specific considerations with respect to treatment. Symptoms of menopause are not generally specific to menopause, and may need to be distinguished from symptoms related to their disease or its treatment.

As commonplace as menopausal symptoms may be, their impact on quality of life can be easily underestimated. Daly *et al* assessed quality of life in a sample of menopausal women, using rating scales and utility values, where 0 is equivalent to death and 1.0 perfect health, found that menopausal women rated their quality of life with mild symptoms as .65, and with severe symptoms 0.3 [43]. These ratings confirm that women with symptoms do experience a substantial deterioration in quality of life, one that has lead to a search for safe and effective means of relief.

Schultz assessed menopausal symptoms in women who had a history of breast cancer and found that hot flashes, painful intercourse, inability to concentrate, fatigue, sleep disturbances and feeling unhappy impacted significantly on quality of life [44]. They found that numerous symptoms common in, but not specifically to menopause, were more severe in women who had undergone chemotherapy and radiotherapy as part of their treatment, including arthritis ($p<0.0007$), dizziness ($p<0.004$) and memory loss ($p<000003$), compared to women who had surgery alone.

Harris, in a case-control survey of 110 breast cancer survivors aged 16 to 69, found that menopausal symptoms were 5.3 times (95% CI 2.7-10.2) more common in breast cancer survivors than in the controls [45]. Gupta also found a very high prevalence of disruptive symptoms; 95% of two hundred women assessed reported symptoms, with significant impact on their quality of life. Severe hot flashes, night sweats and symptoms of vaginal dryness were particularly troublesome [46]. Older post-menopausal women on tamoxifen had somewhat less severe somatic symptoms, but no difference in vasomotor symptoms. Morales on the other hand, noted increase in the severity of vasomotor symptoms with both tamoxifen and with aromatase inhibitors ($p<0.0001$ and $p=0.014$) [47]. In this series of 184 patients, tamoxifen was also associated with decreased libido ($p< 0.0001$) , where aromatase inhibitors were associated with an increase in musculo-skeletal symptoms, and in vaginal dryness and dyspareunia ($p=0.0039$ and $p=0.001$).

Menopause Related Symptoms

Menopause is associated with a typical constellation of symptoms. Longitudinal community-based surveys in many countries all record increases in reports of disruptive symptoms, including hot flashes and sweats, depressed mood, sleep disturbances, sexual concerns or problems, cognitive symptoms, vaginal dryness, urinary incontinence, and somatic or bodily pain with menopause. The prevalence of specific symptoms varies somewhat between national and ethnic groups, but are universal phenomena. These observational studies have been well summarized in a recent review by Fugate-Woods [48].

Vasomotor Symptoms

The hot flash, or hot flush, is a subjective sensation of warmth, that maybe accompanied by other symptoms, including anxiety, irritability, sweating, palpitations, and panic. Hot flashes are the popular hallmark symptom of menopause, and are experienced by up to 80% of women, of whom 10-20% report severe symptoms [49]. In the general population the peak of symptoms occurs in the late menopausal transition, to the early postmenopausal years, but symptoms can persist for decades thereafter. Approximately 10% of women still complain of hot flushes into their seventies [50].

The hot flash can last from a few seconds, to several minutes (typically 3-5 minutes), but can last for hours [51]. Physiologic changes associated with the hot flash include blood flow increases to the skin, and there is an increase in skin temperature, sweating and skin conductance. A feeling of being chilled, and shivering may follow hot flashes [52]. Some women experience a sense of anxiety or apprehension with the hot flash.

The hot flash can be a nonspecific response to many physiologic challenges, but the menopausal hot flash, is only a part of the vaso-motor disturbance; women report as a difficulty maintaining a comfortable temperature, alternately feeling too hot, or shivering with cold. Increases in ambient temperature or exercise are able to provoke hot flashes. These symptoms are thought to be due to alteration in the CNS thermoregulatory set point located in the anterior portion of the hypothalamus. Freedman has observed that threshold between sweating and shivering (thermo neutral zone) is wider in asymptomatic menopausal women (0.4°) than in symptomatic and in women with severe symptoms is virtually absent, 0° [53]. Freedman has also documented the circadian rhythm that women report, demonstrating an increase frequency in hot flashes in the evening and night. Sweating is more commonly associated with nocturnal flashes, the reason for night sweats is not known.

Complementary and Alternative Management of Vasomotor Symptoms

Women with a history of cancer are likely to be interested in non-hormonal alternative treatments for vasomotor symptoms, Harris found breast cancer survivors were 25 (95% CI 8.3-100) times less likely to use estrogen, and 7.4 (95% CI 2.5-21.9) times more likely to use alternatives than non-affected women. Women with a history of breast cancer are seven times more likely to report the use of soy based phytoestrogens, vitamin E and herbal remedies [45,64].

The challenge becomes to find effective alternatives to offer. Assessment of effective therapies for hot flashes can only be made by placebo-controlled trials, as the placebo effect is considerable, and the natural spontaneous resolution of hot flashes is also substantial. A 58% reduction in hot flashes was noted for placebo in a recent Cochrane review [54], stressing the need for well-designed studies with sufficient power to accurately detect a treatment effect.

Much recent attention has been paid to environmental, lifestyle and behavioural techniques that can reduce the discomfort of hot flushes, and to herbal and botanical remedies.

Environmental factors Hot flashes can be provoked by high ambient temperature, leading to advice to dress in light clothing, and in layers. Moisture wicking material is commercially available in nightwear designed with cancer patients in mind [55]. The use a fan is also helpful, particularly for sleep, as is reducing room temperature.

Physical activity Women who are physically active tend to report fewer hot flashes, but exercise *per se* has not been found to be effective in reducing vasomotor symptoms [56], and in fact increased the frequency of hot flashes, presumable as a manifestation of the reduced thermo-neutral zone [52]. Women should be advised to exercise in moderation, and early in the day for maximum benefit to vasomotor symptoms. Women with cancer may be de-conditioned or less active with exercise because of fatigue, pain or complications of treatment. Maintaining some level of physical fitness may be helpful.

Paced respiration There is some evidence for the benefit of paced respiration [52,57,58,59]. Paced respiration reduced hot flashes by as much as 50%, and was more effective than relaxation therapy.

Herbal and botanical remedies have been the subject of popular interest and scientific study [60,61,62]. Six trials have found evidence for benefit of Black Cohosh; these studies have methodological flaws, but nonetheless have consistent results. There have been isolated case reports of hepatotoxicity with black cohosh [63]; a consideration of particular importance in women who may be receiving other medications with potential hepatotoxicity. Dong quai, vitamin E and Evening Primrose Oil have not been found to be effective [63]

The phytoestrogens Harris found greatly increased use of soy amongst breast cancer survivors, both for menopausal symptoms, and in hope of preventing recurrence [45]. The isoflavones (soy or red clover derived) have not proven to be as effective as might have been hoped; clinical outcomes have been modest, and studies have not shown consistent benefit [65,66]. In a recent meta-analysis by Nelson [67] a non-statistically significant benefit was noted for red clover siofalvones, of –0.44 hot flushes per day (95% CI, -1.47 to 0.58). A small benefit was noted for the soy isofalvones of – 0.97 after 6 weeks (95% CI, -1.82 to – 0.12). Findings were inconsistent, and drop out rates in some trials are quite substantial, due to bloating and gas. There is ongoing research and considerable individual variation in response to phyto-estrogens, so it is reasonable to give these alternatives a therapeutic trial [68].

Drug-Herb Interaction

The potential for drug-herb interactions is relevant. Recent reviews catalogue some of the potential interaction [69,70]. There are a number of herbal remedies that have potential interactions with warfarin, including several that are popular with menopausal women, including red clover, don quai, ginseng and vitamin, chamomile and green tea [69,70,71]. The potential for interaction with chemotherapeutic drugs is particularly important, as menopausal women use a variety of complementary and alternative remedies. Six of the top ten best-selling herbal preparations in the United States are frequently used by menopausal women, including ginseng, soy, black cohosh, St John's Wort and valerian [72]. Cancer patients are more likely than the general population to use complementary therapies. Most users do not inform their physicians of this. Because of the narrow therapeutic index of many chemotherapeutic agents, a subtle interaction may lead to a significant clinical effect. Many interactions are described in animal models, and their human impact remains potential. Thus women and their physicians need to be aware of these concerns.

Soy is commonly used by menopausal women, as a supplement, in the form of a phytoestrogenic extract, as well as a foodstuff. There is evidence of stimulation of breast tissue by phytoestrogens [73,74,75]. Moreover, there may be an interaction between phytoestrogens and the selective estrogen receptor modulator tamoxifen [76]. Safety data on the use of phytoestrogen supplements, in medicinal amounts, as opposed to their use as a dietary component, is needed. There is some basic science to suggest that some tumors may grow in response to Phytoestrogens [77]. Interactions *in vitro* have been observed that might impair the efficacy of adjuvant therapy [78,79]. Authors advise women to refrain from use of phytoestrogens, at least during active therapy. Prudence, and use of these compounds as a food rather than in pharmacologic doses should be advised.

Black Cohosh, one of the most frequently used preparations by menopausal women has no known drug interaction. A table listing herbal preparations with potential interaction is provided in Table 2.

Table 1. Top Selling Herbal Supplements in the United States

Table 1. Top-Selling Herbal Supplements in the United States

2002 Rank	Herb	Plant Name	Primary Clinical Indications	Retail Sales in 2002* ($US)	2001 Rank
1	Garlic	*Allium sativum*	Hypercholesterolemia	34,509,288	3
2	Ginkgo	*Ginkgo biloba*	Dementia, intermittent claudication	32,998,528	1
3	Echinacea	*Echinacea purpurea*†	Prevention of common cold	32,448,966	2
4	Soy	*Glycine max*	Menopausal symptoms	28,252,518	5
5	Saw palmetto	*Serenoa repens*	Benign prostate hyperplasia	23,053,036	6
6	Ginseng	*Panax ginseng*	Physical and mental fatigue	21,686,192	4
7	St. John's wort	*Hypericum perforatum*	Mild depression	14,969,575	7
8	Black cohosh	*Actaea racemosa*‡	Menopausal symptoms	12,333,188	10
9	Cranberry	*Vaccinium macrocarpon*	Urinary tract infection	11,857,782	9
10	Valerian	*Valeriana officinalis*	Insomnia, stress	8,120,329	8
11	Milk thistle	*Silybum marianum*	Alcoholic cirrhosis and hepatitis	7,762,350	12
12	Evening primrose	*Oenothera biennis*	Premenstrual syndrome	6,024,896	13
13	Kava	*Piper methysticum*	Anxiety	4,423,427	11
14	Bilberry	*Vaccinium myrtillus*	Diabetic retinopathy	3,381,351	15
15	Grape seed	*Vitis vinifera*	Allergic rhinitis	3,054,816	14

*Data obtained from Blumenthal[12].
†Other species include *E. angustifolia*, and *E. pallida*.
‡Formerly *Cimicifuga racemosa*.

Table 2. Specific Herbal Remedies to Avoid During Chemotherapy

Herb	Concurrent Chemotherapy/Condition (suspected effect)
Garlic	Avoid with decarbazine (CYP2E1 inhibition); caution with other concurrent chemotherapy (inconclusive data)
Ginkgo	Caution with camptothecins, cyclophosphamide, EGFR-TK inhibitors, epipodophyllotoxins, taxanes, and vinca alkaloids (CYP3A4 and CYP2C19 inhibition); discourage with alkylating agents, antitumor antibiotics, and platinum analogues (free-radical scavenging)
Echinacea	Avoid with camptothecins, cyclophosphamide, EGFR-TK inhibitors, epipodophyllotoxins, taxanes, and vinca alkaloids (CYP3A4 induction)
Soy	Avoid with tamoxifen (antagonism of tumor growth inhibition), and treatment of patients with estrogen-receptor positive breast cancer and endometrial cancer (stimulation of tumor growth)
Saw palmetto	No significant interactions expected
Ginseng	Caution with camptothecins, cyclophosphamide, EGFR-TK inhibitors, epipodophyllotoxins, taxanes, and Vinca alkaloids (CYP3A4 inhibition); discourage in patients with estrogen-receptor positive breast cancer and endometrial cancer (stimulation of tumor growth)
St. John's wort	Avoid with all concurrent chemotherapy (CYP2B6, CYP2C9, CYP2C19, CYP2E1, CYP3A4, and P-glycoprotein induction)
Black cohosh	No significant interactions expected
Cranberry	No significant interactions expected
Valerian	Caution with tamoxifen (CYP2C9 inhibition), cyclophosphamide, and teniposide (CYP2C19 inhibition), cyclophosphamide, and teniposide (CYP2C19 inhibition)
Milk thistle	No significant interactions expected
Evening primrose	No significant interactions expected, but caution with highly extracted drugs (serum-binding displacement)
Kava	Avoid in all patients with pre-existing liver disease, with evidence of hepatic injury (herb-induced hepatotoxicity), and/or in combination with hepatotoxic chemotherapy; caution with camptothecins, cyclophosphamide, EGFR-TK inhibitors, epipodophyllotoxins, taxanes, and vinca alkaloids (CYP3A4 induction)
Bilberry	No significant interactions expected
Grape seed	Caution with camptothecins, cyclophosphamide, EGFR-TK inhibitors, epipodophyllotoxins, taxanes, and vinca alkaloids (CYP3A4 induction), and with alkylating agents, antitumor antibiotics, and platinum analogues (free-radical scavenging)

Abbreviation: EGFR-TK, epidermal growth factor receptor tyrosine-kinase.

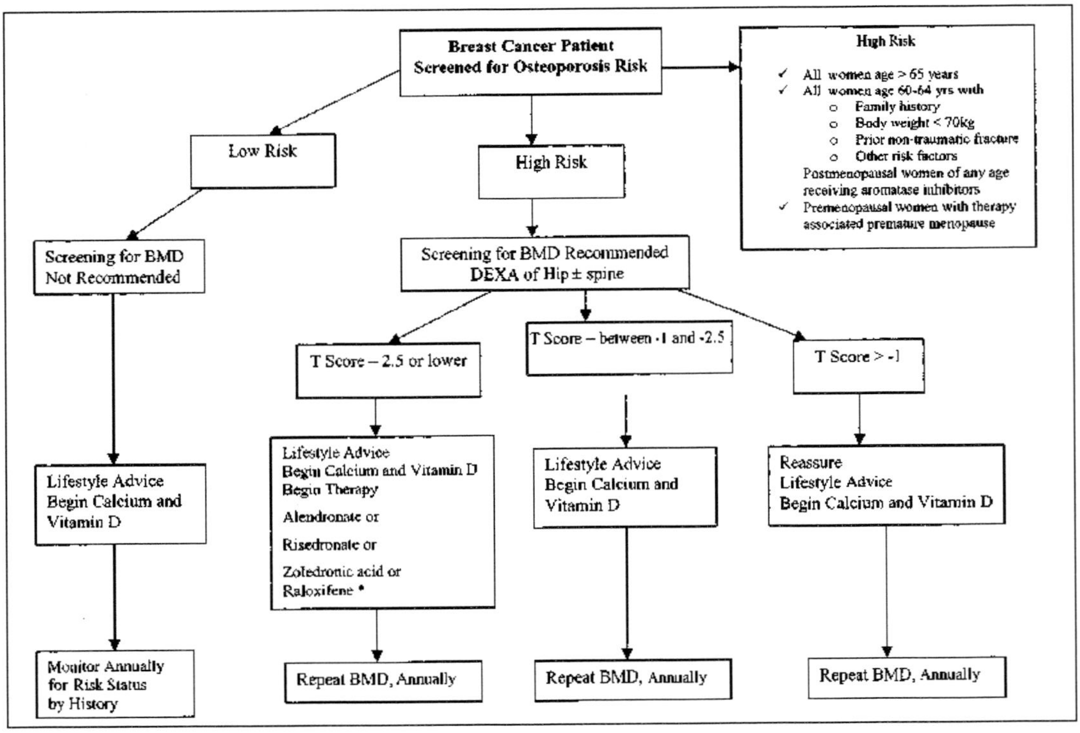

Figure 1. Recommended management strategy for patients with diagnosed breast cancer. This management strategy is largely based on influence from results in non-breast cancer populations. BMD, bone mass density; DEXA, dual energy x-ray absorptiometry bone scan.

Non-Hormonal Medical Treatments

A variety of non-hormonal medical treatments have been evaluated, either for use in menopause, or more specifically, for use in women with a history of breast cancer [80,81]. Clonidine, a centrally acting α agonist, has been in use for the management of menopausal symptoms for many years [82]. Evidence for its use is derived from small trials with mixed result. It has been investigated in tamoxifen-induced hot flashes, where it showed a modest benefit, a 20 to 38% reduction with substantial placebo effect [83,84]. Sleeplessness, constipation drowsiness and dry mouth are common side effects. Goldberg noted that while statistically impressive, the results of a 20% reduction in symptoms were not clinically important, noting that patients did not prefer Clonidine over placebo because of adverse effects, and concluded that better means of relief were needed. In practice the clinical experience with Clonidine has not been particularly favourable. Freedman showed that Clonidine raised the sweating threshold in symptomatic, but not asymptomatic women [85]. This is consistent with the clinical observation that Clonidine seems particularly helpful to patients with the complaint of night sweats.

While Clonidine retains a place in the options available, Interest has turned to selective seratonin re-uptake inhibitors (SSRI's) paroxetine [86,87] and the seratonin and norepinephrine re-uptake inhibitors (SNRIS), Venlafaxine, both of which have RCT evidence of efficacy for VMS. Recent evidence that Paroxetine has the potential of reducing the levels of an active metabolite of tamoxifen [88,89] would favour the use of Venlafaxine, although there is no clinical data to suggest that this is clinically significant. Biglia used a lower dose of Venlafaxine, 37.5 mgm extended release formulation with good success. The benefit was gradual, with further improvement noted over eight weeks of treatment of up to a 59% improvement in the hot flush score (a composite of frequency and severity). Even with the low dose, 15% of women reported nausea and vomiting, though this subsided after the first week of treatment [90]. Other side effects include decreased appetite, decreased libido, dry mouth and constipation.

In Nelson's meta-analysis of SSRIs and SNRI's based on 6 trials, there was a significant reduction in hot flashes compared to placebo of –1.13 (95% CI –1.70 to -0.57) hot flashes/day [35]. When breast cancer patients who were treated with tamoxifen were considered separately, the reduction increased to –1.40 (95% CI -1.97 to –0.82). This may or may not be deemed clinically significant.

In a head to head trial with depo-medroxyprogesterone acetate (MPA), better control of symptoms with fewer side effects was achieved with MPA. However until the role of Progestin in breast caner is clarified, it is likely that a SNRI would be preferred over a Progestin [91].

There have been two trials of Gabapentin. The 300 mgm dose was not effective, while with 900 mgm day there was a significant reduction in hot flash frequency and severity by 67% [92,93]. Side effects include fatigue, dizziness, rash, palpitations, but overall drop outs on treatment were few. Reduction in pain was a positive side effect of treatment.

Hormone Therapy

For women able to use hormone therapy, it remains the single most effective modality for dealing with menopausal symptoms. Estrogen therapy has been used for hot flashes since the 1950's; its effectiveness has recently been reassessed and confirmed. The Cochrane review calculated a 75% reduction in hot flash frequency, and a significant decrease in symptom severity (OR 0.13, 95% CI 0.06-0.27).

All types of estrogen (conjugated oral estrogens, oral estradiol) and routes (oral vs. transdermal) have been found to be equally efficacious for relief of hot flashes [94] Transdermal estrogens are particularly appropriate for women who wish to avoid first pass- hepatic metabolism of estrogen, by smokers, and by women who prefer a transdermal to an oral route of administration. There is some evidence to suggest that they have a lesser impact on blood coagulability [95,96,97] and they appear to have a lesser impact on mammographic breast density [98].

After the publication of WHI there has been heightened interest in low dose hormone therapy. Lower doses for estrogen therapy to control hot flashes has been found to be less effective in reducing frequency and severity of hot flashes, but with fewer adverse effects than conventional doses. Recent reviews of data [99,100] have concluded that there is an approximately 65% reduction in hot flashes with low dose HT, against a 75-90% reduction with conventional, and a 35% reduction in placebo arms. The time to maximum effect is also much longer in lower dose therapy, taking 8-12 weeks for maximal effect, compared to four weeks with conventional doses.

Low dose HT has been found to be associated with fewer reported side effects, such as breast tenderness, and fewer adverse events, In the Nurse's Health Study long term use of Premarin 0.625mgm was associated with an increased risk of stroke (OR 1.35 95%CI 1.08-1.68). The risk was higher for higher doses of Premarin. This was not seen in women on low dose (0.3 mgm) of Premarin. Both groups had an equal reduction in cardiovascular disease risk [101]. There is, as yet, no evidence for increased safety with respect to breast cancer risk [102] Paganini- Hill recently reported on apparent benefit of low-dose, rather than moderate dose hormone therapy in a long-term follow-up of the Leisure World cohort.

Specific Consideration: Hormone Replacement in Women with Cancer

There are two broad categories of women in whom consideration of hormones may arise, those with an early menopause induced by treatment, regardless of their symptomatology, and those with menopausal symptoms, regardless of their age at menopause [103]. Young women with induced menopause are at risk for premature atherosclerosis, osteoporosis, decreased libido and increased severity of menopausal symptoms. There is consensus that women with premature menopause, in the absence of contra-indication, should be offered physiologically appropriate hormone replacement. Controversy arises in management of women with a history of an estrogen dependent tumor. This has been the subject of several recent reviews, with authors expressing a range of opinion, from strongly advising against HT to others finding the evidence to be less compelling [104,105,106]. There have also been meta-analyses addressing this controversy [107,108].

In women with a history of early stage endometrial cancer, there is somewhat more consensus, as the cancer can be completely surgically removed, and epidemiological studies have consistently shown reduced, or no increased risk of recurrence [109,110,111,112]. There is an overall benefit in treated women. Unfortunately, there is no RCT data, and the trial that was underway was halted shortly after the release of the WHI findings. Thus, there is potential for selection bias to have affected the outcome. Since endometrial cancer is more common in older postmenopausal women in whom symptoms typically have abated, the question of use of hormones to manage symptoms is less likely to arise.

Breast cancer is often diagnosed in younger women, in whom the question of hormone therapy is more likely to arise. Since publication of WHI patients are themselves more likely to avoid the use of hormone therapy, and pursue alternative therapies [45]; however controversy remains. The concerns regarding use of hormone therapy is supported by the fact that, unlike endometrial cancer, breast cancer may not be completely surgically removed, with breast cancer patients having an ongoing risk of recurrence even twenty years or longer post diagnosis. As well, a reduced recurrence rate is seen in patients treated with tamoxifen or aromatase inhibitors. The studies of women treated with hormone therapy are less clear. The eight observational studies of women treated with hormone therapy include over 1200 breast cancer patients, and more than 2800 controls, and have shown a reduced recurrence risk with hormone therapy. In the meta-analysis by Col this RR was 0.64 (95% CI 0.50 –0.82) [107]. Treated women have tended to be younger and with less advanced disease, and the possibility of selection bias exists. There have been two randomized of hormone therapy, neither of which were completed, and which raise some further questions. The HABITS trial was halted prior to completion when an interim analysis found an increased risk of recurrence at 2.1 years; the RR was 3.3 (95% CI 1.5 -7.4)[113]. The Stockholm trial was halted shortly after HABITS, even though it had shown a reduced risk in women followed to 4.1 years (RH 0.82, 95% C! 0.35-1.9) [114]. Many fewer women in the HABITS trail used tamoxifen (21% vs. 52% in the Stockholm trial) The HABITS did not utilize a standard approach to hormone therapy, but randomized women to be treated according to local practice. An important difference between these two trials was the use of progestin. In the HABITS trail, the majority of women with an intact uterus were prescribed combined continuous HT. In the Stockholm trial the HT regimen was standardized, with a protocol designed to reduce exposure to progestin, and to administer it sequentially. Older women received a long cycle progestin, and all were prescribed a hormone free interval. Accumulating evidence on the increased risk of breast cancer associated with estrogen progestin, compared to estrogen alone is very consistent with the differences noted in these two trials [115], and is supported by our understanding of the biologic response of the breast vs. the endometrium to progestins. Progestins are classified on the basis of their ability to induce secretory change in estrogen primed (rabbit) endometrium, however the breast cells are known to be proliferating during the luteal phase. Apoptosis in breast tissue is maximal 48 hours after progestin withdrawal. Finally, progestational agents show differing profiles with respect to breast proliferation vs apoptosis in vitro, and clinical evidence will be helpful in providing clinical advice.

In the absence of unequivolcal evidence for safety, current practice is to avoid hormone therapy in women with a history of breast cancer. Individual consideration can be given to women whose symptoms are intractable, unresponsive to alternative approaches and impairing quality of life. In these cases, the lowest effective dose for the shortest time needed to manage symptoms is prudent. Currently there is no consensus that favours any particular hormone therapy regimen or progestational agent, however, it is an area of ongoing research, as clinicians seek to identify patients who would be at risk, and those who might benefit from the option of hormone therapy [116,117].

Sleep Disturbance

Sleep disturbances are a very common symptom in the menopausal transition, and are particularly common in survivors of cancer, in whom they are associated with a significantly decreased quality of life. Gupta found that 86% of women reported sleep disturbance, and 65% reported moderate to sever symptoms [46]. This contrasts with the SWAN study [118], which surveyed women in the community from early menopausal transition, through to post menopausal, and found sleep disturbance was reported by approximately 30%.

The most common complaints of menopausal women are of difficulty falling asleep, and of frequent awakenings, with difficulty falling back to sleep. The most symptomatic women were those with surgical menopause, 43.5% or those in the late transition, at 43.5%. In the early menopause 40.6% reported sleep disturbance. Hot flashes were strongly associated with sleep disturbance, as indicated by an OR 1.99 (95%CI 1.81–2.19). Physical activity was inversely associated with sleep disturbance, only 31.2% of active women, compared to 60.8% of the least active women reported symptoms [119].

Common sleep disturbances that increase with age include increased sleep latency, increased nocturnal awakening, and early awakening with difficulty returning to sleep. These disturbances are increased with poor health [120]. Although sleep disturbance is strongly associated with vasomotor flushes, insomnia can occur in the absence of any reported hot flushes, and may be the only menopausal complaint.

Sleep complaints cannot be assumed to be as a result of hot flashes, but deserve to be investigated for other factors. Potential contributors to sleep disruption are medical illness, such as hyperthyroidism or Cushing's, psychiatric illness, obstructive sleep apnea, medications or substances such as caffeine or alcohol, and restless leg syndrome. Behavioural and environmental factors include poor sleep hygiene, stress, disturbance by a spouse, and shift work. Poor sleep conditions include old mattresses, high ambient noise, light or temperature.

Management of Sleep Disturbances

Sleep disturbances are common, and are particularly common in cancer survivors, but should only be attributed to menopause after excluding other possible causes. Sleep hygiene and behavioural changes are the first strategy in managing sleep problems. While there has been some dispute as to the causative role of the hot flash in sleep disruption, there has been consistent evidence that hormone therapy does improve sleep quality

After ruling out other causes of sleep disruption, sleep hygiene and behavioural changes should be addressed. Education about normal changes in sleep, including the shift in circadian rhythm towards earlier awakening may be helpful in setting realistic expectations.

Basic sleep hygiene includes avoidance of heavy evening meals and stimulants, sleeping in a dark, quiet room, restricting the bedroom to sleep, relaxing activity or warm milk at bedtime. Behavioural therapy includes bedtime routines, relaxation therapy and cognitive behavioural therapy

Physical activity levels are associated with better sleep quality, and there is evidence that adopting a regular exercise habit may be beneficial. Both regular walking and stretching appear beneficial, but vigorous exercise should be avoided close to retiring, because of an increase in hot flashes associated with increases in core body temperature [121].

Hormone therapy has long been used for improvement of sleep at menopause, and the WHI has confirmed the beneficial effect [122] the improvement in sleep appears to be only partially associated with reduction in reported hot flashes [123,124]. Suggesting that estrogen may be acting through other neural means to improve sleep quality.

Depressed Mood

Feeling sad or blue is a commonly reported symptom of women in the menopausal transition; in population studies 19-29% of women report such feelings. There is little longitudinal follow-up data to track the resolution or persistence of these symptoms, but cross sectional studies indicate that reporting of sad feelings peaks in the transition, and is less frequent in older post menopausal women. Clinical depression is far less common affecting 4-6% of women [125,126,127]. Depression is not considered a normal part of menopause. In the SWAN study, depressive symptoms were far more common in women reporting sleep disturbance (39.7% of women with sleep problems, vs. 15.4% of those without) and a similar association was noted for vasomotor symptoms (36.6% vs. 18%) [128]. This study noted a peak of symptoms with 28.9% in the menopausal transition, vs. 22% in the post menopause, against a baseline of 20% pre-menopausal. Menopausal status (peri menopausal vs. post menopausal) was independently significantly associated with risk of psychological distress, independent of all co-variates, and race/ethnicity.

Risk factors for development of depression during the peri-menopausal period include a history of depressive disorders, poor physical heath and life stressors (lack of employment and social support), history of surgical menopause, and a long peri-menopausal transition [129]. Avis, in a longitudinal study of women in the state of Massachusetts, found no association between depressive symptoms and circulating estrogen levels. A definite association was found between the incidence of depression and reports of other menopausal symptoms, notably hot flushes and sleep disturbance [130]. This study supports the "domino" theory, which proposes that depression is a result of vasomotor symptoms leading to sleep disturbance, which in turn leads to irritability and depression. In the Melbourne study, negative mood was significantly predicted by a history of premenstrual complaints, negative attitudes towards menopause and aging, and low parity. Menopausal symptoms, poor self-health, negative feelings towards partner, smoking, stress and sedentary life style [131].

Management of Mood Symptoms

Women with predominantly mood complaints need to be carefully evaluated to rule out clinical depression, and managed accordingly. Conventional modalities for treatment of clinical depression, as in any other phase of life, include psychotherapy (cognitive behavioural therapy or interpersonal therapy), anti-depressant medication, and other therapies as indicated.

For women in whom there is no contra-indication, there may be a therapeutic role for estrogen therapy. The role of estrogen therapy in the management of mood disorders at menopause has been the subject of recent reviews [132,133,134]. Estrogen therapy has shown significant benefit for women with mild to moderate depressive symptoms in the late menopausal transition and early post menopause. A quantitative review of 26 studies examining the effect of hormones on mood using broad inclusion criteria and including non-placebo controls [132], found the overall mean effect size of hormone replacement therapy (HT) to improve mood was 0.68 (variance = 0.14, $p< 0.00$).

Hormone therapy appears of particular benefit to women in the transition or early post menopause. Women who were 5-10 years postmenopausal did not benefit from the administration of estrogen [135]. There is a placebo effect, and there may be an adverse impact on mood for women receiving MPA in addition to estrogen. Relief of depressive symptoms in peri-menopausal women treated with HT has been noted independent of a reduction in vasomotor symptoms, and benefits were observed in women with or without vasomotor symptoms, suggesting that the mechanism of action of estrogen is at multiple levels in the CNS [136]. Estradiol has also been found to be effective in treating peri-menopausal women meeting criteria for major depressive disorder [137].

Vulvo-vaginal Symptoms

Vulvo-vaginal symptoms are among the most commonly reported in menopausal women. Unlike vasomotor or mood symptoms, that spontaneously resolve, vaginal symptoms are progressive with prolonged hypo-estrogenism in menopause. Vulvo vagainl symptoms are more pronounced in women who are being treated with aromatase inhibitors, and in women who have had vaginal irradiation.

Vaginal dryness is reported by from 27% to 55% of healthy menopausal women [138], and dyspareunia from 32% to 41%. Women may complain of decreased sensitivity to touch, and decreased sensitivity has been objectively documented [139]. It is thought that only one fifth of women suffering from vulvo vaginal complaints will actually seek help from a physician [140], placing the onus on the physician to enquire into vaginal health. The detection and management changes associated with urogenital aging are the subject of recent reviews [141,142].

Estrogen is not the only contributor to the changes noted at menopause; aging in and of itself contributes to atrophy. Over time, the vagina undergoes shortening and narrowing, with loss of the vaginal fornices, and loses distensability. These progressive changes can culminate in a rigid and contracted vagina; the vaginal walls may become adherent with synechiae from chronic inflammation. In end stage atrophy, sexual intercourse becomes impossible. Women with irradiated vaginas or with surgical foreshortening and hypoestrogenism need to be monitored to avoid this complication.

Prevention

The risk of vaginal atrophy is higher in women who smoke, in women who are sexually inactive [143], and in women who have never had a vaginal birth [144]. Vaginal health is better maintained, in women with higher circulating levels of androgen, and in women who are more frequently sexually active [143].

Treatment of gynecologic cancer can affect vaginal health through reduction of vaginal length, surgical remodeling of the introitus, radiation changes to soft tissues and their blood supply, or surgical disruption of nerves or blood vessels. Early institution of vaginal estrogen, as a cream or ring, and teaching women to use dilators from an early stage in treatment is helpful.

If possible, regular sexual activity with intercourse will help to maintain vaginal health. In addition to the increased blood flow associated with sexual arousal, and the mechanical distension provided, the seminal fluid itself, rich in prostaglandins, sex steroids, and essential fatty acids, is postulated to benefit the vaginal epithelium [144].

Management of Atrophic Vaginitis

Atrophic vaginitis is most effectively treated with the use of exogenous estrogen, (particularly vaginal estrogen). For women in whom estrogen therapy is contra-indicated or not acceptable to all, symptomatic management can reduce the symptoms of dryness and irritation, or supply lubrications for vaginal intercourse.

Vaginal moisturizers, containing a non-hormonal moisturizing vaginal gel containing water, glycerin, mineral oil, polycarbophil, carbopol, hydrogenated palm oil glyceride and sorbic acid (Replens®) used three times a week has been found effective to relieve symptoms of atrophic vaginitis, by adhering to the vaginal epithelium and retaining moisture [145,146] but does not reverse atrophic changes. Water-soluble lubricants can improve comfort with intercourse.

Atrophic vaginitis can develop in women on low dose systemic therapy [147]. In these women, as well as women who have only vaginal symptoms, vaginal delivery systems of estrogen provide a low dose that effectively reverses atrophic change, and relieves symptoms [148].

A recent Cochrane review of sixteen studies, which involved a total of 2129 participants [149]. All formulations of local estrogen, cream, ring or low dose tablet, had efficacy in both relieving symptoms of dryness and pruritis or burning, as well as improving scores for vaginal moisture, vaginal elasticity, and fluid volume.

Vaginal estrogens in doses sufficient to relieve atrophic symptoms do not raise circulating levels of estrogen beyond post-menopausal levels making them available for women in whom estrogen replacement would be otherwise contra-indicated [150]. The comparative studies between the newer silicone impregnated rings or tablets and vaginal estrogen cream to employ higher doses of estrogen cream that are currently recommended, making comparison difficult. Low dose vaginal estrogen appears to have a safe endometrial profile [151,152,153,154].

In the Cochrane review no cases of endometrial cancer were reported, though rare cases of endometrial hyperplasia were noted with low dose vaginal estrogens. Johnston [155] has concluded that there is no evidence to support annual surveillance of women on low does of local vaginal therapy (estradiol 25 mcg tablet twice weekly, estradiol ring replaced q 3 monthly, or CEE 0.5 grams 3/week). Other authors have noted that there may still be a need for caution [156] as some women may exhibit a greater endometrial response than others. The reports are on a relatively small number of women. Thus it seems reasonable to individualize surveillance, taking into account endogenous estrogen production in heavier women, or increased absorption in women with a thin atrophic vaginal epithelium. In women in whom estrogens are contraindicated, using vaginal products strictly as prescribed is important. Part of the achievement of low circulating levels is believed to come from thickening of the vaginal epithelium, women who increase the interval between application of vaginal estrogen may theoretically increase their exposure. There are limited clinical studies looking at recurrence rates, but to date their appears to be no risk, or increased risk of breast cancer in women using vaginal estrogen [157].

Aches and Pain

One of the most troubling symptoms that women experience is of joint pain and stiffness, or generalized aches and pains; symptoms that make women 'feel old" and may hamper physical activity. Patients who have had chemotherapy appear to be at greatly increased risk of arthritis and joint pain; this common symptom is not specific to menopause [158].

Joint pain is among the most commonly reported symptoms of menopause, experienced by up to 67% of peri-menopausal women [159]. In the SWAN study the odds ratio of joint pain and stiffness in the menopausal transition was 1.48 (CI 1.35-1.62) and even higher in women who had undergone surgical menopause (OR 1.5, CI 1.33-1.69). Joint symptoms were the most commonly reported symptom in the Melbourne longitudinal study of the menopausal transition [160].

Management of Joint Pain and Stiffness

Physical activity may help pain and stiffness, particularly exercise that promotes flexibility and stretching [161]. In the SWAN study, joint stiffness was much more common in women who reported little to no physical activity, compared to those reporting the highest level of activity, (73.1% vs. 46.8%). These were associations, and it is not possible to determine if increased pain and soreness contributed to being less physically active, or vice versa. In the Melbourne women associations between pain and lower mood, and higher BMI were noted, but the authors noted that it was not possible to tease out the relationship between these observations.

Menopausal hormone therapy appears to improve musculo-skeletal symptoms. In the WHI, women assigned to E+P were more likely than women assigned to placebo to report relief of joint pain and stiffness, and from generalized aches and pains (47.1 vs. 38.4%, OR 1.43, CI 1.24-1.64, $p<0.01$, and 49.3 vs. 43.7%, OR 1.25, CI 1.05-1.44, $p=0.02$ respectively).

Women assigned to E+P were also less likely to develop new onset of joint pain (OR 0.68, CI 0.61-0.76, $p<0.01$), or general aches and pains (OR 0.73, CI 0.66-0.82, $p<0.01$).

There appears to be little known about how to mitigate these symptoms specifically in the cancer survivor.

Sexuality

Sexual concerns are among the most frequent in women attending menopause clinics [162] and the most common complaint amongst women in the menopausal transition is of decreased interest. Women with cancer, particularly cancers that have affected body image (the breast or genital tract) or who have undergone treatment that diminishes the blood supply or innervation of the genitals, or in whom estrogen therapy is contra indicated.

Changes in sexual function appear normal with age and menopause, and sexual concerns are very common. In the Melbourne study of women aged 45-55, the frequency of self-reported sexual dysfunction rose from 42% in the early menopausal transition, to 88% after 8 years, in the post-menopause. Sexual concerns included lowered interest, responsiveness, frequency, and change in feelings toward the partner. Vaginal dryness and discomfort increased with age.

Sexual function is affected by both age and estradiol levels. Dennerstien has conducted one of the few longitudinal studies of sexual function. The Melbourne Women's Midlife Health Project study involved a cohort of women aged 45-55 was followed for nine years [163]. In A decline in sexual function was noted with age, and duration of relationship, but an additional negative impact was associated with menopause, and the declining levels of estradiol (not androgens). The changes that women experience in their sexual function can impact their self-identity, their relationships, and their sense of connectedness to a highly sexualized society.

A decrease in sexual function that is not distressing to the woman is not classified as a dysfunction. In a study of American women aged 20-65, 25% reported marked distress about their sexuality, with younger women being more troubled than older women by a lack of sexual interest, $p=0.01$ [163].It is important that clinicians obtain a sexual history, and determine what the impact is to the patient. In the WISHes study, hypoactive sexual desire disorder was accompanied by significant psychological, emotional and interpersonal distress, lower sexual and partner satisfaction, and decreased general health status, both mental and physical health [165].Basson notes that mental well being, health and feelings towards one's partner are the most important predictors of sexual function, with biological factors modulating the response. She further notes that in women with distressing loss of sexual function in menopause, both menopausal interest and response tend to be suppressed [166]. Lack of interest is experienced as an absence of sexual thoughts and fantasies, little attraction to others, and rare initiation of any sexual activity.

Management

Anticipation of changes in sexuality, and letting women know help is available should issues arise is very helpful. Women with body image concerns after cancer surgery or treatment may require counseling to re-discover their sexual identity. Relationship issues and past sexual concerns need to be addressed. Fatigue may be a particular concern for women who have undergone treatment for cancer. Improved physical conditioning, achieved by an exercise program and healthy diet may ameliorate some of the fatigue. Behavioural changes in patterns of sexual activity, to avoid times when fatigue may be more pronounced, may be effective.

Vaginal estrogen and moisturizers can improve sexual satisfaction, and lubricants can assist with dryness. Androgen replacement has been shown to be effective for women who have undergone surgical menopause, however, these trials have not included women with breast cancer. The potential for testosterone being metabolized to estrogen is an unresolved concern.

Conclusion

With increasing numbers of cancer survivors, and earlier diagnosis, unprecedented number of women are going through menopause with a history of cancer. Menopause poses unique challenges to these women and to their health care providers. There are specific considerations for younger women, related both to the implications of a premature "menopause", with loss of fertility, psychosexual impact, and significant health risks for cardiovascular disease and osteoporosis. Women going through the menopausal transition in association with cancer treatment, particularly women who are treated with radiation or chemotherapy in addition to surgery, appear to be at increased risk of severe menopausal symptoms. The more severe symptoms are particularly difficult to manage in women in whom hormone therapy is contraindicate, but a variety of non-hormonal options do offer some relief. The role of hormone therapy in women with a history of an estrogen sensitive breast cancer remains controversial. Hormones are only offered for the most severely symptomatic women if other approaches have failed.

References

[1] World Health Organization 1996 Research on the Menopause in the 1990s. *Technical report* 866, Geneva, Switzerland

[2] Meister LA, Meadows AT. Late effects of childhood cancer. *Curr Probl Pediatr* 1993;23: 102-31

[3] Goodwin PJ, Ennis M, Pritchard KI, Trudeau M, Hood N. Risk of menopause during the first year after breast cancer diagnosis. *J Clin Oncol.* 1999 Aug;17(8):2365-70

[4] Bokemeyer C, Schmoll HJ, van Rhee J, Kuczyk M, Schuppert F, Poliwoda H. ong-term gonadal toxicity after therapy for Hodgkin's and non-Hodgkin's lymphoma. *Ann Hematol.* 1994 Mar;68(3):105-10.

[5] C. L. Shapiro and A. Recht Side Effects of Adjuvant Treatment of Breast Cancer. *N. Engl. J. Med., June 28,* 2001;344(26): 1997 - 2008.

[6] Wallace WH, Thomson AB, Kelsey TW. The radiosensitivity of the human oocyte. *Hum Reprod.* 2003 Jan;18(1):117-21

[7] Wallace WH, Thomson AB, Saran F, Kelsey TW. Predicting age of ovarian failure after radiation to a field that includes the ovaries. *Int J Radiat Oncol Biol Phys.* 2005 Jul 1;62(3):738-44.

[8] Hendrix SL.Bilateral oophorectomy and premature menopause. *Am J Med.* 2005 Dec 9;118(12 Suppl 2):131-5

[9] Oldenhave A, Jaszmann LJ, Everaerd WT, Haspels AA. Hysterectomized women with ovarian conservation report more severe climacteric complaints than do normal climacteric women of similar age. *Am J Obstet Gynecol.* 1993 Mar;168(3 Pt 1):765-71

[10] Riedel HH, Lehmann-Willenbrock E, Semm K. Ovarian failure phenomena after hysterectomy. *J Reprod Med.* 1986 Jul;31(7):597-600.

[11] Szlachter BN, Nachtigall LE, Epstein J, et al. Premature ovarian failure: A reversible entity? *Obstet Gynecol* 1979;54:396–398

[12] Rebar RW, Connolly HV. Clinical features of young women with hypergonadotropic amenorrhea. *Fertil Steril* 1990;53:804–810

[13] Elit L, Esplen MJ, Butler K, Narod S. Quality of life and psychosexual adjustment after prophylactic oophorectomy for a family history of ovarian cancer. *Fam Cancer.* 2001;1(3-4):149-56

[14] Ganz PA. Menopause and breast cancer: symptoms, late effects, and their management. *Semin Oncol.* 2001 Jun;28(3):274-83. Review

[15] Berg G, Gottwall T, Hammar M, Lindgren R. Climacteric symptoms among women aged 60-62 in Linkoping, Sweden, in 1986.Maturitas. 1988 Oct;10(3):193-9. Erratum in: *Maturitas* 1988 Dec;10(4):363. Gottgall T [corrected to Gottwall T

[16] Judd HL, Lucas WE, Yen SS. Serum 17 beta-estradiol and estrone levels in postmenopausal women with and without endometrial cancer. *J Clin Endocrinol Metab.* 1976 Aug;43(2):272-8.

[17] Laughlin GA, Barrett-Connor E, Kritz-Silverstein D, von Muhlen D. Hysterectomy, oophorectomy, and endogenous sex hormone levels in older women: the Rancho Bernardo Study. *J Clin Endocrinol Metab.* 2000 Feb;85(2):645-51

[18] Bancroft J, Loftus J, Long JS. Distress about sex: a national survey of women in heterosexual relationships. *Arch Sex Behav.* 2003 Jun;32(3):193-208.

[19] Crandall C, Petersen L, Ganz PA, Greendale GA. Association of breast cancer and its therapy with menopause-related symptoms. *Menopause.* 2004 Sep-Oct;11(5):519-30

[20] Knobf MT. Carrying on: the experience of premature menopause in women with early stage breast cancer. *Nurs Res.* 2002 Jan-Feb;51(1):9- 17

[21] Jacobsen BK, Heuch I, Kvale G. Age at natural menopause and all-cause mortality: a 37-year follow-up of 19,731 Norwegian women. *Am J Epidemiol* 2003;157:923–929

[22] Kannel WB, Hjortland MC, McNamara PM, Gordon T. Menopause and risk of cardiovascular disease: the Framingham study. *Ann Intern Med.* 1976 Oct;85(4):447-52

[23] Colditz GA, Willett WC, Stampfer MJ, Rosner B, Speizer FE, Hennekens CH. Menopause and the risk of coronary heart disease in women. *N Engl J Med.* 1987 Apr 30;316(18):1105-10

[24] van der Schouw YT, van der Graaf Y, Steyerberg EW, Eijkemans JC, Banga JD. Age at menopause as a risk factor for cardiovascular mortality. *Lancet.* 1996 Mar 16;347(9003):714-8

[25] BRIEF REPORT: Coronary Heart Disease Events Associated with Hormone Therapy in Younger and Older Women. A Meta-Analysis Shelley R Salpeter MD, Judith ME Walsh MD, MPH, Elizabeth Greyber MD, Edwin E Salpeter PhD *Journal of General Internal Medicine* 2006 21:4 363

[26] Mack WJ, Slater CC, Xiang M, Shoupe D, Lobo RA, Hodis HN. Elevated subclinical atherosclerosis associated with oophorectomy is related to time since menopause rather than type of menopause. *Fertil Steril.* 2004 Aug;82(2):391-7.

[27] Joakimsen O, Bonaa KH, Stensland-Bugge E, Jacobsen BK. Population-based study of age at menopause and ultrasound assessed carotid atherosclerosis: The Tromso Study. *J Clin Epidemiol.* 2000 May;53(5):525-30.

[28] Ouyang P, Michos ED, Karas RH. Hormone replacement therapy and the cardiovascular system lessons learned and unanswered questions. *J Am Coll Cardiol.* 2006 May 2;47(9):1741-53. Epub 2006 Apr 17. Review

[29] Molina JR, Barton DL, Loprinzi CL. Chemotherapy-induced ovarian failure: manifestations and management. *Drug Saf.* 2005;28(5):401-16. Review.

[30] Ramaswamy B, Shapiro CL. Osteopenia and osteoporosis in women with breast cancer. *Semin Oncol.* 2003 Dec;30(6):763-75. Review

[31] Chlebowski RT. Bone health in women with early-stage breast cancer. *Clin Breast Cancer.* 2005 Feb;5 Suppl(2):S35-40. Review

[32] Mackey JR, Joy AA. Skeletal health in postmenopausal survivors of early breast cancer. *Int J Cancer.* 2005 May 10;114(6):1010-5. Review.

[33] Kelly J, Damron T, Grant W, Anker C, Holdridge S, Shaw S, Horton J, Cherrick I, Spadaro J. Cross-sectional study of bone mineral density in adult survivors of solid pediatric cancers. *J Pediatr Hematol Oncol.* 2005 May;27(5):248-53

[34] Shapiro CL, Manola J, Leboff M. Ovarian failure after adjuvant chemotherapy is associated with rapid bone loss in women with early-stage breast cancer. *J Clin Oncol.* 2001 Jul 15;19(14):3306-11

[35] Lester J, Dodwell D, McCloskey E, Coleman R. The causes and treatment of bone loss associated with carcinoma of the breast. *Cancer Treat Rev.* 2005 Apr;31(2):115-42. Review

[36] Kanis JA, McCloskey EV, Powles T, et al. A high incidence of vertebral fracture in women with breast cancer. *Br J Cancer* 1999; 79: 1179-81

[37] Howell A, Cuzick J, Baum M, Buzdar A, Dowsett M, Forbes JF, Hoctin-Boes G, Houghton J, Locker GY, Tobias JS; ATAC Trialists' Group. Results of the ATAC (Arimidex, Tamoxifen, Alone or in Combination) trial after completion of 5 years' adjuvant treatment for breast cancer. *Lancet.* 2005 Jan 1-7;365(9453):60-2.

[38] Goss PE, Ingle JN, Martino S, Robert NJ, Muss HB, Piccart MJ, Castiglione M, Tu D, Shepherd LE, Pritchard KI, Livingston RB, Davidson NE, Norton L, Perez EA, Abrams JS, Cameron DA, Palmer MJ, Pater JL. Randomized trial of letrozole following tamoxifen as extended adjuvant therapy in receptor-positive breast cancer: updated findings from NCIC CTG MA.17. *J Natl Cancer Inst.* 2005 Sep 7;97(17):1262-71

[39] Early Breast Cancer Trialists' Collaborative Group. Tamoxifen benefits of estrogen plus progestin in healthy postmenopausal for early breast cancer: an overview of the randomized trials. *Lancet* 1998; 351: 1451-67

[40] McCune JS, Games DM, Espirito JL. Assessment of ovarian failure and osteoporosis in premenopausal breast cancer survivors. *J Oncol Pharm Pract*. 2005 Jun;11(2):37-43

[41] McCune JS, Games DM, Espirito JL. Assessment of ovarian failure and osteoporosis in premenopausal breast cancer survivors. *J Oncol Pharm Pract*. 2005 Jun;11(2):37-43.

[42] Hillner BE, Ingle JN, Chlebowski RT, Gralow J, Yee GC, Janjan NA, Cauley JA, Blumenstein BA, Albain KS, Lipton A, Brown S; American Society of Clinical Oncology. American Society of Clinical Oncology 2003 update on the role of bisphosphonates and bone health issues in women with breast cancer. J Clin Oncol. 2003 Nov 1;21(21):4042-57. Epub 2003 Sep 8. Erratum in: *J Clin Oncol*. 2004 Apr 1;22(7):1351

[43] Daly E, Gray A, Barlow D, McPherson K, Roche M, Vessey M Measuring the impact of menopausal symptoms on quality of life. *BMJ*. 1993 Oct 2;307(6908):836-40

[44] Schultz PN, Klein MJ, Beck ML, Stava C, Sellin RV. Breast cancer: relationship between menopausal symptoms, physiologic health effects of cancer treatment and physical constraints on quality of life in long-term survivors. *J Clin Nurs*. 2005 Feb;14(2):204-11

[45] Harris PF, Remington PL, Trentham-Dietz A, Allen CI, Newcomb PA. Prevalence and treatment of menopausal symptoms among breast cancer survivors. *J Pain Symptom Manage*. 2002 Jun;23(6):501-9

[46] Gupta P, Sturdee DW, Palin SL, Majumder K, Fear R, Marshall T, Paterson I. Menopausal symptoms in women treated for breast cancer: the prevalence and severity of symptoms and their perceived effects on quality of life. *Climacteric*. 2006 Feb;9(1):49-58

[47] Morales L, Neven P, Timmerman D, Christiaens MR, Vergote I, Van Limbergen E, Carbonez A, Van Huffel S, Ameye L, Paridaens R. Acute effects of tamoxifen and third-generation aromatase inhibitors on menopausal symptoms of breast cancer patients. *Anticancer Drugs*. 2004 Sep;15(8):753-60

[48] Nancy Fugate Woods, PhD, RN, Ellen Sullivan Mitchell, PhD, RN Symptoms during the menopausal transition: prevalence, severity, trajectory, and significance in women's lives. *The American Journal of Medicine* (2005) Vol 118 (12B), 14S–24S

[49] Stearns V, Ullmer L, Lopez JF, Smith Y, Isaacs C, Hayes D. Hot flushes. *Lancet*. 2002 Dec ;360(9348):1851-61.

[50] Rodstrom K, Bengtsson C, Lissner L, Milsom I, Sundh V, Bjorkelund C. A longitudinal study of the treatment of hot flushes: the population study of women in Gothenburg during a quarter of a century. *Menopause*. 2002 May-Jun;9(3):156-61

[51] Freedman RR. Physiology of hot flashes. Am J Hum Biol 2001;13:453–64.

[52] Freedman RR. Hot flashes: behavioral treatments, mechanisms, and relation to sleep. *Am J Med*. 2005 Dec 19;118(12 Suppl 2):124-30.

[53] Freedman RR, Krell W. Reduced thermoregulatory null zone in postmenopausal women with hot flashes. *Am J Obstet Gynecol* 1999; 181: 66–70.

[54] MacLennan AH, Broadbent JL, Lester S, Moore V. Oral oestrogen and combined oestrogen/progestogen therapy versus placebo for hot flushes. The Cochrane Database of Systematic Reviews 2004, Issue 4. Art. No.: CD002978. DOI: 10.1002/14651858.CD002978.pub2

[55] http://www.coolfemme.ca

[56] Wilbur J, Miller AM, McDevitt J, Wang E, Miller J. Menopausal status, moderate-intensity walking, and symptoms in midlife women. *Res Theory Nurs Pract*. 2005 Summer;19(2):163-80.

[57] Germaine LM, Freedman RR. Behavioral treatment of menopausal hot flashes: evaluation by objective methods. *J Consult Clin Psychol*. 1984;52:1072–1079.

[58] Freedman RR, Woodward S. Behavioral treatment of menopausal hot flushes: evaluation by ambulatory monitoring. *Am J Obstet Gynecol*. 1992;167:436–439

[59] Freedman RR, Woodward S, Brown B, Javaid JI, Pandey GN. Biochemical and thermoregulatory effects of behavioral treatment for menopausal hot flashes. *Menopause*. 1995;2:211–218

[60] Low Dog, Tieraona Menopause: a review of botanical dietary supplements. *Amer. J Med* 2005 118 (12) Suppl Dec pp. 98-108

[61] Desindes, S, Belisle, S, Graves, G. SOGC Consensus on Menopause JOGC 2006 *in press*

[62] Geller SE, Studee L. Botanical and dietary supplements for menopausal symptoms: what works, what does not. *J Womens Health* 2005 Sep;14(7):634-49.

[63] Whiting PW, Clouston A, Kerlin P. Black cohosh and other herbal remedies associated with acute hepatitis. *Med J Aust*. 2002 Oct 21;177(8):440-3.

[64] Newton KM, Buist DS, Keenan NL, Anderson LA, LaCroix AZ. Use of alternative therapies for menopause symptoms: results of a population-based survey. Obstet Gynecol. 2002 Jul;100(1):18-25. Erratum in: *Obstet Gynecol* 2003 Jan;101(1):205

[65] Krebs EE, Ensrud KE, MacDonald R, Wilt TJ. Phytoestrogens for treatment of menopausal symptoms: a systematic review. *Obstet Gynecol*. 2004 Oct;104(4):824-36

[66] Phipps WR, Duncan AM, Kurzer MS. Isoflavones and postmenopausal women: a critical review. *Treat Endocrinol*. 2002;1(5):293-311

[67] Nelson HD, Vesco KK, Haney E, Fu R, Nedrow A, Miller J, Nicolaidis C, Walker M, Humphrey L. Nonhormonal therapies for menopausal hot flashes: systematic review and meta-analysis. *JAMA*. 2006 May 3;295(17):2057-71

[68] Barentsen R. Red clover isoflavones and menopausal health. *J Br Menopause Soc*. 2004 Mar;10 Suppl 1:4-7

[69] Huntley A. Drug-herb interactions with herbal medicines for menopause. *J Br Menopause Soc*. 2004 Dec;10(4):162-5

[70] Woodward KN. The potential impact of the use of homeopathic and herbal remedies on monitoring the safety of prescription products. *Hum Exp Toxicol*. 2005 May;24(5):219-33.

[71] Heck AM, DeWitt BA, Lukes AL. Potential interactions between alternative therapies and warfarin *Am J Health Syst Pharm*. 2000 Jul 1;57(13):1221-7

[72] Sparreboom A, Cox MC, Acharya MR, Figg WD. Herbal remedies in the United States: potential adverse interactions with anticancer agents. *J Clin Oncol.* 2004 Jun 15;22(12):2489-503

[73] Petrakis NL, Barnes S, King EB, et al: Stimulatory influence of soy protein isolate on breast secretion in pre- and postmenopausal women. *Cancer Epidemiol Biomarkers Prev 5*:785-794, 1996

[74] Hargreaves DF, Potten CS, Harding C, et al: Two-week dietary soy supplementation has an estrogenic effect on normal premenopausal breast. *J Clin Endocrinol Metab 84*:4017-4024, 1999

[75] Allred CD, Allred KF, Ju YH, et al: Soy diets containing varying amounts of genistein stimulate growth of estrogen-dependent (MCF-7) tumors in a dose-dependent manner. *Cancer Res 61*:5045-5050, 2001

[76] Ju YH, Doerge DR, Allred KF, et al: Dietary genistein negates the inhibitory effects of tamoxifen on growth of estrogen-dependent human breast cancer (MCF-7) cells in athymic mice. *Cancer Res 62*:2474-2477, 2002

[77] Limer JL, Parkes AT, Speirs V. Differential response to phytoestrogens in endocrine sensitive and resistant breast cancer cells in vitro.*Int J Cancer*. 2006 Aug 1;119(3):515-21

[78] Ju YH, Doerge DR, Allred KF, Allred CD, Helferich WG. Dietary genistein negates the inhibitory effect of tamoxifen on growth of estrogen-dependent human breast cancer (MCF-7) cells implanted in athymic mice. *Cancer Res*. 2002 May 1;62(9):2474-7

[79] Wesierska-Gadek J, Schreiner T, Gueorguieva M, Ranftler C. Phenol red reduces ROSC mediated cell cycle arrest and apoptosis in human MCF-7 cells. *J Cell Biochem*. 2006 Jun 1; [Epub ahead of print]

[80] Loprinzi CL, Stearns V, Barton D. Centrally active nonhormonal hot flash therapies. *Am J Med*. 2005 Dec 19;118(12 Suppl 2):118-23

[81] Fugate SE, Church CO. Nonestrogen treatment modalities for vasomotor symptoms associated with menopause. *Ann Pharmacother*. 2004 Sep;38(9):1482-99. Epub 2004 Aug 3.

[82] Nagamani M, Kelver ME, Smith ER. Treatment of menopausal hot flashes with transdermal administration of clonidine. *Am J Obstet Gynecol*. 1987 Mar;156(3):561-5.

[83] Pandya KJ, Raubertas RF, Flynn PJ, Hynes HE, Rosenbluth RJ, Kirshner JJ, Pierce HI, Dragalin V, Morrow GR. Oral clonidine in postmenopausal patients with breast cancer experiencing tamoxifen-induced hot flashes: a University of Rochester Cancer Center Community Clinical Oncology Program study. *Ann Intern Med*. 2000 May 16;132(10):788-93

[84] Goldberg RM, Loprinzi CL, O'Fallon JR, Veeder MH, Miser AW, Mailliard JA, Michalak JC, Dose AM, Rowland KM Jr, Burnham NL. Transdermal clonidine for ameliorating tamoxifen-induced hot flashes. *J Clin Oncol*. 1994 Jan;12(1):155-8. Erratum in: J Clin Oncol 1996 Aug;14(8):2411

[85] Freedman RR, Dinsay R. Clonidine raises the sweating threshold in symptomatic but not in asymptomatic postmenopausal women. *Fertil Steril*. 2000 Jul;74(1):20-3

[86] Stearns V, Beebe KL, Iyengar M, Dube E. Paroxetine controlled release in the treatment of menopausal hot flashes: a randomized controlled trial. *JAMA* 2003;289:2827–34.

[87] Weitzner MA, Moncello J, Jacobsen PB, Minton S. A pilot trial of paroxetine for the treatment of hot flashes and associated symptoms in women with breast cancer. *J Pain Symptom Manage* 2002;23:337– 45.

[88] Stearns V, Johnson MD, Rae JM, Morocho A, Novielli A, Bhargava P, Hayes DF, Desta Z, Flockhart DA. Active tamoxifen metabolite plasma concentrations after coadministration of tamoxifen and the selective serotonin reuptake inhibitor paroxetine. *J Natl Cancer Inst.* 2003 Dec 3;95(23):1758-64.

[89] Jin Y, Desta Z, Stearns V, Ward B, Ho H, Lee KH, Skaar T, Storniolo AM, Li L, Araba A, Blanchard R, Nguyen A, Ullmer L, Hayden J, Lemler S, Weinshilboum RM, Rae JM, Hayes DF, Flockhart DA. CYP2D6 genotype, antidepressant use, and tamoxifen metabolism during adjuvant breast cancer treatment. *J Natl Cancer Inst.* 2005 Jan 5;97(1):30-9.

[90] Biglia N, Torta R, Roagna R, Maggiorotto F, Cacciari F, Ponzone R, Kubatzki F, Sismondi P. Evaluation of low-dose venlafaxine hydrochloride for the therapy of hot flushes in breast cancer survivors. *Maturitas.* 2005 Sep 16;52(1):78-85

[91] Loprinzi CL, Levitt R, Barton D, Sloan JA, Dakhil SR, Nikcevich DA, Bearden JD 3rd, Mailliard JA, Tschetter LK, Fitch TR, Kugler JW. Phase III comparison of depomedroxyprogesterone acetate to venlafaxine for managing hot flashes: North Central Cancer Treatment Group Trial N99C7. *J Clin Oncol.* 2006 Mar 20;24(9):1409-14. Epub 2006 Feb 27

[92] Guttuso T Jr, Kurlan R, McDermott MP, Kieburtz K. Gabapentin's effects on hot flashes in postmenopausal women: a randomized controlled trial. *Obstet Gynecol.* 2003 Feb;101(2):337-45

[93] Pandya KJ, Morrow GR, Roscoe JA, Zhao H, Hickok JT, Pajon E, Sweeney TJ, Banerjee TK, Flynn PJ. Gabapentin for hot flashes in 420 women with breast cancer: a randomised double-blind placebo-controlled trial. *Lancet.* 2005 Sep 3-9;366(9488):818-24.

[94] Nelson HD. Commonly used types of postmenopausal estrogen for treatment of hot flashes: scientific review. *JAMA.* 2004 Apr 7;291(13):1610-20

[95] Post MS, van der Mooren MJ, van Baal WM, Blankenstein MA, Merkus HM, Kroeks MV, Franke HR, Kenemans P, Stehouwer CD. Effects of low-dose oral and transdermal estrogen replacement therapy on hemostatic factors in healthy postmenopausal women: a randomized placebo-controlled study. *Am J Obstet Gynecol.* 2003 Nov;189(5):1221-7.

[96] Scarabin PY, Oger E, Plu-Bureau G; EStrogen and THromboEmbolism Risk Study Group. Differential association of oral and transdermal oestrogen-replacement therapy with venous thromboembolism risk. *Lancet.* 2003 Aug 9;362(9382):428-32.

[97] Eilertsen AL, Hoibraaten E, Os I, Andersen TO, Sandvik L, Sandset PM. The effects of oral and transdermal hormone replacement therapy on C-reactive protein levels and other inflammatory markers in women with high risk of thrombosis. *Maturitas.* 2005 Oct 16;52(2):111-8.

[98] Harvey J, Scheurer C, Kawakami FT, Quebe-Fehling E, de Palacios PI, Ragavan VV. ormone replacement therapy and breast density changes. *Climacteric*. 2005 Jun;8(2):185-92

[99] Ettinger B. Vasomotor symptom relief versus unwanted effects: role of estrogen dosage. *Am J Med*. 2005 Dec 19;118(12 Suppl 2):74-8

[100] Crandall C. Low-dose estrogen therapy for menopausal women: a review of efficacy and safety. *J Womens Health (Larchmt)*. 2003 Oct;12(8):723-47

[101] Grodstein F, Manson JE, Colditz GA, Willett WC, Speizer FE, Stampfer MJ. A prospective, observational study of postmenopausal hormone therapy and primary prevention of cardiovascular disease. *Ann Intern Med*. 2000 Dec 19;133(12):933-41

[102] Collins JA, Blake JM, Crosignani PG. Breast cancer risk with postmenopausal hormonal treatment. *Hum Reprod Update*. 2005 Nov-Dec;11(6):545-60. Epub 2005 Sep 8.

[103] Clemons M, Clamp A, Anderson B. Management of the menopause in cancer survivors. *Cancer Treat Rev*. 2002 Dec;28(6):321-33. Review

[104] Pritchard KI, Khan H, Levine M; Steering Committee on Clinical Practice Guidelines for the Care and Treatment of Breast Cancer. Clinical practice guidelines for the care and treatment of breast cancer: 14. The role of hormone replacement therapy in women with a previous diagnosis of breast cancer. *CMAJ*. 2002 Apr 16;166(8):1017-22. Review

[105] Creasman WT. Hormone replacement therapy after cancers. *Curr Opin Oncol*. 2005 Sep;17(5):493-9. Review

[106] Biglia N, Gadducci A, Ponzone R, Roagna R, Sismondi P. Hormone replacement therapy in cancer survivors. *Maturitas*. 2004 Aug 20;48(4):333-46. Review

[107] Col NF, Kim JA, Chlebowski RT. Menopausal hormone therapy after breast cancer: a meta-analysis and critical appraisal of the evidence. *Breast Cancer Res*. 2005;7(4):R535-40. Epub 2005 May 19

[108] Meurer LN, Lena S. Cancer recurrence and mortality in women using hormone replacement therapy: meta-analysis. *J Fam Pract*. 2002 Dec;51(12):1056-62.

[109] Suriano KA, McHale M, McLaren CE, Li KT, Re A, DiSaia PJ. Estrogen replacement therapy in endometrial cancer patients: a matched control study.*Obstet Gynecol*. 2001 Apr;97(4):555-60

[110] Chapman JA, DiSaia PJ, Osann K, Roth PD, Gillotte DL, Berman ML. Estrogen replacement in surgical stage I and II endometrial cancer survivors. *Am J Obstet Gynecol*. 1996 Nov;175(5):1195-200

[111] Lee RB, Burke TW, Park RC. Estrogen replacement therapy following treatment for stage I endometrial carcinoma. *Gynecol Oncol*. 1990 Feb;36(2):189-91

[112] Creasman WT, Henderson D, Hinshaw W, Clarke-Pearson DL. Estrogen replacement therapy in the patient treated for endometrial cancer. *Obstet Gynecol*. 1986 Mar;67(3):326-30.

[113] Holmberg L, Anderson H; HABITS steering and data monitoring committees. ABITS (hormonal replacement therapy after breast cancer--is it safe?), a randomised comparison: trial stopped. *Lancet*. 2004 Feb 7;363(9407):453-5

[114] von Schoultz E, Rutqvist LE; Stockholm Breast Cancer Study Group. Menopausal hormone therapy after breast cancer: the Stockholm randomized trial. *J Natl Cancer Inst*. 2005 Apr 6;97(7):533-5.

[115] Chlebowski RT, Anderson GL. Progestins and recurrence in breast cancer survivors. *J Natl Cancer Inst*. 2005 Apr 6;97(7):471-2.

[116] Kwan K, Ward C, Marsden J. Is there a role for hormone replacement therapy after breast cancer? *J Br Menopause Soc*. 2005 Dec;11(4):140-4. Review.

[117] Batur P, Blixen CE, Moore HC, Thacker HL, Xu M. Menopausal hormone therapy (HT) in patients with breast cancer. *Maturitas*. 2006 Jan 20;53(2):123-32. Review.

[118] Gold EB, Sternfeld B, Kelsey JL, et al. Relation of demographic and lifestyle factors to symptoms in a multi-racial/ethnic population of women 40–55 years of age. *Am J Epidemiol*. 2000;152:463– 473.

[119] Moe KE. Hot flashes and sleep in women. *Sleep Med Rev*. 2004 Dec;8(6):487-97

[120] Dzaja A, Arber S, Hislop J, Kerkhofs M, Kopp C, Pollmacher T, Polo-Kantola P, Skene DJ, Stenuit P, Tobler I, Porkka-Heiskanen T. Women's sleep in health and disease. *J Psychiatr Res*. 2005 Jan;39(1):55-76

[121] Tworoger SS, Yasui Y, Vitiello MV, Schwartz RS, Ulrich CM, Aiello EJ, Irwin ML, Bowen D, Potter JD, McTiernan A. Effects of a yearlong moderate-intensity exercise and a stretching intervention on sleep quality in postmenopausal women. *Sleep*. 2003 Nov 1;26(7):830-6

[122] Brunner RL, Gass M, Aragaki A, Hays J, Granek I, Woods N, Mason E, Brzyski R, Ockene J, Assaf A, LaCroix A, Matthews K, Wallace R; Women's Health Initiative Investigators. Effects of conjugated equine estrogen on health-related quality of life in postmenopausal women with hysterectomy: results from the Women's Health Initiative Randomized Clinical. *Arch Intern Med*. 2005 Sep 26;165(17):1976-86

[123] Polo-Kantola P, Erkkola R, Helenius H, Irjala K, Polo O. When does estrogen replacement therapy improve sleep quality? *Am J Obstet Gynecol*. 1998 May;178(5):1002-9

[124] Gambacciani M, Ciaponi M, Cappagli B, Monteleone P, Benussi C, Bevilacqua G, Vacca F, Genazzani AR. Effects of low-dose, continuous combined hormone replacement therapy on sleep in symptomatic postmenopausal women. *Maturitas*. 2005 Feb 14;50(2):91-7

[125] Kaufert PA, Gilbert P, Tate R. The Manitoba Project: a re-examination of the link between menopause and depression. *Maturitas*. 1992;14:143–155

[126] Avis NE, Crawford S, Stellato R, et al. Longitudinal study of hormone levels and depression among women transitioning through menopause.Climacteric. 2001;4:243–249

[127] Woods NF, Mariella A, Mitchell E. Patterns of depressed mood across the MT: approaches to studying patterns in longitudinal data. *Acta Obstet Gynecol Scand*. 2002;81:623– 632.

[128] Brornberger, Joyce T. Meyer, Peter M. Kravitz, Howard M. Sommer, Barbara Cordal, Adriana Powell, Lynda Ganz, Patricia A. Sutton-Tyrrell, Kim, Psychologic Distress and Natural Menopause. *American Journal of Public Health*; Sep2001, 91; (9), p1435-43

[129] Avis NE, Brambilla D, McKinlay SM, Vass K. A longitudinal analysis of the association between menopause and depression: results from the Massachusetts women's health survey. *Ann Epidemiol* 1994;4:214-2

[130] Avis NE, Crawford S, Stellato R, Longcope C. Longitudinal study of hormone levels and depression among women transitioning through menopause. *Climacteric.* 2001 Sep;4(3):243-9

[131] Guthrie JR, Dennerstein L, Taffe JR, Lehert P, Burger HG. The menopausal transition: a 9-year prospective population-based study. The Melbourne Women's Midlife Health Project. *Climacteric.* 2004 Dec;7(4):375-89

[132] Zweifel JE, O'Brien WH. A meta-analysis of the effect of hormone replacement therapy upon depressed mood. Psychoneuroendocrinology. 1997 Apr;22(3):189-212. Erratum in: *Psychoneuroendocrinology* 1997 Nov;22(8):655

[133] Schmidt, Peter J Mood, depression, and reproductive hormones in the menopausal transition. *The American Journal of Medicine* 2005 Volume: 118, Issue: 12, Supplement 2 December 19 pp 54-58

[134] Grigoriadis S, Sherwin, B Mood and Memory Disorders JOGC 2006 *in press*

[135] Morrison MF, Kallan MJ, Ten Have T, Katz I, Tweedy K, Battistini M. Lack of efficacy of estradiol for depression in postmenopausal women: a randomized, controlled. *Biol Psychiatry.* 2004 Feb 15;55(4):406-12

[136] Schmidt PJ, Nieman L, Danaceau MA, Tobin MB, Roca CA, Murphy JH et al. Estrogen replacement in perimenopause-related depression: A preliminary report. *Am J Obstet Gynecol* 2000;183:414-20

[137] De Noaves Soares C, Almeida OP, Joffee H, Cohen LS. Efficacy of estradiol for the treatment of depressive disorders in perimenopausal women. *Arch Gen Psychiatry* 2001;58:529-34

[138] Stenberg A, Heimer G, Ulmsten U, Cnattingus S. Prevalence of genitourinary and other climacteric symptoms in 61-year-old women. *Maturitas* 1996;24:31–6

[139] Romanzi LJ, Groutz A, Feroz F, Blaivas JG. Evaluation of female external genitalia sensitivity to pressure/touch: a preliminary prospective study using Semmes-Weinstein monofilaments. *Urology* 2001;57(6):1145-50

[140] Berg G, Gottqall T, Hammar M, Lindgren R. Climacteric symptoms among women aged 60-62 in Linkoping, Sweden in 1986. *Maturitas* 1988;10:193-9

[141] Johnston, SL, Farrell, SA, Bouchard, C et al SOGC Joint Committee – Clinical Practice Gynaecology and Urogynaecology. Detection and management of urogenital atrophy. *JOGC* 2004; 26 (%): 503-15

[142] Castelo-Branco C, Cancelo MJ, Villero J, Nohales F, Julia MD. Management of post-menopausal vaginal atrophy and atrophic vaginitis. *Maturitas.* 2005 Nov 15;52 Suppl 1:S46-52. Epub 2005 Sep 1.

[143] Leiblum S, Bachmann G, Kemmann E, Colburn D, Swartzman L Vaginal atrophy in the postmenopausal woman. The importance of sexual activity and hormones. *JAMA.* 1983 Apr 22-29;249(16):2195-8

[144] Pandit L, Ouslander JG. Postmenopausal vaginal atrophy and atrophic vaginitis. *Am J Med Sci.* 1997 Oct;314(4):228-31

[145] Bygdeman M, Swah ML. Replens versus dlienoestrol cream in symptomatic treatment of vaginal atrophy in postmenopausal women. *Maturitas* 1996;23:259–63

[146] Nachtigall LE. Comparative study: Replens versus local estrogen in menopausal women. *Fertil Steril* 1994;61:178–80

[147] Palacios S, Castelo-Branco C, Cancelo MJ, Vazquez F. Low-dose, vaginally administered estrogens may enhance local benefits of systemic therapy in the treatment of urogenital atrophy in postmenopausal women on hormone therapy. *Maturitas.* 2005 Feb 14;50(2):98-104

[148] Cardozo L, Bachmann G, McClish D, Fonda D, Birgerson L. Meta-analysis of estrogen therapy in the management of urogenital atrophy in postmenopausal women: second report of the Hormones and Urogenital Therapy Committee. *Obstet Gynecol.* 1998 Oct;92(4 Pt 2):722-7

[149] Suckling J, Lethaby A, Kennedy R. Local oestrogen for vaginal atrophy in postmenopausal women. *Cochrane Database Syst Rev.* 2003;(4):CD001500

[150] Weisberg E, Ayton R, Darling G, Farrell E, Murkies A, O'Neill S, Kirkegard Y, Fraser IS. Endometrial and vaginal effects of low-dose estradiol delivered by vaginal ring or vaginal tablet. *Climacteric.* 2005 Mar;8(1):83-92

[151] Gabrielsson, Johan; Wallenbeck, Ingrid; Larsson, Gregor; Birgerson, Lars; Heimer, Gun Studies of the low dose ring have shown negligible serum levels New kinetic data on estradiol in light of the vaginal ring concept. *Maturitas* pp. S35-S39 and have not showm any endometrial response

[152] Bachmann G. The estradiol vaginal ring--a study of existing clinical data. *Maturitas.* 1995 Dec;22 Suppl:S21-9

[153] Bakos O, Smith P, Heimer G, Ulmsten U. Transvaginal sonography of the internal genital organs in postmenopausal women on low-dose estrogen treatment. *Ultrasound Obstet Gynecol.* 1994 Jul 1;4(4):326-9.

[154] Rioux JE, Devlin C, Gelfand MM, Steinberg WM, Hepburn DS 17beta-estradiol vaginal tablet versus conjugated equine estrogen vaginal cream to relieve menopausal atrophic vaginitis. *Menopause.* 2000 May-Jun;7(3):156-61

[155] Johnston, S. SOGC *Canadian Consensus on Menopause* 2006 JOGC *in press*

[156] Ballagh SA. Vaginal hormone therapy for urogenital and menopausal symptoms. *Semin Reprod Med.* 2005 May;23(2):126-40

[157] Dew JE, Wren BG, Eden JA. A cohort study of topical vaginal estrogen therapy in women previously treated for breast cancer. *Climacteric.* 2003 Mar;6(1):45-52

[158] Maccormick RE. Possible acceleration of aging by adjuvant chemotherapy: A cause of early onset frailty? *Med Hypotheses.* 2006;67(2):212-5. Epub 2006 Mar 20

[159] Xu J, Bartoces M, Neale AV, Dailey RK, Northrup J, Schwartz KL Natural history of menopause symptoms in primary care patients: a MetroNet study. *J Am Board Fam Pract.* 2005 Sep-Oct;18(5):374-82.

[160] Szoeke CE, Cicuttini F, Guthrie J, Dennerstein L. Self-reported arthritis and the menopause. *Climacteric.* 2005 Mar;8(1):49-55

[161] Sherman KJ, Cherkin DC, Erro J, Miglioretti DL, Deyo RA. Comparing yoga, exercise, and a self-care book for chronic low back pain: a randomized, controlled trial. *Ann Intern Med.* 2005 Dec 20;143(12):849-56

[162] Dennerstein L, Alexander JL, Kotz K The menopause and sexual functioning: a review of the population-based studies. *Annu Rev Sex Res.* 2003;14:64-82

[163] Lorraine Dennerstein, PhD, Philippe Lehert, PhD, Henry Burger, MD, Janet Guthrie, PhD Sexuality. *The American Journal of Medicine* (2005) Vol 118 (12B), 59S–63S

[164] Bancroft J, Loftus J, Long JS. Distress about sex: a national survey of women in heterosexual relationships. *Arch Sex Behav.* 2003 Jun;32(3):193-208.

[165] Leiblum, Sandra R PhD Koochaki, Patricia E PhD ; Rodenberg, Cynthia A PhD Barton, Ian P BSc Rosen, Raymond C PhD Hypoactive sexual desire disorder in postmenopausal women: US results from the Women's International Study of Health and Sexuality (WISHeS). *Menopause. 13(1)*:46-56, January/February 2006

[166] Basson, R; Graves, G, Johnston, S. SOGC Canadian Consensus on Menopause. *JOGC* 2006 *in press*

SECTION 7: WOMEN WITH CANCER AND THE RISKS OF OTHER MEDICAL DISORDERS

In: Women and Cancer
Editor: Laurie Elit, pp. 293-313

ISBN: 978-1-60021-494-3

Chapter I

Diagnosis and Treatment of Venous Thromboembolism in Women with Cancer

*Agnes Y. Y. Lee**
Department of Medicine, McMaster University, Hamilton, Ontario, Canada.

Abstract

Objective: VTE is a common complication of patients with cancer.

Results: There are several techniques for diagnosing DVT: Doppler U/S is the preferred method due to low cost, high accuracy and high availability. There are several techniques for diagnosing PE: spiral CT scan is the preferred method. Treatment with LMWH or UFH in cancer is acceptable. Use of coumadin or long term LMWH is the subject of investigations.

Conclusion: VTE is a common complication in women with a diagnosis of cancer. Research continues into the optimal management strategy.

Introduction

Venous thromboembolism (VTE) is a common complication in patients with cancer. For women with cancer, the incidence of VTE is increased during treatment with hormonal agents, such as tamoxifen. Pelvic malignancy, with or without nodal involvement, can also increase the risk of VTE. This chapter will review the current standard of care in managing VTE in patients with cancer, focusing on diagnosis and treatment. Aspects that are unique to women with gynecological malignancies are highlighted.

* Correspondence concerning this article should be addressed to Agnes Lee MD, Henderson Hospital, 711 Concession Street Hamilton, Ontario, Canada L8V 1C3. Phone 905 527-4322 ext 42484; Fax 905 574-7625; E-mail: leeagnes@HHSC.CA

Diagnosis of Venous Thromboembolism

Fewer than 25% of patients presenting with symptoms compatible with thrombosis are confirmed to have deep vein thrombosis (DVT) or pulmonary embolism (PE) on objective testing. Therefore, clinical features alone are neither sufficiently sensitive nor specific to diagnose acute thrombosis. However, clinical assessment remains the corner stone for diagnosis and a careful history and physical examination are essential in estimating the clinical probability of DVT/PE to guide diagnostic strategies. In general, patients are first stratified into high, moderate or low risk categories using a validated clinical prediction rule and then undergo objective testing to confirm or refute the presence of thrombus in the leg veins or pulmonary vasculature. For radiological imaging, venous compression ultrasonography has replaced contrast venography for diagnosing proximal DVT because of its high sensitivity and specificity [1]; whereas, spiral or helical computed tomography (CT) or CT angiography has surpassed ventilation-perfusion (VQ) lung scanning as the diagnostic test of choice for PE because of its availability and accuracy in detecting emboli in the main and lobar pulmonary arteries [2]. D-dimer testing is an important and useful investigation for excluding acute DVT or PE in the general population but its accuracy in patients with cancer is somewhat uncertain [3].

In women with cancer, the approaches to diagnosing DVT or PE are similar to the usual strategies but specific risk factors can alter the clinical probability and may influence the accuracy of some of the tests. In women with breast cancer, the use of tamoxifen is a unique extrinsic factor that places them at a higher risk of VTE. Tamoxifen increases the risk of VTE by approximately 4-fold and acts synergistically with chemotherapy. For example, in women with node-negative breast cancer, the risk of VTE over 5 years is 0.2% on placebo, 0.9% on tamoxifen and 4% on tamoxifen combined with chemotherapy [4,5]. The thrombotic effect of tamoxifen is also highest in postmenopausal women [6,7]. Recently, aromatase inhibitors are found to be more efficacious than tamoxifen in the treatment of receptor-positive breast cancer in postmenopausal women [8,9]. These agents are also associated with half the risk of thrombosis.

Another group of women with a high risk of VTE appears to be those with cervical cancer who are receiving concurrent chemotherapy, radiation and recombinant erythropoietin. A risk of VTE as high as 23% has been reported in some series [10,11]. The use of erythropoietin was also reported to be associated with a high incidence of thrombosis in a trial in women with advanced breast cancer [12]. However, it remains uncertain whether erythropoietin is thrombogenic and mechanisms of action have not been identified.

Lastly, injury or extrinsic compression of the pelvic veins will increase the risk of VTE. Women with extensive pelvic tumours or lymphadenopathy experience significant venous stasis in the legs and pelvic surgery to debulk disease with or without nodal dissection can lead to significant endothelial injury. Because both of these mechanisms are potent stimuli for activation of coagulation, physicians caring for such patients must maintain a high clinical suspicion for VTE in these clinical scenarios.

Diagnosis of Deep Vein Thrombosis

Rigorously performed management studies have demonstrated that diagnostic strategies incorporating clinical pretest probability, venous ultrasonography, and D-dimer testing are safe and reliable for diagnosing DVT in unselected patients who present with a first episode of suspected DVT [13]. The success of these algorithms is dependent on the appropriate stratification of patients into different risk groups, the sensitivity and specificity of venous ultrasonography, and the negative predictive value of a sensitive D-dimer assay.

Clinical Assessment

The typical signs and symptoms of DVT are leg pain, tenderness, swelling, and occasionally, discolouration. These clinical manifestations are non-specific and can be found in patients with superficial thrombophlebitis, cellulitis, lymphedema, traumatic hematoma, Baker's cyst and other musculoskeletal conditions [14]. In women with cancer of the pelvis, these symptoms are often present despite the absence of a DVT.

The first step in evaluating a patient with suspected DVT is to establish the clinical likelihood of thrombosis using a validated clinical prediction rule. Based on clinical symptoms and signs and the presence of risk factors, patients are triaged as having a "high", "moderate" or "low" probability of DVT, or classified as "likely" or "unlikely" to have DVT (Table 1) [15-17]. The presence of active cancer alone usually places the patient in the moderate probability or likely group, but the final risk category is determined by the overall score, which is influenced by whether the clinical features could be due to an alternative diagnosis. Based on numerous studies evaluating the Well's prediction rule for DVT, the prevalence of DVT in the low, moderate, and high clinical probability groups is 5%, 17% and 53%, respectively [17]. Consequently, a low score in combination with a negative test result (either D-dimer assay or ultrasonography) effectively and safely excludes acute DVT.

Table 1. Well's Clinical Prediction Rule for Diagnosis of DVT [15]

	Score
Active cancer (treatment ongoing or within previous 6 months or palliative)	1
Paralysis, paresis or recent plaster immobilization of the lower extremities	1
Recently bedridden > 3 days or major surgery within 4 weeks	1
Localized tenderness along the distribution of the deep venous system	1
Entire leg swollen	1
Calf swelling 3 cm > asymptomatic side (measured 10 cm below tibial tuberosity)	1
Pitting edema confined to the symptomatic leg	1
Collateral superficial veins (non-varicose)	1
Alternative diagnosis as likely or greater than that of DVT	-2

Note: In patients with symptoms in both legs, the more symptomatic leg is used.
Pretest probability calculated as: high ≥ 3; moderate 1 or 2; low ≤ 0

It should be noted that although validated clinical prediction rules are useful, they are not designed specifically for patients with cancer. For example, the prediction rules do not distinguish between a cancer patient with metastatic disease who is on chemotherapy and a patient with early-stage disease who is not receiving active treatment; the former patient is at much higher risk of VTE than the latter but most rules do not differentiate the risks of these patients.

Venous Ultrasonography

Venous ultrasonography is the radiological test of choice for the diagnosis of DVT. A noncompressible segment in the popliteal or more proximal veins is considered diagnostic for proximal DVT. Compression or duplex ultrasonography has a sensitivity of 95% and a specificity of 96% for diagnosing symptomatic proximal thrombosis and a sensitivity and specificity of about 60% to 70% for isolated calf vein thrombosis [18]. Aside from its accuracy in diagnosing proximal DVT, compression ultrasonography is a good diagnostic test because it is inexpensive, noninvasive and readily available. Consequently, ultrasonography has largely replaced venography in the clinical setting. However, its accuracy is limited for diagnosing distal DVT.

It is unknown if the accuracy of ultrasonography differs in patients with cancer. It is possible that extrinsic venous obstruction from tumour or nodal masses could cause reduced flow and lack of compressibility that are characteristic of DVT.

Magnetic Resonance Imaging

MRI has several advantages over traditional imaging techniques. Compared with venography, it is non-invasive, more readily available, less technically demanding, and does not expose patients to contrast or radiation. Compared with ultrasonography, it is more sensitive and specific for diagnosing distal DVT and provides better visualization of the pelvis. Also, unlike most imaging techniques that identify thrombus as filling defects, magnetic resonance direct thrombus imaging (MRDTI) visualizes thrombus against a suppressed background [19]. Moreover, MRI has the potential to diagnose PE as well as DVT using a single scan. The major limitations of MR techniques are cost and it cannot be done in patients with claustrophobia or metal devices. Patients must also be able to lie flat for about 15 minutes.

Small accuracy studies comparing it with venography have shown that MRDTI has a sensitivity of 95% and a specificity of 96% for any DVT, a sensitivity of 88% and a specificity of 95% for isolated distal DVT and a sensitivity of 100% and specificity of 100% for ileofemoral DVT [20-22]. Although these results are very promising, validation in management studies is needed before MRDTI can be recommended for general use in diagnosing DVT.

Constrast Venography

Contrast venography remains the reference standard for diagnosing DVT [23]. A thrombus is diagnosed by the presence of a constant intraluminal filling defect detected by radiography after injection of iodinated contrast dye into the leg veins. Because it can visualize the iliac vessels and the entire venous system in the legs, venography can detect pelvic thrombi and small, distal calf clots that are usually missed by noninvasive studies. However, venography is invasive and can be painful. It can be technically difficult to perform, which can lead to inadequate imaging and misinterpretation of the results. Even when it is preformed by experienced radiologists, there is a 5% to 12% frequency of inadequate venograms [23]. Other disadvantages include cost and limited accessibility. Rarely, the contrast medium can precipitate phlebitis and anaphylaxis. It is contraindicated in patients with advanced renal insufficiency.

D-dimer Testing

D-dimer testing was introduced as an alternative or adjunctive test to ultrasonography about 2 decades ago. D-dimer assays measure the level of D-dimer present in a blood sample using quantitative or qualitative methods. Because D-dimer is a degradation product of cross-linked fibrin, it is elevated in acute thrombosis as well as in malignancy, pregnancy, and infection.

Different D-dimer assays vary in their sensitivity and specificity; therefore, the performance of one assay cannot be extrapolated to another [24]. Enzyme-linked immunosorbent assays (ELISAs) have the highest sensitivities, but their specificity is low. Therefore, a negative result using a highly sensitive ELISA is useful in excluding DVT, but a positive result cannot confirm a diagnosis. Studies have now shown that if an ELISA is negative, DVT can be excluded safely without further testing in patients with a low or moderate probability [25]. The major disadvantage of most ELISAs is their cost.

Another D-dimer assay that has been extensively studied is a whole-blood, red cell agglutination assay. This test is unique among D-dimer assays because it can be performed at the bedside using a drop of blood from a fingerstick, and the result is ready in 2 minutes. In contrast to ELISAs, a negative result alone with the whole blood assay cannot rule out acute DVT because the sensitivity is only 85% to 90% [25]. However, acute DVT can be excluded with a negative result in a patient who also has a low clinical probability or a negative ultrasound result [26,27].

One other type of D-dimer assays is based on latex agglutination. In general, these semi-quantitative assays lack sensitivity and specificity and should not be used for diagnosing DVT. However, recent reports show that a new quantitative latex D-dimer assay does have sufficiently high negative predictive value to rule out acute DVT and that a negative result can safely eliminate the need for further testing in patients with low or moderate pretest clinical probability [28,29].

Compared with the performance of D-dimer testing in patients without cancer, the accuracy of D-dimer assays in cancer patients is less certain [3]. To-date, studies have shown inconsistent results. The reduced accuracy of a D-dimer assay in cancer patients was demonstrated in a meta-analysis in which the false-negative rate rose from 3% in non-cancer patients to 21% in cancer patients due to substantial differences in the prevalence of thrombosis and the specificity of the assay between the two patient groups [30]. However, another study evaluating the same assay found no reduction in the negative predictive value [31]. D-dimer testing is also limited in cancer patients because cancer alone can produce a positive result, thereby lowering the specificity and usefulness of the test. Therefore, until D-dimer assays are shown to be accurate and reliable in excluding DVT in cancer patients, D-dimer testing should be used with caution to manage patients with cancer and suspected DVT.

Overall Approach to Diagnosing DVT in Women with Cancer

All women with cancer presenting with symptoms suggestive of DVT should be objectively investigated. After determining the clinical probability using a validated prediction rule, ultrasonography of the involved leg(s) should be performed. In general, when the ultrasound is positive in a cancer patient with a moderate or high clinical probability, acute DVT is confirmed; when the ultrasound result is negative in a patient with low clinical probability, proximal DVT is excluded [32]. In all other cases, when the clinical probability is discordant with the ultrasound result, further testing is required. For example, in a patient with a high clinical probability but a negative ultrasound result, repeat or serial ultrasonography in 1 week should be performed. This will help to detect extension of a calf vein thrombus that might have been missed on initial testing [33]. In addition, because isolated iliac vein thrombosis can be found in those who have pelvic malignancies or have recently undergone abdominopelvic surgery, it is important to image the pelvic vasculature using ultrasonography at initial presentation if routine leg ultrasonography failed to demonstrate DVT. If iliac vein thrombosis is not seen on initial testing, patients with a moderate or high clinical suspicion should be brought back for serial ultrasonography or contrast venography because the risk of PE from an iliac vein or more proximal thrombosis is substantial.

Diagnosis of Pulmonary Embolism

Making a diagnosis of PE remains a challenge. The clinical presentation is variable, and a battery of investigations is often necessary to confirm or refute a diagnosis of PE [34]. Although clinical prediction rules have been validated for diagnosing PE, they are more difficult to apply than models for DVT because of the nonspecific nature of the symptoms and the prevalence of these symptoms in patients with cancer or other medical conditions.

Clinical Assessment

Depending on the severity of the PE, patients may present with complaints ranging from mild shortness of breath to circulatory collapse or sudden death. Physical findings range from an essentially normal exam to tachycardia, arrhythmia, loud S_2, and pleural rub, to an elevated JVP with right heart failure, to hypotension and shock. The classical and most prevalent symptom is shortness of breath, while pleuritic chest pain and hemoptysis are infrequent. All of these features are commonly found in other cardiorespiratory disorders, such as viral or bacterial pneumonia, exacerbation of asthma or chronic obstructive lung disease, ischemic coronary events, and congestive heart failure. In cancer patients, other differential diagnoses include pleural effusions, primary pulmonary malignancy, pulmonary metastases, and lymphangitic carcinomatosis.

Most physicians rely on a history, a physical examination, and some basic laboratory investigations (such as a chest x-rayand an electrocardiogram) to form an impression of the likelihood of PE. This was the approach used in the landmark Prospective Investigation of Pulmonary Embolism Diagnosis (PIOPED) study, in which clinical judgment was found to correlate well with the findings of VQ lung scanning [35]. Since then, many studies evaluating formal clinical assessment models or prediction rules have been published [36-38]. These rules in complexity and, in general, categorize patients into having a low, moderate or high probability of PE (Table 2). The major criticism of these prediction rules is the subjectivity of the judgment about alternative diagnoses. However, they are useful when the result is combined with one or more objective tests to confirm or exclude PE.

Table 2. Well's Clinical Prediction Rule for Diagnosing PE [37]

	Score*
Clinical signs and symptoms of deep venous thrombosis	3.0
Alternative diagnosis deemed less likely than pulmonary embolism	3.0
Heart rate > 100 beats/min	1.5
Immobilization or surgery in the previous 4 weeks	1.5
Previous deep venous thrombosis or pulmonary embolism	1.5
Hemoptysis	1.0
Active cancer (treatment ongoing or within previous 6 months or palliative)	1.0

*Pretest probability is calculated as the sum of the scores: high $\geq$ 6.0; moderate = 2.0 – 6.0; low $\leq$ 2.0.

Ventilation-Perfusion Lung Scanning

VQ lung scanning is the traditional test of choice but it has been replaced by spiral CT in most clinical centres because lung scanning is not widely available and it is nondiagnostic in up to 70% of those who present with suspected PE. In the PIOPED study, the combined use of clinical probability and lung scanning was found to be effective in diagnosing PE [35]. In patients with both a high-probability VQ scan interpretation and a high-probability pretest assessment, the prevalence of PE was 96%. When the VQ scan and clinical assessment indicated a low probability of PE, the prevalence of PE was only 4%. If the VQ scan was normal, PE is ruled out. However, when the VQ scan interpretation and clinical likelihood were discordant, the probability of PE ranged from 16% to 88%. Venous ultrasonography of the legs is often used in these latter cases to help diagnose PE because about 6% of patients with a nondiagnostic VQ scan will have ultrasound evidence of DVT [37]. If the ultrasound result confirms a diagnosis of DVT and the VQ scan is abnormal, then the patient can be treated with anticoagulant therapy. Alternatively, if the ultrasound result is negative, it is safe to withhold anticoagulant therapy in patients without a high probability for PE on both clinical assessment and VQ scanning and follow them with serial ultrasonography [39,40].

Spiral Computed Tomography

Because of the practical and accuracy limitations of VQ scanning, spiral CT has gained wide acceptance because it is readily available in most centers and can provide an alternative diagnosis in one-quarter of cases [41]. However, spiral CT is contraindicated in renal and cardiac failure because patients are exposed to a substantial dose of contrast medium.

Management studies and meta-analyses have shown that spiral CT has a sensitivity of about 70% and a specificity of about 90% for detecting PE [42-44]. It is highly sensitive and specific for PE when an intraluminal filling defect is seen in the central pulmonary vasculature, but it does not have a high sensitivity for emboli in subsegmental and smaller vessels. Therefore, unlike a normal VQ scan, a negative result with spiral CT is not sufficient to exclude a diagnosis of PE because up to 30% of patients with PE are missed [43]. Modern scanners with multi-detectors now provide improved resolution for evaluating subsegmental pulmonary veins but studies confirming the accuracy of spiral CT in diagnosing subsegmental PE are lacking [45].

Outcome studies have demonstrated that it is safe to withhold anticoagulant therapy in patients with a negative spiral CT and negative ultrasound of the legs, particularly in those who do not have a high clinical probability of PE [41,46-49]. Large randomized trials also showed that a diagnostic strategy using a clinical decision rule, D-dimer testing and multi-detector spiral CT is effective and safe for diagnosing PE, without the routine use of leg ultrasonography [43,50].

Magnetic Resonance Imaging

Magnetic resonance angiography (MRA) has been evaluated against pulmonary angiography in diagnosing PE. Based on the limited data available, MRA has a sensitivity of 75 – 90% and specificity of 77 – 100% for PE [51,52]. Similar to spiral CT, it is not sensitive enough to detect isolated subsegmental PE and thus cannot be a stand alone test in ruling out PE.

Pulmonary Angiography

Pulmonary angiography is the reference standard for diagnosing PE but it is technically demanding and invasive. It is associated major complication rate of 0.5% and a mortality rate of 0.1% [53,54]. It involves catheter-directed injection of iodinated contrast into the pulmonary arteries, which allows visualization of emboli to the subsegmental level. Persistent intraluminal filling defects or an abrupt cut-off in an artery with a diameter of greater than 2 mm are diagnostic of PE. Approximately 4% of the results are nondiagnostic and about 10% to 20% of patients are unable to undergo angiography [55,56]. It is contraindicated when pulmonary artery pressures are high and if the patient has a history of allergy to contrast medium. Because of these limitations, pulmonary angiography is usually reserved for patients in whom an appropriate decision about management cannot be made when less invasive approaches are used.

D-dimer Testing

As an adjunct to imaging studies, D-dimer testing has been evaluated in diagnostic and management studies. Although the exact role of D-dimer testing in the diagnosis of PE is still under investigation, the current evidence does support the finding that a negative result using a sensitive ELISA D-dimer assay is safe and reliable in excluding acute PE [43,50]. However, D-dimer testing may be unreliable and less useful in diagnosing PE in hospitalized patients [57]. Studies addressing the use of D-dimer in diagnosing PE in cancer patients have not been performed.

Overall Approach to Diagnosing PE in Women with Cancer

The limitations of the available tests to diagnose PE can be even more problematic in patients with cancer. Of the testing available to diagnose PE, algorithms using a combination of clinical prediction rule, spiral CT and ultrasonography are likely the most prudent. Spiral CT is preferable over VQ scanning because of its availability and its capability of detecting an alternative diagnosis in approximately 25% of patients. Many cancer patients have pulmonary abnormalities, such as metastases and pneumonia, which can render the VQ scan nondiagnostic, and so even fewer patients can be diagnosed using this test. However, VQ scanning would be the imaging technique of choice in patients with poor renal or cardiac function because of their intolerance to contrast dye.

As in diagnosing DVT, it is important to correlate the clinical likelihood of PE with the results of objective tests. In a patient with a low clinical probability of PE, negative results from spiral CT and leg ultrasound exclude a diagnosis of PE. In a patient with a high clinical probability, positive result on spiral CT or ultrasonography confirms a diagnosis of PE. In those with a high or moderate clinical probability but negative results on spiral CT and ultrasonography, serial leg ultrasonography or pulmonary angiography should be done. Patients with poor cardiorespiratory reserve should undergo angiography since they are less able to tolerate recurrent PE. To date, there are no published studies addressing the accuracy of objective testing for diagnosing PE in patients with cancer.

Treatment of Venous Thromboembolism

Treatment of cancer patients with VTE is difficult because these patients have an increased risk of recurrent VTE and anticoagulant-induced bleeding compared to patients without cancer [58,59]. In addition, many cancer patients have a compromised quality of life and the occurrence of thrombosis has an additional negative impact on their quality of life. Furthermore, cancer patients who develop VTE have shortened survival compared to cancer patients without VTE [60,61].

Initial Therapy

The standard regimen for the treatment of acute VTE consists of initial therapy with UFH or LMWH followed by long-term therapy with a coumarin derivative for secondary prophylaxis. To-date, multiple randomized trials and meta-analyses of these trials have confirmed that for initial therapy LMWHs are more efficacious than UFH in reducing recurrent thrombosis and are associated with a lower risk of major bleeding [62]. Furthermore, LMWHs can be given in an outpatient setting without the need for laboratory monitoring and has a lower risk of heparin-induced thrombocytopenia. In many developed countries, outpatient LMWH has become the standard of care for the initial treatment in patients with DVT.

Few trials have compared LMWH with UFH in patients with acute PE. In a study that compared the LMWH tinzaparin with intravenous UFH in hospitalized patients with PE, no difference was detected in recurrent VTE and bleeding [63]. In the trial performed by the Columbus Investigators, which found no difference in these outcomes between the LMWH reviparin and UFH, the majority of patients were treated at home and 27% of all patients had PE [64]. In these two trials, 10% and 23% of patients had cancer, respectively. In a prospective cohort study, 108 patients with PE were treated as outpatients with a LMWH dalteparin; 22% had cancer [65]. The rate of recurrent thrombosis was 5.6%, and major bleeding occurred in 2.9% of the patients. Based on this evidence and the large experience with LMWHs in DVT, it is reasonable to manage patients with acute PE who are hemodynamically stable by treating them with outpatient LMWH. However, in patients who are hemodynamically unstable, intravenous UFH should be used because such patients were excluded from the clinical trials that compared LMWH with UFH.

Whether LMWHs and UFH perform comparably in patients with cancer and acute VTE has not been formally investigated. Cancer patients were included in randomized trials but they represented only 10 – 15% of the total population. Furthermore, many cancer patients with VTE would not have been included in these trials because of poor performance status. Based on published data extracted from trials that reported on the outcomes of the subgroup of cancer patients, it appears that LMWHs and UFH have similar efficacy in patients with and without cancer. Cohort studies have shown that cancer patients can be treated safely at home with LMWH [66-69].

For several LMWHs, both once-daily versus twice-daily injections are available or approved for use but there is a paucity of data that have directly compared the two regimens. In a 3-arm randomized controlled trial, intravenous UFH was compared with subcutaneous enoxaparin at 1.0 mg per kg of body weight given twice daily or 1.5 mg per kg injected once daily for the initial treatment of DVT [70]. No difference in symptomatic recurrent VTE or bleeding was detected among the three treatment groups for all patients. However, among the subgroups of patients with cancer, patients receiving once-daily enoxaparin had a two-fold risk of recurrent VTE compared with patients on twice-daily injections (12.2% vs 6.4%). This difference was not statistically significant. Of note, patients in the once-daily group received only 75% of the total daily doses received by those in the twice-daily group, so that the observed difference in recurrent VTE in this study could have been related to dose rather than frequency of injections. Twice-daily administration of the LMWH reviparin also appeared to be more efficacious than once-daily injections in another randomized trial [71]. The results of patients with cancer were not reported separately in this study. Given the hypercoagulable status of cancer patients, it is possible that twice-daily administration of a LMWH is required to provide a more steady state of anticoagulation, but this hypothesis has not been properly tested.

Long-term Therapy

Coumarin derivatives are the mainstay of long-term anticoagulant treatment for preventing recurrent VTE [72]. These vitamin K antagonists are started within the first 24 hours of diagnosis and are continued for a minimum of 3 months. Due to differences in the anticoagulant response between patients and within patients over time, dose adjustments are needed based on the international normalized ratio (INR). For the majority of patients with VTE, the target therapeutic range is 2.0 to 3.0 [73]. Unpredictable anticoagulant response can result from drug interactions, changes in vitamin K status, liver dysfunction, gastrointestinal disturbances such as vomiting and diarrhea, and consumption of alcohol. Furthermore, because vitamin K antagonists have a delayed onset of action and prolonged clearance of the anticoagulant effect, it is difficult to manage in patients who require frequent interruption of their anticoagulant therapy. Thus, for cancer patients who require periodic invasive procedures (e.g., therapeutic paracentesis) or experience frequent episodes of chemotherapy-induced thrombocytopenia, treatment with warfarin is very problematic. Switching to or bridging with heparins may be indicated in these circumstances to provide more thorough and flexible coverage when invasive procedures are necessary [74-76].

Although standard vitamin K antagonist therapy is highly effectively in most patients, warfarin is associated with frequent recurrent VTE in the oncology population. Treatment failures may be related to subtherapeutic anticoagulation but recurrent VTE also occurs commonly while the INR is maintained within the therapeutic range. In a prospective cohort study of 181 cancer and 661 non-cancer patients on oral anticoagulant therapy, the 12-month cumulative incidence of recurrent VTE was 20.7% in cancer patients versus 6.8% in patients without cancer [59]. The higher incidence of recurrence in cancer patients is also evident regardless of the INR achieved [58]. For example, for INRs within the therapeutic range, the recurrence incidence is 18.9 per 100 patient-years in cancer patients versus 7.2 per 100 patient-years in patients without cancer. Overall, based on the available literature, the risk of recurrent VTE in cancer patients is 2- to 3-fold higher than in patients without cancer [77].

Cancer patients on vitamin K antagonist therapy also have a high risk for major bleeding. In a prospective study, the 12-month cumulative incidence for major bleeding was 12.4% versus 4.9% for patients with and without cancer, respectively [59]. In another study, the incidence of major bleeding in these patient groups were 13.3 per 100 patient-years and 2.1 per 100 patient-years, respectively. In contrast to the INR-related increase in bleeding observed in patients without cancer, the incidence of bleeding in patients with malignancy was independent of the INR.

LMWH therapy has now been investigated as an alternative to vitamin K antagonist therapy for secondary prophylaxis to prevent recurrent VTE. The majority of these studies are small and included primarily patients without cancer [78-85]. Two meta-analyses of these studies have found a statistically non-significant reduction of approximately 30% in the risk of recurrent VTE favoring LMWH [86,87], while one of these reviews found a significant reduction of 62% in the risk of bleeding with LMWH [87].

To-date, two published clinical trials have examined the use of long-term LMWH as an alternative to warfarin therapy in cancer patients with acute VTE [88,89]. The CLOT trial evaluated the use of long-term dalteparin [89]. In this multicentre, randomized, open-label study, 676 cancer patients with proximal DVT, PE or both were randomized to usual treatment with dalteparin initially followed by 6 months of vitamin K antagonist therapy or dalteparin alone for 6 months. In the dalteparin group, patients received therapeutic doses at 200 U/kg once daily for the first month and then 75 – 80% of the full dose for the next 5 months. Patients were followed for the primary outcome of symptomatic, recurrent VTE and secondary outcomes of bleeding and survival. Over the 6-month treatment period, a total of 80 patients had a confirmed, symptomatic recurrent thromboembolic event: 27 of 338 in the dalteparin group and 53 of 338 in the oral anticoagulant group. The cumulative risk of recurrent VTE at 6 months was reduced from 17% in the vitamin K antagonist group to 9% in the dalteparin group, resulting in a statistically significant risk reduction of 52% (P=0.002). In the vitamin K antagonist group, the INR was therapeutic or higher for 70% of the total treatment time and 25 of the 53 recurrences occurred while the INR was 2.0 or above. Accordingly, one episode of recurrent VTE is prevented for every 13 patients treated with dalteparin. Overall, there were no differences in major or any bleeding between the groups; major bleeding was reported in 6% in the dalteparin arm and 4% in the vitamin K antagonist arm. By 6 months, 39% of the patients had died in each group; 90% were due to progressive cancer. At one year, over 60% of the patients were dead. These figures are not surprising given that 67% of the patients had metastatic cancer at the time of study enrolment. The mean duration of treatment time in both groups was approximately 120 days.

In a similar patient population, the CANTHANOX trial compared 3 months of standard warfarin therapy with enoxaparin therapy in cancer patients with proximal DVT, PE or both [88]. All patients were treated initially for at least 4 days with therapeutic doses of enoxaparin at 1.5 mg/kg once daily and were randomized to either continue with enoxaparin at the same dose or warfarin therapy. After 147 patients were randomized, the study was terminated prematurely because of poor recruitment. A total of 75 patients in the warfarin group and 71 patients in the enoxaparin group were evaluable for the primary endpoint of treatment failure, defined as symptomatic, recurrent VTE and/or major bleeding within the 3-month treatment period. About 52% of the study patients had metastatic malignancy at randomization and these patients were equally distributed between the treatment groups. By 3 months, 15 patients had recurrent VTE or major bleeding in the warfarin group compared with 7 patients assigned to enoxaparin. The difference was not statistically significant (P=0.09). The majority of the outcome events were major bleeding, reported in 12 and 5 patients, respectively. Of these, 6 patients in the warfarin group died of bleeding. At 6-month follow-up, 38.7% of the warfarin patients and 31.0% of the enoxaparin patients had died. Based on these results, the investigators concluded that warfarin is associated with a high bleeding risk in cancer patients with VTE and that prolonged treatment with LMWH may be as effective and safer than oral anticoagulant therapy. Two unpublished studies have also evaluated LMWH for long-term use in cancer patients and the results have been presented in abstract form. A subgroup analysis of the LITE study reported improved efficacy with tinzaparin over warfarin in the 167 patients with cancer [90]. Tinzaparin reduced the rate of recurrent VTE by half but this was not statistically significant because of the small number of patients. Also, a difference in recurrent VTE was not found for the two treatment groups overall (3% in both groups) [83]. Similarly, in the ONCENOX study, enoxaparin was compared with warfarin in cancer patients with VTE. Again, no differences in efficacy or bleeding were observed because the study was prematurely terminated after 101 patients were randomized [91].

In summary, there is strong evidence that long-term LMWH is efficacious and safe for preventing recurrent VTE in cancer patients. Bleeding does not appear to be increased compared with warfarin therapy. The 2004 American College of Chest Physicians guidelines has endorsed the use of LMWH dalteparin or tinzaparin for the treatment of acute DVT in cancer patients for the first 3 to 6 months [72].

Use of Caval Filters

There is little evidence to support the routine insertion of caval filters in cancer patients with acute VTE. A large randomized trial has shown that filters will reduce the short-term risk of PE at the expense of an increased risk of recurrent DVT over the long term, despite concurrent warfarin therapy [92]. Other studies have also suggested that thrombosis at the insertion site is a common complication of filter placement [93]. Although cancer patients have a higher risk of bleeding, particularly during periods of thrombocytopenia during chemotherapy, there is no evidence that filters should be used as first-line treatment of acute VTE in these patients. Filters should be reserved for patients who are actively bleeding and cannot receive anticoagulant therapy. Retrievable IVC filters are preferred over permanent devices because they can be removed after the bleeding has stopped and, thus, avoid the long-term potential complications of IVC filters [94]. Further studies are required to determine the optimal role, if any, of caval filters in the management of VTE.

Acknowledgement

We would like to thank all of the chapter authors for their hard work in preparing the chapters. We would like to acknowledge Sherri Ellis for her role in editing the document.

Proceeds from this work will go to the Juravinski Cancer Centre Foundation, Hamilton, Canada. The Cancer Centre Foundation was established in 1997 with a Mission is to develop, manage and distribute charitable resources to support and enhance patient care, research and education related to cancer at the Juravinski Cancer Centre. The Regional Cancer Centre is a place of healing and compassion. But most of all, it's a place of hope. For nearly 50 years, patients from across Central West Ontario have been coming to the Hamilton Regional Cancer Centre (HRCC) after being diagnosed with cancer. The centre is internationally recognized for its leading-edge programs in cancer treatment, education and research. It is one of nine regional cancer centres in Ontario. It provides treatment to more than 7,000 new patients each year. The Centre is affiliated with Hamilton Health Sciences, a network of five hospitals serving Central West Ontario.

References

[1] Kearon, C; Julian, JA; Newman, TE; Ginsberg, JS. Noninvasive diagnosis of deep venous thrombosis. McMaster Diagnostic Imaging Practice Guidelines Initiative [published erratum appears in Ann Intern Med, 1998 Sep 1 129(5), 425] [see comments]. *Ann Intern Med*, 1998 128(8), 663-677.

[2] Hull, RD. Diagnosing pulmonary embolism with improved certainty and simplicity. *JAMA*, 2006 295(2), 213-215.

[3] Gomes, MP; Deitcher, SR. Diagnosis of venous thromboembolic disease in cancer patients. *Oncology (Huntingt)*, 2003 17(1), 126-35, 139.

[4] Fisher, B; Costantino, J; Redmond, C; Poisson, R; Bowman, D; Couture, J; et al. A randomized clinical trial evaluating tamoxifen in the treatment of patients with node-negative breast cancer who have estrogen-receptor- positive tumors. *N Engl J Med*, 1989 320(8), 479-484.

[5] Fisher, B; Dignam, J; Wolmark, N; DeCillis, A; Emir, B; Wickerham, DL; et al. Tamoxifen and chemotherapy for lymph node-negative, estrogen receptor- positive breast cancer. *J Natl Cancer Inst*, 1997 89(22), 1673-1682.

[6] Fisher, B; Costantino, JP; Wickerham, DL; Redmond, CK; Kavanah, M; Cronin, WM; et al. Tamoxifen for prevention of breast cancer: report of the National Surgical Adjuvant Breast and Bowel Project P-1 Study [see comments]. *J Natl Cancer Inst*, 1998 90(18), 1371-1388.

[7] Saphner, T; Tormey, DC; Gray, R. Venous and arterial thrombosis in patients who received adjuvant therapy for breast cancer. *J Clin Oncol*, 1991 9(2), 286-294.

[8] Bonneterre, J; Buzdar, A; Nabholtz, JM; Robertson, JF; Thurlimann, B; von Euler, M; et al. Anastrozole is superior to tamoxifen as first-line therapy in hormone receptor positive advanced breast carcinoma. *Cancer*, 2001 92(9), 2247-2258.

[9] Baum, M; Budzar, AU; Cuzick, J; Forbes, J; Houghton, JH; Klijn, JG; et al. Anastrozole alone or in combination with tamoxifen versus tamoxifen alone for adjuvant treatment of postmenopausal women with early breast cancer: first results of the ATAC randomised trial. *Lancet*, 2002 359(9324), 131-2139.

[10] Wun, T; Law, L; Harvey, D; Sieracki, B; Scudder, SA; Ryu, JK. Increased incidence of symptomatic venous thrombosis in patients with cervical carcinoma treated with concurrent chemotherapy, radiation, and erythropoietin. *Cancer*, 2003 98(7), 1514-1520.

[11] Lavey, RS; Liu, PY; Greer, BE; Robinson, WR III; Chang, PC; Wynn, RB; et al. Recombinant human erythropoietin as an adjunct to radiation therapy and cisplatin for stage IIB-IVA carcinoma of the cervix: a Southwest Oncology Group study. *Gynecol Oncol*, 2004 95(1), 145-151.

[12] Rosenzweig, MQ; Bender, CM; Lucke, JP; Yasko, JM; Brufsky, AM. The decision to prematurely terminate a trial of R-HuEPO due to thrombotic events. *J Pain Symptom Manage*, 2004 27(2), 185-190.

[13] Hull, RD. Revisiting the past strengthens the present: an evidence-based medicine approach for the diagnosis of deep venous thrombosis. *Ann Intern Med*, 2005 142(7), 583-585.

[14] Weinmann, EE; Salzman, EW. Deep-vein thrombosis [see comments]. *N Engl J Med*, 1994 331(24), 1630-1641.

[15] Wells, PS; Anderson, DR; Bormanis, J; Guy, F; Mitchell, M; Gray, L; et al. Value of assessment of pretest probability of deep-vein thrombosis in clinical management. *Lancet*, 1997 350(9094), 1795-1798.

[16] Wells, PS; Anderson, DR; Ginsberg, J. Assessment of deep vein thrombosis or pulmonary embolism by the combined use of clinical model and noninvasive diagnostic tests. *Semin Thromb Hemost*, 2000 26(6), 643-656.

[17] Wells, PS; Owen, C; Doucette, S; Fergusson, D; Tran, H. Does this patient have deep vein thrombosis? *JAMA*, 2006 295(2), 199-207.

[18] Kearon, C; Ginsberg, JS; Hirsh, J. The role of venous ultrasonography in the diagnosis of suspected deep venous thrombosis and pulmonary embolism. *Ann Intern Med*, 1998 129(12), 1044-1049.

[19] Moody, AR; Pollock, JG; O'Connor, AR; Bagnall, M. Lower-limb deep venous thrombosis: direct MR imaging of the thrombus. *Radiology*, 1998 209(2), 349-355.

[20] Carpenter, JP; Holland, GA; Baum, RA; Owen, RS; Carpenter, JT; Cope, C. Magnetic resonance venography for the detection of deep venous thrombosis: comparison with contrast venography and duplex Doppler ultrasonography. *J Vasc Surg*, 1993 18(5), 734-741.

[21] Fraser, DG; Moody, AR; Morgan, PS; Martel, AL; Davidson, I. Diagnosis of lower-limb deep venous thrombosis: a prospective blinded study of magnetic resonance direct thrombus imaging. *Ann Intern Med*, 2002 136(2), 89-98.

[22] Spritzer, CE; Norconk, JJ, Jr; Sostman, HD; Coleman, RE. Detection of deep venous thrombosis by magnetic resonance imaging. *Chest*, 1993 104(1), 54-60.

[23] Lensing, AW; Buller, HR; Prandoni, P; Batchelor, D; Molenaar, AH; Cogo, A; et al. Contrast venography, the gold standard for the diagnosis of deep-vein thrombosis: improvement in observer agreement. *Thromb Haemost*, 1992 67(1), 8-12.

[24] Kelly, J; Rudd, A; Lewis, RR; Hunt, BJ. Plasma D-dimers in the diagnosis of venous thromboembolism. *Arch Intern Med*, 2002 162(7), 747-756.

[25] Stein, PD; Hull, RD; Patel, KC; Olson, RE; Ghali, WA; Brant, R; et al. D-dimer for the exclusion of acute venous thrombosis and pulmonary embolism: a systematic review. *Ann Intern Med*, 2004 140(8), 589-602.

[26] Wells, PS; Anderson, DR; Rodger, M; Forgie, M; Kearon, C; Dreyer, J; et al. Evaluation of D-dimer in the diagnosis of suspected deep-vein thrombosis. *N Engl J Med*, 2003 349(13), 1227-1235.

[27] Kraaijenhagen, RA; Piovella, F; Bernardi, E; Verlato, F; Beckers, EA; Koopman, MM; et al. Simplification of the diagnostic management of suspected deep vein thrombosis. *Arch Intern Med*, 2002 162(8), 907-911.

[28] Bates, SM; Grand'Maison, A; Johnston, M; Naguit, I; Kovacs, MJ; Ginsberg, JS. A latex D-dimer reliably excludes venous thromboembolism. *Arch Intern Med*, 2001 161(3), 447-453.

[29] Bates, SM; Kearon, C; Crowther, M; Linkins, L; O'Donnell, M; Douketis, J; et al. A Diagnostic Strategy Involving a Quantitative Latex d-Dimer Assay Reliably Excludes Deep Venous Thrombosis. *Ann Intern Med*, 2003 138(10), 787-794.

[30] Lee, AY; Julian, JA; Levine, MN; Weitz, JI; Kearon, C; Wells, PS; et al. Clinical utility of a rapid whole-blood D-dimer assay in patients with cancer who present with suspected acute deep venous thrombosis. *Ann Intern Med*, 1999 131(6), 417-423.

[31] ten Wolde, M; Kraaijenhagen, RA; Prins, MH; Buller, HR. The clinical usefulness of D-dimer testing in cancer patients with suspected deep venous thrombosis. *Arch Intern Med*, 2002 162(16), 1880-1884.

[32] Stevens, SM; Elliott, CG; Chan, KJ; Egger, MJ; Ahmed, KM. Withholding anticoagulation after a negative result on duplex ultrasonography for suspected symptomatic deep venous thrombosis. *Ann Intern Med*, 2004 140(12), 985-991.

[33] Kearon, C; Ginsberg, JS; Douketis, J; Crowther, MA; Turpie, AG; Bates, SM; et al. A randomized trial of diagnostic strategies after normal proximal vein ultrasonography for suspected deep venous thrombosis: D-dimer testing compared with repeated ultrasonography. *Ann Intern Med*, 2005 142(7), 490-496.

[34] Fedullo, PF; Tapson, VF. Clinical practice. The evaluation of suspected pulmonary embolism. *N Engl J Med*, 2003 349(13), 1247-1256.

[35] PIOPED. Value of the ventilation/perfusion scan in acute pulmonary embolism. Results of the prospective investigation of pulmonary embolism diagnosis (PIOPED). The PIOPED Investigators [see comments]. *JAMA*, 1990 263(20), 2753-2759.

[36] Miniati M, Monti, S; Bottai, M. A structured clinical model for predicting the probability of pulmonary embolism. *Am J Med*, 2003 114(3), 173-179.

[37] Wells, PS; Ginsberg, JS; Anderson, DR; Kearon, C; Gent, M; Turpie, AG; et al. Use of a clinical model for safe management of patients with suspected pulmonary embolism. *Ann Intern Med*, 1998 129(12), 997-1005.

[38] Wicki, J; Perneger, TV; Junod, AF; Bounameaux, H; Perrier, A. Assessing clinical probability of pulmonary embolism in the emergency ward: a simple score. *Arch Intern Med*, 2001 161(1), 92-97.

[39] Hull, RD; Raskob, GE; Ginsberg, JS; Panju, AA; Brill-Edwards, P; Coates, G; et al. A noninvasive strategy for the treatment of patients with suspected pulmonary embolism. *Arch Intern Med*, 1994 154(3), 289-297.

[40] Stein, PD; Hull, RD; Pineo, G. Strategy that includes serial noninvasive leg tests for diagnosis of thromboembolic disease in patients with suspected acute pulmonary embolism based on data from PIOPED. Prospective Investigation of Pulmonary Embolism Diagnosis. *Arch Intern Med*, 1995 155(19), 2101-2104.

[41] van Strijen, MJ; de Monye, W; Schiereck, J; Kieft, GJ; Prins, MH; Huisman, MV; et al. Single-detector helical computed tomography as the primary diagnostic test in suspected pulmonary embolism: a multicenter clinical management study of 510 patients. *Ann Intern Med*, 2003 138(4), 307-314.

[42] Mullins, MD; Becker, DM; Hagspiel, KD; Philbrick, JT. The role of spiral volumetric computed tomography in the diagnosis of pulmonary embolism. *Arch Intern Med*, 2000 160(3), 293-298.

[43] Perrier, A; Roy, PM; Sanchez, O; Le Gal, G; Meyer, G; Gourdier, AL; et al. Multidetector-row computed tomography in suspected pulmonary embolism. *N Engl J Med*, 2005 352(17), 1760-1768.

[44] Rathbun, SW; Raskob, GE; Whitsett, TL. Sensitivity and specificity of helical computed tomography in the diagnosis of pulmonary embolism: a systematic review. *Ann Intern Med*, 2000 132(3), 227-232.

[45] Perrier A, Bounameaux H. Validation of helical computed tomography for suspected pulmonary embolism: a near miss? *J Thromb Haemost*, 2005 3(1), 14-16.

[46] Goodman, LR; Lipchik, RJ; Kuzo, RS; Liu, Y; McAuliffe, TL; O'Brien, DJ. Subsequent pulmonary embolism: risk after a negative helical CT pulmonary angiogram--prospective comparison with scintigraphy. *Radiology*, 2000 215(2), 535-542.

[47] Moores, LK; Jackson, WL Jr; Shorr, AF; Jackson, JL. Meta-analysis: outcomes in patients with suspected pulmonary embolism managed with computed tomographic pulmonary angiography. *Ann Intern Med*, 2004 141(11), 866-874.

[48] Musset, D; Parent, F; Meyer, G; Maitre, S; Girard, P; Leroyer, C; et al. Diagnostic strategy for patients with suspected pulmonary embolism: a prospective multicentre outcome study. *Lancet*, 2002 360(9349), 1914-1920.

[49] Perrier, A; Howarth, N; Didier, D; Loubeyre, P; Unger, PF; de Moerloose, P; et al. Performance of helical computed tomography in unselected outpatients with suspected pulmonary embolism. *Ann Intern Med*, 2001 135(2), 88-97.

[50] van Belle, A; Buller, HR; Huisman, MV; Huisman, PM; Kaasjager, K; Kamphuisen, PW; et al. Effectiveness of managing suspected pulmonary embolism using an algorithm combining clinical probability, D-dimer testing, and computed tomography. *JAMA*, 2006 295(2), 172-179.

[51] Erdman, WA; Peshock, RM; Redman, HC; Bonte, F; Meyerson, M; Jayson, HT; et al. Pulmonary embolism: comparison of MR images with radionuclide and angiographic studies. *Radiology*, 1994 190(2), 499-508.

[52] Oudkerk, M; van Beek, EJ; Wieloploski, P; van Ooijen, PMA; Brouwers-Kuyper; EMJ; Bongaerts, AHH; et al. Comparison of contrast-enhanced magnetic resonance agiography and conventional pulmonary angiography for the diagnosis of pulmonary embolism: a prostective study. *Lancet*, 2002 (359), 1643-1647.

[53] Hudson, ER; Smith, TP; McDermott, VG; Newman, GE; Suhocki, PV; Payne, CS; et al. Pulmonary angiography performed with iopamidol: complications in 1,434 patients. *Radiology*, 1996 198(1), 61-65.

[54] Nilsson, T; Carlsson, A; Mare, K. Pulmonary angiography: a safe procedure with modern contrast media and technique. *Eur Radiol*, 1998 8(1), 86-89.

[55] Stein, PD; Athanasoulis, C; Alavi, A; Greenspan, RH; Hales, CA; Saltzman, HA; et al. Complications and validity of pulmonary angiography in acute pulmonary embolism. *Circulation*, 1992 85(2), 462-468.

[56] van Beek, EJ; Reekers, JA; Batchelor, DA; Brandjes, DP; Buller, HR. Feasibility, safety and clinical utility of angiography in patients with suspected pulmonary embolism. *Eur Radiol*, 1996 6(4), 415-419.

[57] Miron, MJ; Perrier, A; Bounameaux, H; de Moerloose, P; Slosman, DO; Didier, D; et al. Contribution of noninvasive evaluation to the diagnosis of pulmonary embolism in hospitalized patients. *Eur Respir J*, 1999 13(6), 1365-1370.

[58] Hutten, BA; Prins, MH; Gent, M; Ginsberg, J; Tijssen, JG; Buller, HR. Incidence of recurrent thromboembolic and bleeding complications among patients with venous thromboembolism in relation to both malignancy and achieved international normalized ratio: a retrospective analysis [see comments]. *J Clin Oncol*, 2000 18(17), 3078-3083.

[59] Prandoni, P; Lensing, AW; Piccioli, A; Bernardi, E; Simioni, P; Girolami, B; et al. Recurrent venous thromboembolism and bleeding complications during anticoagulant treatment in patients with cancer and venous thrombosis. *Blood*, 2002 100(10), 3484-3488.

[60] Sorensen, HT; Mellemkjaer, L; Olsen, JH; Baron, JA. Prognosis of cancers associated with venous thromboembolism. *N Engl J Med*, 2000 343(25), 1846-1850.

[61] Levitan, N; Dowlati, A; Remick, SC; Tahsildar, HI; Sivinski, LD; Beyth, R; et al. Rates of initial and recurrent thromboembolic disease among patients with malignancy versus those without malignancy. Risk analysis using Medicare claims data. *Medicine (Baltimore)*, 1999 78(5), 285-291.

[62] van Dongen, CJ; van den Belt, AG; Prins, MH; Lensing, AW. Fixed dose subcutaneous low molecular weight heparins versus adjusted dose unfractionated heparin for venous thromboembolism. *Cochrane Database Syst Rev* 2004 (4):CD001100.

[63] Simonneau, G; Sors, H; Charbonnier, B; Page, Y; Laaban, JP; Azarian, R; et al. A comparison of low-molecular-weight heparin with unfractionated heparin for acute pulmonary embolism. The THESEE Study Group. Tinzaparine ou Heparine Standard: Evaluations dans l'Embolie Pulmonaire. *N Engl J Med*, 1997 337(10), 663-669.

[64] Columbus Investigators. Low-molecular-weight heparin in the treatment of patients with venous thromboembolism. The Columbus Investigators. *N Engl J Med*, 1997 337(10), 657-662.

[65] Kovacs, MJ; Anderson, D; Morrow, B; Gray, L; Touchie, D; Wells, PS. Outpatient treatment of pulmonary embolism with dalteparin. *Thromb Haemost*, 2000 83(2), 209-211.

[66] Wells, PS; Kovacs, MJ; Bormanis, J; Forgie, MA; Goudie, D; Morrow, B; et al. Expanding eligibility for outpatient treatment of deep venous thrombosis and pulmonary embolism with low-molecular-weight heparin: a comparison of patient self-injection with homecare injection [see comments]. *Arch Intern Med*, 1998 158(16), 1809-1812.

[67] Harrison, L; McGinnis, J; Crowther, M; Ginsberg, J; Hirsh, J. Assessment of outpatient treatment of deep-vein thrombosis with low- molecular-weight heparin [see comments]. *Arch Intern Med*, 1998 158(18), 2001-2003.

[68] O'Shaughnessy, D; Miles, J; Wimperis, J. UK patients with deep-vein thrombosis can be safely treated as out-patients. *QJM*, 2000 93(10), 663-667.

[69] Ageno, W; Steidl, L; Marchesi, C; Dentali, F; Mera, V; Squizzato, A; et al. Selecting patients for home treatment of deep vein thrombosis: the problem of cancer. *Haematologica*, 2002 87(3), 286-291.

[70] Merli, G; Spiro, TE; Olsson, CG; Abildgaard, U; Davidson, BL; Eldor. A; et al. Subcutaneous enoxaparin once or twice daily compared with intravenous unfractionated heparin for treatment of venous thromboembolic disease. *Ann Intern Med*, 2001 134(3), 191-202.

[71] Breddin, HK; Hach-Wunderle, V; Nakov, R; Kakkar, VV. Effects of a low-molecular-weight heparin on thrombus regression and recurrent thromboembolism in patients with deep-vein thrombosis. *N Engl J Med*, 2001 344(9), 626-631.

[72] Buller, HR; Agnelli, G; Hull, RD; Hyers, TM; Prins, MH; Raskob, GE. Antithrombotic therapy for venous thromboembolic disease: the Seventh ACCP Conference on Antithrombotic and Thrombolytic Therapy. *Chest*, 2004 126(3 Suppl), 401S-428S.

[73] Ansell, J; Hirsh, J; Poller, L; Bussey, H; Jacobson, A; Hylek, E. The pharmacology and management of the vitamin K antagonists: the Seventh ACCP Conference on Antithrombotic and Thrombolytic Therapy. *Chest*, 2004 126(3 Suppl), 204S-233S.

[74] Dunn, AS; Turpie, AG. Perioperative management of patients receiving oral anticoagulants: a systematic review. *Arch Intern Med*, 2003 163(8), 901-908.

[75] Kearon, C. Management of anticoagulation before and after elective surgery. Hematology 2003 *American Society of Hematology Educational Program Book*. 2003; 528-539.

[76] Kearon, C; Hirsh, J. Perioperative management of patients receiving oral anticoagulants. *Arch Intern Med*, 2003 163(20), 2532-2533.

[77] Lee, AY; Levine, MN. Venous thromboembolism and cancer: risks and outcomes. *Circulation*, 2003 107(23 Suppl 1), I17-I21.

[78] Gonzalez-Fajardo, JA; Arreba, E; Castrodeza, J; Perez, JL; Fernandez, L; Agundez, I; et al. Venographic comparison of subcutaneous low-molecular weight heparin with oral

anticoagulant therapy in the long-term treatment of deep venous thrombosis. *J Vasc Surg*, 1999 30(2), 283-292.

[79] Veiga, F; Escriba, A; Maluenda, MP; Lopez, RM; Margalet, I; Lezana, A; et al. Low molecular weight heparin (enoxaparin) versus oral anticoagulant therapy (acenocoumarol) in the long-term treatment of deep venous thrombosis in the elderly: a randomized trial [In Process Citation]. *Thromb Haemost*, 2000 84(4), 559-564.

[80] Lopaciuk, S; Bielska-Falda, H; Noszczyk, W; Bielawiec, M; Witkiewicz, W; Filipecki, S; et al. Low molecular weight heparin versus acenocoumarol in the secondary prophylaxis of deep vein thrombosis. *Thromb Haemost*, 1999 81(1), 26-31.

[81] Das, SK; Cohen, AT; Edmondson, RA; Melissari, E; Kakkar, VV. Low-molecular-weight heparin versus warfarin for prevention of recurrent venous thromboembolism: a randomized trial. *World J Surg*, 1996 20(5), 521-526.

[82] Pini, M; Aiello, S; Manotti, C; Pattacini, C; Quintavalla, R; Poli T; et al. Low molecular weight heparin versus warfarin in the prevention of recurrences after deep vein thrombosis. *Thromb Haemost*, 1994 72(2), 191-197.

[83] Hull, RD; Pineo, GF; Mah, AF; Brant, RF; for the LITE Study Investigators. A randomized trial evaluating long-term low-molecular-weight heparin therapy for three months versus intravenous heparin followed by warfarin sodium. *Blood* 100, 148a. 2002. Abstract

[84] Lopez-Beret, P; Orgaz, A; Fontcuberta, J; Doblas, M; Martinez, A; Lozano, G; et al. Low molecular weight heparin versus oral anticoagulants in the long-term treatment of deep venous thrombosis. *J Vasc Surg*, 2001 33(1), 77-90.

[85] Hamann, H. Low molecular weight heparin versus coumarin in the prevention of recurence after deep vein thrombosis. Rezidivprophylaxe nach Phlebothrombose - orale antikoagulation oder niedermolekulares heparin subkutan. *Vasemed,* 1998 10, 133-136.

[86] Iorio A, Guercini F, Pini M. Low-molecular-weight heparin for the long-term treatment of symptomatic venous thromboembolism: meta-analysis of the randomized comparisons with oral anticoagulants. *J Thromb Haemost*, 2003 1(9), 1906-1913.

[87] van der Heijden, JF; Hutten, BA; Buller, HR; Prins, MH. Vitamin K antagonists or low-molecular-weight heparin for the long term treatment of symptomatic venous thromboembolism. *Cochrane Database Syst Rev* 2003;(1):CD002001.

[88] Meyer, G; Marjanovic, Z; Valcke, J; Lorcerie, B; Gruel, Y; Solal-Celigny, P; et al. Comparison of low-molecular-weight heparin and warfarin for the secondary prevention of venous thromboembolism in patients with cancer: a randomized controlled study. *Arch Intern Med*, 2002 162(15), 1729-1735.

[89] Lee, AY; Levine, MN; Baker, RI; Bowden, C; Kakkar, AK; Prins, M; et al. Low-molecular-weight heparin versus a coumarin for the prevention of recurrent venous thromboembolism in patients with cancer. *N Engl J Med*, 2003 349(2), 146-153.

[90] Hull, R; Pineo, GF; Mah, AF; Brant, RF; for the LITE Investigators. A randomized trial evaluating long-term low-molecular-weight heparin therapy for three months vs. intravenous heparin followed by warfarin sodium in patients with current cancer. *J Thromb Haemost* 1[suppl 1], P1373. 2003. Abstract

[91] Deitcher, SR; Kessler, CM; Merli, G; Rigas, J; Lyons, RM; Cort, S. Secondary prevention of venous thromboembolic events (VTE) in patients with active malignancy:

a randomized study of enoxaparin sodium alone vs. initial enoxaparin sodium followed by warfarin for a 180-day period. *J Thromb Haemost 1[suppl 1], OC* 194. 2003. Abstract.

[92] Decousus, H; Leizorovicz, A; Parent, F; Page, Y; Tardy, B; Girard, P; et al. A clinical trial of vena caval filters in the prevention of pulmonary embolism in patients with proximal deep-vein thrombosis. Prevention du Risque d'Embolie Pulmonaire par Interruption Cave Study Group [see comments]. *N Engl J Med*, 1998 338(7), 409-415.

[93] Streiff, MB. Vena caval filters: a comprehensive review. *Blood*, 2000 95(12), 3669-3677.

[94] Millward, SF; Oliva, VL; Bell, SD; Valenti, DA; Rasuli, P; Asch, M; et al. Gunther Tulip Retrievable Vena Cava Filter: results from the Registry of the Canadian Interventional Radiology Association. *J Vasc Interv Radiol*, 2001 12(9), 1053-1058.

INDEX

A

B

C

D

E

F

G

H

I

J

K

L

M

N

O

P

Q

R

S

T

U

V

W

X

Y